Innovations in the Integrated Management of Breast Cancer

Innovations in the Integrated Management of Breast Cancer

Editors

Gianluca Franceschini
Alejandro Martin Sanchez
Riccardo Masetti

MDPI • Basel • Beijing • Wuhan • Barcelona • Belgrade • Manchester • Tokyo • Cluj • Tianjin

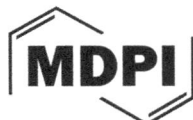

Editors
Gianluca Franceschini
Multidisciplinary Breast Center
Fondazione Policlinico
Universitario A. Gemelli IRCCS
Rome
Italy

Alejandro Martin Sanchez
Multidisciplinary Breast Center
Fondazione Policlinico
Universitario A. Gemelli IRCCS
Rome
Italy

Riccardo Masetti
Multidisciplinary Breast Center
Fondazione Policlinico
Universitario A. Gemelli IRCCS
Rome
Italy

Editorial Office
MDPI
St. Alban-Anlage 66
4052 Basel, Switzerland

This is a reprint of articles from the Special Issue published online in the open access journal *Journal of Personalized Medicine* (ISSN 2075-4426) (available at: www.mdpi.com/journal/jpm/special_issues/technological_innovations).

For citation purposes, cite each article independently as indicated on the article page online and as indicated below:

LastName, A.A.; LastName, B.B.; LastName, C.C. Article Title. *Journal Name* **Year**, *Volume Number*, Page Range.

ISBN 978-3-0365-3802-0 (Hbk)
ISBN 978-3-0365-3801-3 (PDF)

© 2022 by the authors. Articles in this book are Open Access and distributed under the Creative Commons Attribution (CC BY) license, which allows users to download, copy and build upon published articles, as long as the author and publisher are properly credited, which ensures maximum dissemination and a wider impact of our publications.

The book as a whole is distributed by MDPI under the terms and conditions of the Creative Commons license CC BY-NC-ND.

Contents

About the Editors . . . . **vii**

Gianluca Franceschini, Alejandro Martin Sanchez, Elena Jane Mason and Riccardo Masetti
Innovations in the Integrated Management of Breast Cancer
Reprinted from: *J. Pers. Med.* **2022**, *12*, 531, doi:10.3390/jpm12040531 . . . . **1**

Stefano Lello, Anna Capozzi, Lorenzo Scardina, Lucia Ionta, Roberto Sorge and Giovanni Scambia et al.
Vitamin D and Histological Features of Breast Cancer: Preliminary Data from an Observational Retrospective Italian Study
Reprinted from: *J. Pers. Med.* **2022**, *12*, 465, doi:10.3390/jpm12030465 . . . . **5**

Chung-Chien Huang, Chia-Lun Chang, Mingyang Sun, Ming-Feng Chiang, Shao-Yin Sum and Jiaqiang Zhang et al.
Adjuvant Radiotherapy Is Associated with an Increase in the Survival of Old (Aged over 80 Years) and Very Old (Aged over 90 Years) Women with Breast Cancer Receiving Breast-Conserving Surgery
Reprinted from: *J. Pers. Med.* **2022**, *12*, 287, doi:10.3390/jpm12020287 . . . . **13**

Paola Fuso, Mariantonietta Di Salvatore, Concetta Santonocito, Donatella Guarino, Chiara Autilio and Antonino Mulè et al.
Let-7a-5p, miR-100-5p, miR-101-3p, and miR-199a-3p Hyperexpression as Potential Predictive Biomarkers in Early Breast Cancer Patients
Reprinted from: *J. Pers. Med.* **2021**, *11*, 816, doi:10.3390/jpm11080816 . . . . **27**

Alessia Romito, Sonia Bove, Ilaria Romito, Drieda Zace, Ivano Raimondo and Simona Maria Fragomeni et al.
Ovarian Reserve after Chemotherapy in Breast Cancer: A Systematic Review and Meta-Analysis
Reprinted from: *J. Pers. Med.* **2021**, *11*, 704, doi:10.3390/jpm11080704 . . . . **45**

Vittoria Barberi, Antonella Pietragalla, Gianluca Franceschini, Fabio Marazzi, Ida Paris and Francesco Cognetti et al.
Oligometastatic Breast Cancer: How to Manage It?
Reprinted from: *J. Pers. Med.* **2021**, *11*, 532, doi:10.3390/jpm11060532 . . . . **59**

Marco Pappalardo, Marta Starnoni, Gianluca Franceschini, Alessio Baccarani and Giorgio De Santis
Breast Cancer-Related Lymphedema: Recent Updates on Diagnosis, Severity and Available Treatments
Reprinted from: *J. Pers. Med.* **2021**, *11*, 402, doi:10.3390/jpm11050402 . . . . **73**

Giacomo Santandrea, Chiara Bellarosa, Dino Gibertoni, Maria C. Cucchi, Alejandro M. Sanchez and Gianluca Franceschini et al.
Hormone Receptor Expression Variations in Normal Breast Tissue: Preliminary Results of a Prospective Observational Study
Reprinted from: *J. Pers. Med.* **2021**, *11*, 387, doi:10.3390/jpm11050387 . . . . **89**

Alba Di Leone, Daniela Terribile, Stefano Magno, Alejandro Martin Sanchez, Lorenzo Scardina and Elena Jane Mason et al.
Neoadjuvant Chemotherapy in Breast Cancer: An Advanced Personalized Multidisciplinary Prehabilitation Model (APMP-M) to Optimize Outcomes
Reprinted from: *J. Pers. Med.* **2021**, *11*, 324, doi:10.3390/jpm11050324 . . . . **97**

Anna D'Angelo, Alessandro Cina, Giulia Macrì, Paolo Belli, Sara Mercogliano and Pierluigi Barbieri et al.
Conventional CT versus Dedicated CT Angiography in DIEP Flap Planning: A Feasibility Study
Reprinted from: *J. Pers. Med.* **2021**, *11*, 277, doi:10.3390/jpm11040277 . . . . **111**

Alfredo Cesario, Irene Simone, Ida Paris, Luca Boldrini, Armando Orlandi and Gianluca Franceschini et al.
Development of a Digital Research Assistant for the Management of Patients' Enrollment in Oncology Clinical Trials within a Research Hospital
Reprinted from: *J. Pers. Med.* **2021**, *11*, 244, doi:10.3390/jpm11040244 . . . . **121**

Andrea Bellieni, Domenico Fusco, Alejandro Martin Sanchez, Gianluca Franceschini, Beatrice Di Capua and Elena Allocca et al.
Different Impact of Definitions of Sarcopenia in Defining Frailty Status in a Population of Older Women with Early Breast Cancer
Reprinted from: *J. Pers. Med.* **2021**, *11*, 243, doi:10.3390/jpm11040243 . . . . **135**

Armando Orlandi, Letizia Pontolillo, Caterina Mele, Mariangela Pasqualoni, Sergio Pannunzio and Maria Chiara Cannizzaro et al.
Liver Metastasectomy for Metastatic Breast Cancer Patients: A Single Institution Retrospective Analysis
Reprinted from: *J. Pers. Med.* **2021**, *11*, 187, doi:10.3390/jpm11030187 . . . . **147**

Alejandro Martin Sanchez, Daniela Terribile, Antonio Franco, Annamaria Martullo, Armando Orlandi and Stefano Magno et al.
Sentinel Node Biopsy after Neoadjuvant Chemotherapy for Breast Cancer: Preliminary Experience with Clinically Node Negative Patients after Systemic Treatment
Reprinted from: *J. Pers. Med.* **2021**, *11*, 172, doi:10.3390/jpm11030172 . . . . **157**

Azzurra Irelli, Maria Maddalena Sirufo, Gina Rosaria Quaglione, Francesca De Pietro, Enrica Maria Bassino and Carlo D'Ugo et al.
Invasive Ductal Breast Cancer with Osteoclast-Like Giant Cells: A Case Report Based on the Gene Expression Profile for Changes in Management
Reprinted from: *J. Pers. Med.* **2021**, *11*, 156, doi:10.3390/jpm11020156 . . . . **171**

Gianluca Franceschini, Lorenzo Scardina, Alba Di Leone, Daniela Andreina Terribile, Alejandro Martin Sanchez and Stefano Magno et al.
Immediate Prosthetic Breast Reconstruction after Nipple-Sparing Mastectomy: Traditional Subpectoral Technique versus Direct-to-Implant Prepectoral Reconstruction without Acellular Dermal Matrix
Reprinted from: *J. Pers. Med.* **2021**, *11*, 153, doi:10.3390/jpm11020153 . . . . **183**

Fabio Marazzi, Valeria Masiello, Carlotta Masciocchi, Mara Merluzzi, Simonetta Saldi and Paolo Belli et al.
The Assisi Think Tank Meeting Breast Large Database for Standardized Data Collection in Breast Cancer—ATTM.BLADE
Reprinted from: *J. Pers. Med.* **2021**, *11*, 143, doi:10.3390/jpm11020143 . . . . **195**

Gianluca Franceschini, Elena Jane Mason, Cristina Grippo, Sabatino D'Archi, Anna D'Angelo and Lorenzo Scardina et al.
Image-Guided Localization Techniques for Surgical Excision of Non-Palpable Breast Lesions: An Overview of Current Literature and Our Experience with Preoperative Skin Tattoo
Reprinted from: *J. Pers. Med.* **2021**, *11*, 99, doi:10.3390/jpm11020099 . . . . **207**

Fabio Marazzi, Luca Tagliaferri, Valeria Masiello, Francesca Moschella, Giuseppe Ferdinando Colloca and Barbara Corvari et al.
GENERATOR Breast DataMart—The Novel Breast Cancer Data Discovery System for Research and Monitoring: Preliminary Results and Future Perspectives
Reprinted from: *J. Pers. Med.* **2021**, *11*, 65, doi:10.3390/jpm11020065 . . . . **221**

Petra Tesarova, David Pavlista and Antonin Parizek
Is It Possible to Personalize the Diagnosis and Treatment of Breast Cancer during Pregnancy?
Reprinted from: *J. Pers. Med.* **2020**, *11*, 18, doi:10.3390/jpm11010018 . . . . **231**

Armando Orlandi, Elena Iattoni, Laura Pizzuti, Agnese Fabbri, Andrea Botticelli and Carmela Di Dio et al.
Palbociclib Plus Fulvestrant or Everolimus Plus Exemestane for Pretreated Advanced Breast Cancer with Lobular Histotype in ER+/HER2 Patients: A Propensity Score-Matched Analysis of a Multicenter Retrospective Patient Series
Reprinted from: *J. Pers. Med.* **2020**, *10*, 291, doi:10.3390/jpm10040291 . . . . **245**

Maria Ida Amabile, Federico Frusone, Alessandro De Luca, Domenico Tripodi, Giovanni Imbimbo and Silvia Lai et al.
Locoregional Surgery in Metastatic Breast Cancer: Do Concomitant Metabolic Aspects Have a Role on the Management and Prognosis in this Setting?
Reprinted from: *J. Pers. Med.* **2020**, *10*, 227, doi:10.3390/jpm10040227 . . . . **257**

About the Editors

Gianluca Franceschini

Dr. Gianluca Franceschini has been a top-level senior physician at the Breast Unit, the Department of Women and Children's Health, Catholic University, "Agostino Gemelli" Hospital, Rome, Italy, since 1 June 2006.

He has headed the unit for integrated therapies for breast cancer at the Department of Women and Children's Health, Catholic University, "Agostino Gemelli" Hospital, Rome, since 1st July 2014. He has been an Associate Professor in General Surgery since July 2016 at the Catholic University of Rome.

He is a lecturer at the PhD School "Technological Innovations in the Integrated Therapies of Breast Tumours" (2010–2013) and at the School of Specialization in General Surgery, Plastic Surgery and Oncology at the Catholic University of Rome (2011–2016). He is the Academic Coordinator for the University Master's Degree Course "Endocrinology and Breast Pathology" at the Catholic University of Rome (2014–2016).

He is a reviewer and member of the Editorial Boards of several scientific journals.

On the 15th February 2016, he was appointed as a Permanent Member of the College of Italian Breast Surgeons.

He has authored numerous scientific articles, books, and book chapters. His present interests include therapy for pathologies of the breast and surgical treatment of breast cancer with oncoplastic techniques.

Alejandro Martin Sanchez

Dr. Alejandro Martin Sanchez is a researcher at Multidisciplinary Breast Center, Dipartimento Scienze della Salute della Donna e del Bambino e di Sanità Pubblica, Fondazione Policlinico Universitario A. Gemelli IRCCS, 00168 Rome, Italy, with expertise in breast surgery, surgery, surgical oncology, breast cancer management, breast cancer screening, senology, breast imaging, mammography, breast cancer, and breast cancer stem cells.

Riccardo Masetti

Riccardo Masetti is an expert breast surgeon. He is the head of the Breast Surgery Unit, Women, Children and Public Health Sciences Department, Fondazione Policlinico Universitario Agostino Gemelli IRCCS, Roma.

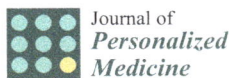

Editorial

Innovations in the Integrated Management of Breast Cancer

Gianluca Franceschini, Alejandro Martin Sanchez *, Elena Jane Mason and Riccardo Masetti

Multidisciplinary Breast Center, Dipartimento Scienze della Salute della Donna e del Bambino e di Sanità Pubblica, Fondazione Policlinico Universitario A. Gemelli IRCCS, 00168 Rome, Italy; gianlucafranceschini70@gmail.com (G.F.); elenajanemason@gmail.com (E.J.M.); riccardo.masetti@policlinicogemelli.it (R.M.)
* Correspondence: martin.sanchez@policlinicogemelli.it; Tel.: +39-06-30156328

Breast cancer is commonly acknowledged as an international priority in healthcare. To date, it is the most common cancer in women worldwide and demographic trends show a steady increase in incidence.

Over the years, increasing efforts and resources have been devoted to a meticulous analysis of risk factors, diagnostic tools and treatment strategies in order to enhance every step of breast cancer management.

Researchers and clinicians strive in search of an optimized, systematic strategy in the diagnosis and treatment of this disease. This effort has led to the creation of the "breast unit model", which is today considered a gold standard to ensure optimal clinical services centered on patients and based on research through multidisciplinary and integrated management [1]. This approach, involving surgical, radiation and medical oncology, allows the optimization of oncological and cosmetic outcomes and the prolonged survival and improvement of patient quality of life; the integrated treatment is tailored to each patient and based on clinical examination, patient status, disease staging, biologic phenotype such as hormone receptor status and human epidermal growth factor receptor 2 (HER2) overexpression, and patient preferences. The decision-making process in the management of breast cancer includes a detailed discussion with the patient about the risks and benefits associated with the selected treatment.

This Special Issue highlights many recent innovations in the integrated management of breast cancer, their potential advantages and the many open issues that still wait to be properly defined and addressed. The authors' interests span every aspect of breast cancer care: from early breast cancer to metastatic patients, and from surgical assessment to artificial intelligence application in data collection.

Cancer biology is addressed in two pre-clinical studies analyzing breast tissue samples. Santandrea et al. focus on hormone receptor expression in normal breast tissue, in search of a pattern that could favor the development of a breast tumor [2], while a study by Fuso et al. examines breast cancer patients treated with neoadjuvant chemotherapy in search of a miRNA expression associated with survival, and therefore acting as a predictive biomarker in women affected by early breast cancer [3].

An accurate and comprehensive preoperative assessment is crucial in order to prepare the patients for surgery, and breast cancer care still holds many issues waiting to be fine-tuned. Nonpalpable lesions can compromise and delay an otherwise smooth operation, and the surgeon should be well-prepared with potential solutions to this common problem. This Special Issue offers a review of current image-guided techniques, highlighting the benefits and controversies of each method [4]. Radiology is also tackled in a study focusing on the best imaging technique to assess patients scheduled to receive breast reconstruction via a DIEP flap, and the researchers advocate conventional CT as an alternative to the traditional but costly CT angiography [5].

During the last decade, the goal in surgery has been to make procedures less and less invasive. Much like breast surgery, which has witnessed a gradual diffusion of breast

Citation: Franceschini, G.; Sanchez, A.M.; Mason, E.J.; Masetti, R. Innovations in the Integrated Management of Breast Cancer. J. Pers. Med. 2022, 12, 531. https://doi.org/10.3390/jpm12040531

Received: 22 February 2022
Accepted: 23 March 2022
Published: 28 March 2022

Publisher's Note: MDPI stays neutral with regard to jurisdictional claims in published maps and institutional affiliations.

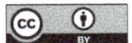

Copyright: © 2022 by the authors. Licensee MDPI, Basel, Switzerland. This article is an open access article distributed under the terms and conditions of the Creative Commons Attribution (CC BY) license (https://creativecommons.org/licenses/by/4.0/).

conserving techniques, axillary surgery has also evolved in an increasingly conservative manner. Where previous surgical approaches tended to favor axillary dissection at all costs, the introduction of sentinel lymph node biopsy (SLNB) has led to the preservation of non-pathological axillary lymph node tissue, and once frequent complications such as post-operative lymphedema have greatly diminished in recent years [6]. In this Special Issue we explore the possibilities of a further evolution in axillary surgery, where treatment with sole SLNB could be extended to include patients downstaged to ycN0 by neoadjuvant chemotherapy [7].

When a breast-conserving approach cannot guarantee both adequate local control and a good aesthetic result, the surgeon has to perform a mastectomy. Innovative surgical procedures called "conservative mastectomies" with immediate prepectoral implant reconstruction have been introduced in order to obtain more favorable aesthetic outcomes and avoid problems caused by manipulation of the pectoralis major muscle, such as breast animation deformity, postoperative pain and injury-induced muscular deficit [8].

The primary goal of management in metastatic disease is the alleviation of symptoms, maintenance or improvement in quality of life and prolongation of survival despite possible treatment toxicity. Patients with metastatic disease receive systemic medical treatments including endocrine therapy, chemotherapy, biologic therapies, targeted and immunotherapy and supportive care measures. However, a subset of patients may benefit from a specific loco-regional treatment [9]: oligometastatic disease has been the object of particular interest because of the possibility to aim for a long-term remission in these patients, and once-discarded options such as liver metastasectomy have been shown to be a possible therapeutic option in selected patients [10,11].

The benefits of a multimodal prehabilitation model are emerging in recent studies, as in this framework patients may be more receptive to health behavior changes in a structured support network. Di Leone et al. shed light on a possible personalized prehabilitation model to enhance patient care in the neoadjuvant setting, which allows each patient to receive the attention of every required specialist in a set frame of time [12,13]. For example, elderly patients can greatly benefit from a preoperative geriatric assessment in order to avoid negative outcomes deriving from otherwise unknown syndromes such as severe sarcopenia [14]. On the other hand, younger women with a new, unexpected diagnosis of breast cancer may face issues related to sexuality and fertility, and studies addressing the impact of treatment on ovarian reserve are paramount to better understand the mechanisms leading to early menopause and subsequent infertility. The clinician's primary objective is to offer a timely oncofertility service, in order to preserve the opportunity for family planning without delaying chemotherapy [15]. Similar strategies must be adopted when confronting pregnancy-associated breast cancer, a rare occurrence that nonetheless threatens the wellbeing of both mother and fetus [16].

Finally, the last few years have seen the creation of new artificial intelligence technologies with the potential to radically change the modern management of breast cancer. Research itself is a viable candidate for the coming high-tech revolution: today, protocol development can be promoted, patient enrollment can be enhanced by a patient-trial matching made possible by the growing diffusion of electronic health records, and patient parameters and adherence to trials can be monitored in real-time by a variety of wearable devices. This Issue witnesses the transformation, thanks to the contribution of authors active in the field of real-world data: Cesario et al. describe the development of a digital research assistant that manages patient enrollment in trials with the employment of an artificial intelligence algorithm [17], while Marazzi et al. exploit text mining to successfully extract data from heterogeneous sources and to generate clinical evidence [18,19].

This Special Issue finds its place in the modern panorama of breast care by promoting a modern, holistic approach to breast disease and encouraging clinicians to tailor patient treatment. The development of appropriate clinical pathways, with a multidisciplinary and standardized approach, is essential for successful, well-rounded treatment in the era of personalized medicine.

Author Contributions: Conceptualization/original draft preparation A.M.S. and E.J.M.; Review and editing/supervision G.F.; final draft conceptualization and approval R.M. All authors have read and agreed to the published version of the manuscript.

Funding: This research received no external funding.

Institutional Review Board Statement: Not applicable.

Informed Consent Statement: Not applicable.

Conflicts of Interest: The authors declare no conflict of interest.

References

1. Franceschini, G.; Sanchez, A.M.; Di Leone, A.; Magno, S.; Moschella, F.; Accetta, C.; Natale, M.; Di Giorgio, D.; Scaldaferri, A.; D'Archi, S.; et al. Update on the surgical management of breast cancer. *Ann. Ital. Chir.* **2015**, *86*, 89–99. [PubMed]
2. Santandrea, G.; Bellarosa, C.; Gibertoni, D.; Cucchi, M.; Sanchez, A.; Franceschini, G.; Masetti, R.; Foschini, M.P. Hormone Receptor Expression Variations in Normal Breast Tissue: Preliminary Results of a Prospective Observational Study. *J. Pers. Med.* **2021**, *11*, 387. [CrossRef] [PubMed]
3. Fuso, P.; Di Salvatore, M.; Santonocito, C.; Guarino, D.; Autilio, C.; Mulè, A.; Arciuolo, D.; Rinninella, A.; Mignone, F.; Ramundo, M.; et al. Let-7a-5p, miR-100-5p, miR-101-3p, and miR-199a-3p Hyperexpression as Potential Predictive Biomarkers in Early Breast Cancer Patients. *J. Pers. Med.* **2021**, *11*, 816. [CrossRef] [PubMed]
4. Franceschini, G.; Mason, E.; Grippo, C.; D'Archi, S.; D'Angelo, A.; Scardina, L.; Sanchez, A.; Conti, M.; Trombadori, C.; Terribile, D.; et al. Image-Guided Localization Techniques for Surgical Excision of Non-Palpable Breast Lesions: An Overview of Current Literature and Our Experience with Preoperative Skin Tattoo. *J. Pers. Med.* **2021**, *11*, 99. [CrossRef] [PubMed]
5. D'Angelo, A.; Cina, A.; Macrì, G.; Belli, P.; Mercogliano, S.; Barbieri, P.; Grippo, C.; Franceschini, G.; D'Archi, S.; Mason, E.; et al. Conventional CT versus Dedicated CT Angiography in DIEP Flap Planning: A Feasibility Study. *J. Pers. Med.* **2021**, *11*, 277. [CrossRef] [PubMed]
6. Pappalardo, M.; Starnoni, M.; Franceschini, G.; Baccarani, A.; De Santis, G. Breast Cancer-Related Lymphedema: Recent Updates on Diagnosis, Severity and Available Treatments. *J. Pers. Med.* **2021**, *11*, 402. [CrossRef] [PubMed]
7. Sanchez, A.; Terribile, D.; Franco, A.; Martullo, A.; Orlandi, A.; Magno, S.; Di Leone, A.; Moschella, F.; Natale, M.; D'Archi, S.; et al. Sentinel Node Biopsy after Neoadjuvant Chemotherapy for Breast Cancer: Preliminary Experience with Clinically Node Negative Patients after Systemic Treatment. *J. Pers. Med.* **2021**, *11*, 172. [CrossRef] [PubMed]
8. Franceschini, G.; Scardina, L.; Di Leone, A.; Terribile, D.; Sanchez, A.; Magno, S.; D'Archi, S.; Franco, A.; Mason, E.; Carnassale, B.; et al. Immediate Prosthetic Breast Reconstruction after Nipple-Sparing Mastectomy: Traditional Subpectoral Technique versus Direct-to-Implant Prepectoral Reconstruction without Acellular Dermal Matrix. *J. Pers. Med.* **2021**, *11*, 153. [CrossRef] [PubMed]
9. Amabile, M.I.; Frusone, F.; De Luca, A.; Tripodi, D.; Imbimbo, G.; Lai, S.; D'Andrea, V.; Sorrenti, S.; Molfino, A. Locoregional Surgery in Metastatic Breast Cancer: Do Concomitant Metabolic Aspects Have a Role on the Management and Prognosis in this Setting? *J. Pers. Med.* **2020**, *10*, 227. [CrossRef] [PubMed]
10. Barberi, V.; Pietragalla, A.; Franceschini, G.; Marazzi, F.; Paris, I.; Cognetti, F.; Masetti, R.; Scambia, G.; Fabi, A. Oligometastatic Breast Cancer: How to Manage It? *J. Pers. Med.* **2021**, *11*, 532. [CrossRef]
11. Orlandi, A.; Pontolillo, L.; Mele, C.; Pasqualoni, M.; Pannunzio, S.; Cannizzaro, M.; Cutigni, C.; Palazzo, A.; Garufi, G.; Vellone, M.; et al. Liver Metastasectomy for Metastatic Breast Cancer Patients: A Single Institution Retrospective Analysis. *J. Pers. Med.* **2021**, *11*, 187. [CrossRef]
12. Di Leone, A.; Terribile, D.; Magno, S.; Sanchez, A.; Scardina, L.; Mason, E.; D'Archi, S.; Maggiore, C.; Rossi, C.; Di Micco, A.; et al. Neoadjuvant Chemotherapy in Breast Cancer: An Advanced Personalized Multidisciplinary Prehabilitation Model (APMP-M) to Optimize Outcomes. *J. Pers. Med.* **2021**, *11*, 324. [CrossRef] [PubMed]
13. Franceschini, G.; Terribile, D.; Fabbri, C.; Magno, S.; D'Alba, P.; Chiesa, F.; Di Leone, A.; Masetti, R. Management of locally advanced breast cancer. Mini-review. *Minerva Chir.* **2007**, *62*, 249–255. [PubMed]
14. Bellieni, A.; Fusco, D.; Sanchez, A.; Franceschini, G.; Di Capua, B.; Allocca, E.; Di Stasio, E.; Marazzi, F.; Tagliaferri, L.; Masetti, R.; et al. Different Impact of Definitions of Sarcopenia in Defining Frailty Status in a Population of Older Women with Early Breast Cancer. *J. Pers. Med.* **2021**, *11*, 243. [CrossRef] [PubMed]
15. Romito, A.; Bove, S.; Romito, I.; Zace, D.; Raimondo, I.; Fragomeni, S.; Rinaldi, P.; Pagliara, D.; Lai, A.; Marazzi, F.; et al. Ovarian Reserve after Chemotherapy in Breast Cancer: A Systematic Review and Meta-Analysis. *J. Pers. Med.* **2021**, *11*, 704. [CrossRef] [PubMed]
16. Tesarova, P.; Pavlista, D.; Parizek, A. Is It Possible to Personalize the Diagnosis and Treatment of Breast Cancer during Pregnancy? *J. Pers. Med.* **2020**, *11*, 18. [CrossRef] [PubMed]

17. Cesario, A.; Simone, I.; Paris, I.; Boldrini, L.; Orlandi, A.; Franceschini, G.; Lococo, F.; Bria, E.; Magno, S.; Mulè, A.; et al. Development of a Digital Research Assistant for the Management of Patients' Enrollment in Oncology Clinical Trials within a Research Hospital. *J. Pers. Med.* **2021**, *11*, 244. [CrossRef] [PubMed]
18. Marazzi, F.; Tagliaferri, L.; Masiello, V.; Moschella, F.; Colloca, G.; Corvari, B.; Sanchez, A.; Capocchiano, N.; Pastorino, R.; Iacomini, C.; et al. GENERATOR Breast DataMart-The Novel Breast Cancer Data Discovery System for Research and Monitoring: Preliminary Results and Future Perspectives. *J. Pers. Med.* **2021**, *11*, 65. [CrossRef] [PubMed]
19. Marazzi, F.; Masiello, V.; Masciocchi, C.; Merluzzi, M.; Saldi, S.; Belli, P.; Boldrini, L.; Capocchiano, N.; Di Leone, A.; Magno, S.; et al. The Assisi Think Tank Meeting Breast Large Database for Standardized Data Collection in Breast Cancer-ATTM.BLADE. *J. Pers. Med.* **2021**, *11*, 143. [CrossRef] [PubMed]

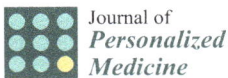

Article

Vitamin D and Histological Features of Breast Cancer: Preliminary Data from an Observational Retrospective Italian Study

Stefano Lello [1], Anna Capozzi [1], Lorenzo Scardina [2,*], Lucia Ionta [2], Roberto Sorge [3], Giovanni Scambia [1] and Gianluca Franceschini [2]

1. Department of Woman and Child Health and Public Health, Institute of Obstetrics and Gynecology, Fondazione Policlinico Universitario Agostino Gemelli IRCCS, Università Cattolica del Sacro Cuore, 00168 Rome, Italy; stefano.lello@policlinicogemelli.it (S.L.); anna.capozzi@policlinicogemelli.it (A.C.); giovanni.scambia@policlinicogemelli.it (G.S.)
2. Department of Woman and Child Health and Public Health, Division of Breast Surgery, Fondazione Policlinico Universitario Agostino Gemelli IRCCS, Università Cattolica del Sacro Cuore, 00168 Rome, Italy; lucia.ionta@guest.policlinicogemelli.it (L.I.); gianlucafranceschini70@gmail.com (G.F.)
3. Laboratory of Biometry, Department of Systems Medicine, University of Rome Tor Vergata, 00187 Rome, Italy; sorge@uniroma2.it
* Correspondence: lorenzoscardina@libero.it

Abstract: Background: Vitamin D (vitD) may be involved in different extraskeletal conditions as well as skeletal muscle diseases. It has been hypothesized that, at least in part, a low level of vitD could contribute to facilitating cancer development. Breast cancer (BC) seems to be associated with low levels of vitD. Materials and methods: This was an observational retrospective evaluation of 87 women (mean age: 54 ± 12 years old) who underwent surgery for the treatment of BC. Our main purpose was to correlate the types of BC and the levels of vitD. Results: A positive significant correlation (R > 0.7) was found between non-invasive carcinoma in situ and 25(OH)D levels and age (R = 0.82, $p < 0.05$). A positive, but nonsignificant, correlation was reported between invasive ductal carcinoma and 25(OH)D and age (R = 0.45, $p > 0.05$). A negative but nonsignificant correlation was found between invasive lobular carcinoma and 25(OH)D and age (R = 0.24, $p > 0.05$). Discussion and Conclusions: We did not find a significant relationship between vitD and BC subtypes. Considering the positive significant correlation between vitD levels and age for in situ BC, although preliminary, our results seem to suggest a possible role of vitD in in situ BC. However, these findings need to be confirmed in larger studies.

Keywords: vitamin D; breast cancer; ductal breast cancer; in situ breast cancer; lobular breast cancer; histology

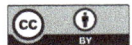

1. Introduction

Breast cancer (BC) is the most common form of female cancer and the second leading cause of death among women worldwide [1]. Many data suggest that several lifestyle and environmental factors—such as a high-fat diet, a lack of physical activity, and chronic alcohol consumption—might play a critical role in the development and risk of recurrence of this cancer [2]. The maintenance of a healthy lifestyle together with regular breast checks, through breast self-examinations, mammography, and/or ultrasonography, represent a cornerstone for primary prevention [3]. Vitamin D (vitD) homeostasis is fundamental for the achievement of bone strength and the prevention of bone and muscle loss [4].

According to the principal international guidelines [5,6], its supplementation is advisable for frail subjects affected by a loss of bone strength and/or hypovitaminosis D. Furthermore, emerging data demonstrate that vitD may produce other important benefits at the extraskeletal level [7]. Hypovitaminosis D is associated with a higher incidence of several cardiovascular, metabolic, autoimmune, endocrine, and neoplastic pathologies [7]. Although large intervention studies about the positive effects of vitD supplementation on these pathologies are limited [8], there is growing interest in the potential involvement of vitD status in the appearance of some of these diseases [7].

An interesting meta-analysis by Hossain et al. [9] showed a direct correlation between vitD deficiency and BC, with a relative risk (RR) of 1.91 (95% confidence interval (CI): 1.51–2.41, $p < 0.001$). At the same time, total vitD intake and supplemental vitD intakes had inverse relationships with BC (RR = 0.99, 95% CI: 0.97–1.00, $p = 0.022$, per 100 IU/day; RR = 0.97, 95% CI: 0.95–1.00, $p = 0.026$, respectively).

Another cohort study [10], evaluating 50,884 women (aged between 35 and 74 years) who had never had BC themselves but had a sister affected by BC, found that high serum 25(OH)D levels and self-reported regular vitD supplementation (≥four times/week) were associated with lower rates of incident BC after menopause over 5 years of follow-up (HR = 0.72 (CI: 0.57–0.93) for high serum 25(OH)D levels, and HR = 0.83 (CI: 0.74–0.93) for regular supplementation).

Our study was an observational retrospective evaluation enrolling 87 women (mean age: 54 ± 12 years old) who underwent surgery for the treatment of BC between December 2019 and March 2020. The objective of this evaluation was to correlate the subtypes of BC with the level of vitD.

2. Materials and Methods

This was an observational retrospective analysis of 87 patients (mean age: 54 ± 12 years old) who had not been supplemented with vitD in the previous 3 months, selected among patients who underwent surgery for the treatment of BC in the Breast Unit Surgery of Fondazione Policlinico Agostino Gemelli IRCCS of Rome. This retrospective analysis included patients without differences in race and/or ethnicity. The exclusion criteria were being a foreign woman and/or being regularly supplemented with vitD analogues in the previous three months before breast surgery and/or being unwilling to be tested for vitD status.

All the enrolled women were screened for serum 25(OH)D levels during the pre-hospitalization stage. The total serum 25(OH)D levels were measured using an automated Abbott Architect 25(OH)D immunoassay (bias ng/mL% = + 0.4/1.7–4.7 between 20 and 40 ng/mL, according to the Vitamin D External Quality Assurance Scheme).

According to the US Endocrine Society Clinical Practice Guidelines, vitamin D sufficiency was defined as serum levels of 25(OH)D ranging between 30 and 100 ng/mL [5].

Twenty-four patients underwent a mastectomy combined with immediate reconstruction, whereas 53 patients were treated through breast-conserving surgery (oncoplastic surgery was performed in nine subjects). In particular, after breast surgery, we collected data about the size, type, and histological features of BC.

All the data were analysed by using SPSS 15.0 version for Windows (SPSS, Chicago, IL, USA). For descriptive statistics, the means ± standard deviations (SDs) for parameters with Gaussian distributions (after confirmation with histograms and Kolmogorov–Smirnov tests), and medians and intervals (minimum–maximum) for non-Gaussian variables, were used.

The comparison among normal variables was performed by using one-way ANOVA or Bonferroni tests. We used chi-square ($\chi 2$) and Fisher tests for comparisons among the variables of frequency. Pearson linear correlation analysis was used for the calculation of R coefficients. A value of $p < 0.05$ was considered statistically significant.

The study was conducted according to the guidelines of the Declaration of Helsinki and approved by the Institutional Review Board and Ethics Committee of Fondazione Policlinico Universitario Agostino Gemelli IRCCS, Università Cattolica del Sacro Cuore, Rome, Italy.

3. Results

The principal characteristics of the study participants are summarized in Table 1.

Table 1. Patients' characteristics and ANOVA correlations between vitamin D levels and tumour type, the type of receptors expressed, and grading.

	Tum	n	Mean	SD	Min	Max	ANOVA	Sum of Squares	df	Mean Square	F	Sig.
Age	1	70	54.2	12.0	36	88	Between Groups	16,861	2	8430	0.054	0.948
	2	6	54.7	15.8	39	77	Within Groups	13,218,403	84	157,362		
	3	11	55.6	14.1	38	77	Total	13,235,264	86			
	Total	87	54.4	12.4	36	88						
Vit D	1	70	24.3	10.2	6.3	55.2	Between Groups	33,251	2	16,625	0.155	0.856
	2	6	22.1	11.8	14.0	45.6	Within Groups	8,984,555	84	106,959		
	3	11	24.9	10.4	15.0	52.1	Total	9,017,806	86			
	Total	87	24.2	10.2	6.3	55.2						
yT (mm)	1	70	13.6	16.0	0	105	Between Groups	1,034,492	2	517,246	2.094	0.130
	2	6	14.0	13.0	1	35	Within Groups	20,752,675	84	247,056		
	3	11	24.0	15.3	4	60	Total	21,787,167	86			
	Total	87	14.9	15.9	0	105						
yN	1	66	0.5	0.9	0	3	Between Groups	1184	2	0.592	0.843	0.435
	2	3	0.0	0.0	0	0	Within Groups	51,985	74	0.702		
	3	8	0.3	0.7	0	2	Total	53,169	76			
	Total	77	0.5	0.8	0	3						
ER	1	70	57.8	40.7	0	100	Between Groups	5,156,117	2	2,578,058	1.687	0.191
	2	6	58.5	37.7	1	90	Within Groups	128,387,286	84	1,528,420		
	3	11	81.0	26.8	1	95	Total	133,543,402	86			
	Total	87	60.8	39.4	0	100						
PR	1	70	28.9	37.6	0	98	Between Groups	7,798,377	2	3,899,189	2.677	0.075
	2	6	44.3	48.2	0	90	Within Groups	122,346,542	84	1,456,506		
	3	11	56.1	36.4	1	90	Total	130,144,920	86			
	Total	87	33.4	38.9	0	98						
Ki67	1	70	34.5	25.7	1	80	Between Groups	3,001,866	2	1,500,933	2.552	0.084
	2	1	20.0	.	20	20	Within Groups	46,465,122	79	588,166		
	3	11	17.2	9.7	5	35	Total	49,466,988	81			
	Total	82	32.0	24.7	1	80						
HER2	1	70	1.4	1.1	0	3	Between Groups	5001	2	2500	1.964	0.147
	2	6	1.5	1.4	0	3	Within Groups	106,953	84	1273		
	3	11	0.7	0.9	0	2	Total	111,954	86			
	Total	87	1.4	1.1	0	3						

The patients were divided into three main subgroups according to the type of cancer: subgroup one (70 women (mean age: 54.2 ± 12 SD) with ductal carcinoma)); subgroup two (six women (mean age: 54.7 ± 15 SD) with carcinoma in situ); and subgroup three (11 women (mean age: 55.6 ± 14 SD) with lobular carcinoma).

We did not find significant differences among groups according to the major analysed variables (i.e., the tumour size, expression of oestrogen receptors (ERs), expression of progesterone receptors (PRs), Ki67, human epidermal growth factor receptor 2 (HER2), and median level of 25(OH)D). In particular, the age did not significantly differ among the subgroups of cancers ($p > 0.05$).

A positive significant correlation ($R > 0.7$) was found between non-invasive carcinoma in situ and 25(OH)D levels and age ($R = 0.82$) (Figure 1).

A positive but nonsignificant correlation was reported between invasive ductal carcinoma and 25(OH)D and age ($R = 0.45$).

A negative but nonsignificant correlation was found between invasive lobular carcinoma and 25(OH)D and age ($R = 0.24$).

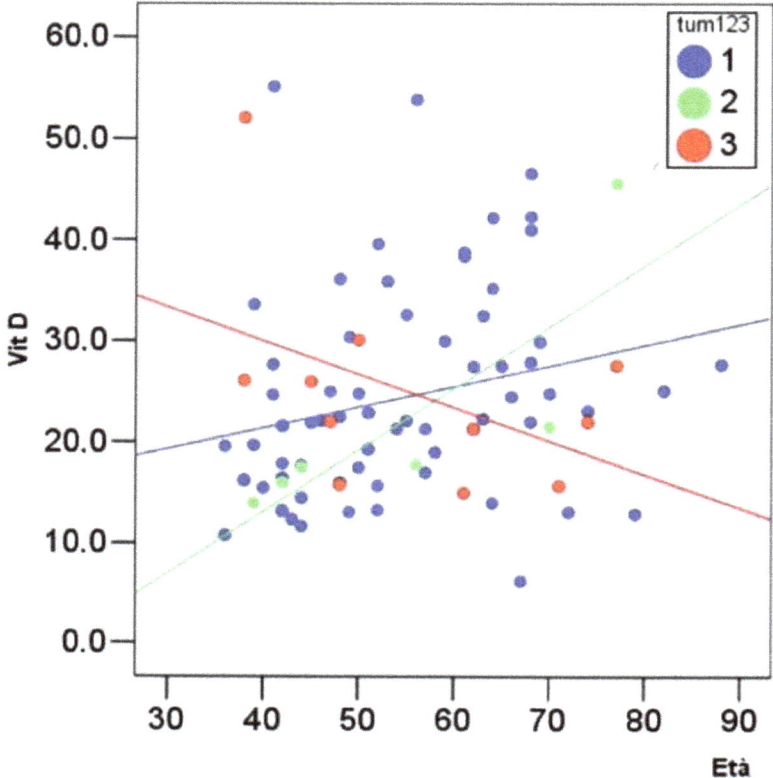

Figure 1. Relationship between age and vitamin D levels in major BC types (tum 1 = ductal BC; tum 2 = in situ BC; and tum 3 = lobular BC).

4. Discussion and Conclusions

Hypovitaminosis D is notably associated with a loss of bone and muscle strength, and major international guidelines recommend maintaining normal 25(OH)D levels (>20 ng/mL) in vitD-deficient elderly institutionalized patients and postmenopausal women at higher risk of fragility fractures through appropriate supplementation [5,11].

Conversely, the benefits of vitD supplementation for skeletal muscle health in community-dwelling, premenopausal women and younger healthy subjects remain questionable [12].

According to some evidence [13], hypovitaminosis D could favour the development of several extraskeletal conditions (i.e., autoimmune, inflammatory, cardiovascular, and metabolic diseases), although the effective role of vitD in the aetiology of these pathologies needs to be further elucidated. In particular, the risks of colon, prostate, ovarian, and breast cancer have been associated with vitD deficiency by many authors [14,15].

Abbas et al. [16] found, in a population-based case–control study including 289 premenopausal women and 595 matched controls (aged between 30 and 50 years), a significant inverse association between BC risk and plasma 25(OH)D concentrations ($p < 0.05$). Compared with the lowest category (<30 nmol/L) (OR = 1 (95% CI)), the ORs for higher plasma concentrations of 30–45, 45–60, and $\geq$ 60 nmol/L were 0.68 (0.43–1.07), 0.59 (0.37–0.94), and 0.45 (0.29–0.70), respectively (p for trend = 0.0006). Interestingly, this association was stronger for progesterone receptor-negative BC (PR-), with evidence suggestive of effect heterogeneity (p for heterogeneity = 0.05, case-only model). Additionally, the authors found a significantly reduced risk of BC, with an OR of 0.90 (0.84–0.96) per 10 nmol/L increment when considering 25(OH)D as a continuous variable. Meanwhile, no significant interactions between plasma 25(OH)D and the first-degree family history of BC, age at menarche, duration of breastfeeding, parity, alcohol intake, or BMI were reported.

It has been hypothesized that vitD may exert direct protective effects against cancer by promoting cellular apoptosis and differentiation and by inhibiting angiogenesis and tissue inflammation. At the same time, different general risk factors that can favour cancer development by themselves could negatively affect vitD metabolism, such as smoking, obesity, low physical activity, and sun exposure [17,18].

Another study by Alipour et al. [19] compared a control group (364 women; mean age: 44.2 years) with a case group (308 women; mean age: 43.2 years; 172 subjects with a benign mass; and 136 subjects with a malignant mass) regarding vitD status. The results of this study show that the median serum 25(OH)D assessed in the case group was lower than that in the control group (7.7 vs. 8.7 ng/mL), and that the median serum 25(OH)D was higher in benign (7.9 ng/mL) than in malignant cases (7 ng/mL). In the comparison between each of these two case groups with controls, the median 25(OH)D was higher in the control group, lower in the group of patients with benign lesions, and the lowest in the group with cancer. However, the differences between the median 25(OH)D in the benign cases and controls, as well as benign cases and cancers, were not statistically significant ($p = 0.3$ and $p = 0.1$, respectively). The histology of four of the 136 BC was in situ ductal carcinoma; the others were invasive ductal carcinomas. In comparison with subjects with euvitaminosis D (25(OH)D > 35 ng/mL), the ORs for BC were 3 (95% CI: 1.11–8.1) in subjects with severe vitD deficiency (25(OH)D < 12.5 ng/mL), 0.96 (95% CI: 0.3- 2.8) in patients with moderate vitD deficiency (25(OH)D between 12.5 and 25 ng/mL), and 1.79 (95% CI: 0.9–3.5) in subjects affected by mild hypovitaminosis D (25(OH)D between 25 and 35 ng/mL), after adjustment of different variables (i.e., age, menarche, parity, menopausal status, breastfeeding, and family history of BC). Thus, for less-severe hypovitaminosis D, the relationship between vitD status and BC risk appeared to be nonsignificant [19].

The main purpose of our retrospective analysis was to find a possible relationship between the biological finding of BC, according to its histological features, and the level of vitD assessed in all the patients before undergoing breast surgery that would have confirmed the suspicious diagnosis of BC. Firstly, we did not find a significant difference among the subgroups with different types of cancer regarding all the analysed variables (age; tumour dimension; expression of ERs, PRs, Ki67, and HER2; and median level of 25(OH)D) ($p > 0.05$). As mentioned above, the available data in the literature highlight the tendency of both benign and malignant breast masses to be associated with lower median levels of 25(OH)D in comparison with those in healthy subjects. However, the difference in terms of vitD status between benign and malignant lesions did not appear to be clearly significant, as also confirmed by our analysis [19]. Additionally, although our study was small, the results seem to be in line with data reporting a decreased frequency of invasive lobular cancers in the last two decades compared with non-invasive in situ and invasive ductal BC [20]. This phenomenon may be explained by the supposed influence of hormonal exposure, which may contribute to facilitating the appearance of invasive lobular BC and may render this type of tumour more susceptible to incidence variation within population studies [21]. Secondly, a positive significant correlation ($R > 0.7$) was found between non-invasive carcinoma in situ and 25(OH)D and age ($R = 0.82$), whereas a nonsignificant but negative correlation was found between invasive lobular carcinoma and 25(OH)D and age ($R = 0.45$). At the same time, a positive but nonsignificant correlation was reported between invasive ductal carcinoma and 25(OH)D and age ($R = 0.45$).

A previous retrospective case–control study by Peppone et al. [22] on 224 women diagnosed with Stage 0–III BC showed that suboptimal vitD levels (<32 ng/mL) were more common in women with later-stage disease, non-Caucasians, and those who received radiation therapy ($p < 0.05$). More specifically, the ORs for suboptimal vitD levels were 3.15 (95 CI%: 1.05–9.49) for triple-negative vs. non-triple-negative, 2.59 (95 CI%: 1.08–6.23) for ER- vs. ER+, 2.35 (95 CI%: 1.14–4.84) for premenopausal vs. postmenopausal status at diagnosis, and 2.29 (95 CI%: 2.05–4.98) for negative family history vs. positive. On the other hand, the OR for suboptimal vitD levels was 2.22 (95 CI%: 0.86–5.71) for invasive vs. non-invasive BC. Our results seem to be consistent with those of the latter study since our evaluation did not show a clear impact of vitD status on the invasiveness of BC.

However, our findings show that vitD status and age could be positively correlated for in situ BC, a type of cancer that is generally associated with lower biological aggressiveness and/or invasiveness than the others. Although the evidence regarding the close correlation between vitD deficiency and in situ BC remains limited, these data show a very interesting picture.

Regarding invasive lobular BC, we observed an inverse, although nonsignificant, correlation between vitD and age, probably due to the small number of patients. These findings may be related, on one hand, to the most frequent biological features of invasive lobular BC, which seem to be influenced more by hormones than by other exogenous and/or endogenous factors, and, on the other hand, to a potentially less-protective role of vitD at the cellular level because of its insufficiency in this type of BC.

According to recent systematic reviews, vitamin D insufficiency is observed in patients with newly diagnosed breast cancer, and supplemental vitamin D intake showed an inverse relationship with this outcome [8,23].

A recent secondary analysis of data from the Women's Health Initiative CaD trial (n = 36,282 cancer-free postmenopausal women aged between 50 and 79 years, randomly assigned to a daily 1000 mg dose of calcium plus 400 IU of vitamin D or to a placebo) found a lower risk of ductal carcinoma in situ (DCIS) throughout approximately 20 years of follow-up (HR = 0.82; 95% CI: 0.70 to 0.96). These results seem to suggest that, since DCIS could be considered a precursor of invasive BC, supplementation with calcium and vitD might reduce BC risk by acting at an early stage in the natural history of the tumour [24]. However, that evaluation has some limitations since it was a post hoc analysis that did not consider calcium and/or vitamin D intake from dietary sources and/or the effects of each supplement separately.

Interestingly, a multicentre randomized, double-blind, placebo-controlled study conducted in the United States in men $\geq$ 50 years and women $\geq$ 55 years without cancer and cardiovascular disease at baseline showed that supplementation with vitamin D3 (cholecalciferol, 2000 IU/d) and marine omega-3 fatty acids (1 g/d) could produce a significant reduction in advanced cancers (metastatic or fatal) compared with placebo (226 of 12,927 assigned to vitamin D (1.7%) and 274 of 12,944 assigned to placebo (2.1%); HR = 0.83 (95% CI: 0.69–0.99); p = 0.04), particularly in subjects with normal BMIs (HR = 0.89; 95% CI: 0.68–1.17) [9].

However, the cancer incidence was similar in the treatment and placebo groups. Thus, a clear conclusion about the favourable impact of vitD supplementation on the cancer risk for the general population cannot be drawn [25].

Moreover, there are many known, and still-unknown, endogenous and exogenous mechanisms involved in tumorigenesis; thus, these results need to be critically evaluated [26].

Our study presents several limitations, as it was a retrospective analysis and may have included some selection biases: the relatively small number of participants, the absence of a control group, and the exclusion of other potential confounding factors, such as body mass index (BMI), dietary and lifestyle habits (smoking, alcohol consumption, and sport activities), family history of BC, comorbidities, and medications.

Taken together, our analysis did not show significant differences among types of BC regarding vitD status. Additionally, we did not find significant differences among subgroups of BC with respect to tumour size and age (p > 0.05).

Despite the small number of cases, since we found a positive significant correlation between vitD levels and age for in situ BC, our results seem to suggest a protective role of baseline endogenous vitD levels in in situ BC, different from that in more invasive types of BC. In other words, vitD, through its putative antiproliferative activity at the cellular level [27], could contribute to reducing the invasiveness of cancer cells.

Therefore, this work provides encouraging data since, even if preliminarily, we can hypothesize that vitD status may affect the occurrence of less-invasive types of BC, rather than others.

Further prospective multicentre trials with larger numbers of patients and longer follow-up are necessary to draw more validated conclusions. Even if clinical studies investigating the synergistic role of vitD in BC treatment are still inconclusive [28], our results could suggest that ensuring an appropriate level of 25(OH)D could become a promising choice in the field of BC cancer prevention. However, these findings need to be confirmed in larger and well-designed intervention studies.

Author Contributions: Conceptualization, S.L. and A.C.; methodology, S.L.; software, R.S.; validation, R.S., G.S. and G.F.; formal analysis, R.S.; investigation, S.L.; resources, L.I.; data curation, R.S.; writing—original draft preparation, A.C. and S.L.; writing—review and editing, G.S. and G.F.; visualization, G.F.; supervision, G.S., L.S.; project administration, A.C. All authors have read and agreed to the published version of the manuscript.

Funding: This research received no external funding.

Institutional Review Board Statement: The study was conducted according to the guidelines of the Declaration of Helsinki and approved by the Institutional Review Board and Ethics Committee of Fondazione Policlinico Universitario Agostino Gemelli IRCCS, Università Cattolica del Sacro Cuore, Rome, Italy.

Informed Consent Statement: Informed consent was obtained from all the subjects involved in the study.

Data Availability Statement: The data presented in this study are available on request from the corresponding author.

Conflicts of Interest: The authors declare no conflict of interest.

References

1. Ghoncheh, M.; Pournamdar, Z.; Salehiniya, H. Incidence and Mortality and Epidemiology of Breast Cancer in the World. *Asian Pac. J. Cancer Prev.* **2016**, *17*, 43–46. [CrossRef] [PubMed]
2. Maumy, L.; Harrissart, G.; Dewaele, P.; Aljaber, A.; Bonneau, C.; Rouzier, R.; Eliès, A. Impact des régimes alimentaires sur la mortalité et le risque de récidive de cancer du sein: Revue de la littérature [Impact of nutrition on breast cancer mortality and risk of recurrence, a review of the evidence]. *Bull. Cancer* **2020**, *107*, 61–71. [CrossRef] [PubMed]
3. Kolak, A.; Kamińska, M.; Sygit, K.; Budny, A.; Surdyka, D.; Kukiełka-Budny, B.; Burdan, F. Primary and secondary prevention of breast cancer. *Ann. Agric. Environ. Med.* **2017**, *24*, 549–553. [CrossRef] [PubMed]
4. Khazai, N.; Judd, S.E.; Tangpricha, V. Calcium and vitamin D: Skeletal and extraskeletal health. *Curr. Rheumatol. Rep.* **2008**, *10*, 110–117. [CrossRef]
5. Holick, M.F.; Binkley, N.C.; Bischoff-Ferrari, H.A.; Gordon, C.M.; Hanley, D.A.; Heaney, R.P.; Murad, M.H.; Weaver, C.M.; Endocrine Society. Evaluation, treatment, and prevention of vitamin D deficiency: An Endocrine Society clinical practice guideline. *J. Clin. Endocrinol. Metab.* **2011**, *96*, 1911–1930, Erratum in *J. Clin. Endocrinol. Metab.* **2011**, *96*, 3908. [CrossRef]
6. Pludowski, P.; Holick, M.F.; Grant, W.B.; Konstantynowicz, J.; Mascarenhas, M.R.; Haq, A.; Povoroznyuk, V.; Balatska, N.; Barbosa, A.P.; Karonova, T.; et al. Vitamin D supplementation guidelines. *J. Steroid Biochem. Mol. Biol.* **2018**, *175*, 125–135. [CrossRef]
7. Bouillon, R.; Marcocci, C.; Carmeliet, G.; Bikle, D.; White, J.H.; Dawson-Hughes, B.; Lips, P.; Munns, C.F.; Lazaretti-Castro, M.; Giustina, A.; et al. Skeletal and Extraskeletal Actions of Vitamin D: Current Evidence and Outstanding Questions. *Endocr. Rev.* **2019**, *40*, 1109–1151. [CrossRef]
8. Chandler, P.D.; Chen, W.Y.; Ajala, O.N.; Hazra, A.; Cook, N.; Bubes, V.; Lee, I.M.; Giovannucci, E.L.; Willett, W.; Buring, J.E.; et al. Effect of Vitamin D3 Supplements on Development of Advanced Cancer: A Secondary Analysis of the VITAL Randomized Clinical Trial. *JAMA Netw. Open.* **2020**, *3*, e2025850, Erratum in *JAMA Netw. Open.* **2020**, *3*, e2032460. [CrossRef]
9. Hossain, S.; Beydoun, M.A.; Beydoun, H.A.; Chen, X.; Zonderman, A.B.; Wood, R.J. Vitamin D and breast cancer: A systematic review and meta-analysis of observational studies. *Clin. Nutr. ESPEN* **2019**, *30*, 170–184. [CrossRef]
10. O'Brien, K.M.; Sandler, D.P.; Taylor, J.A.; Weinberg, C.R. Serum Vitamin D and Risk of Breast Cancer within Five Years. *Environ. Health Perspect.* **2017**, *125*, 077004. [CrossRef]
11. Ross, A.C.; Manson, J.E.; Abrams, S.A.; Aloia, J.F.; Brannon, P.M.; Clinton, S.K.; Durazo-Arvizu, R.A.; Gallagher, J.C.; Gallo, R.L.; Jones, G.; et al. The 2011 report on dietary reference intakes for calcium and vitamin D from the Institute of Medicine: What clinicians need to know. *J. Clin. Endocrinol. Metab.* **2011**, *96*, 53–58. [CrossRef] [PubMed]

12. US Preventive Services Task Force; Grossman, D.C.; Curry, S.J.; Owens, D.K.; Barry, M.J.; Caughey, A.B.; Davidson, K.W.; Doubeni, C.A.; Epling, J.W., Jr.; Kemper, A.R.; et al. Vitamin D, Calcium, or Combined Supplementation for the Primary Prevention of Fractures in Community-Dwelling Adults: US Preventive Services Task Force Recommendation Statement. *JAMA* **2018**, *319*, 1592–1599.
13. Marino, R.; Misra, M. Extra-Skeletal Effects of Vitamin D. *Nutrients* **2019**, *11*, 1460. [CrossRef] [PubMed]
14. De La Puente-Yagüe, M.; Cuadrado-Cenzual, M.A.; Ciudad-Cabañas, M.J.; Hernández-Cabria, M.; Collado-Yurrita, L. Vitamin D: And its role in breast cancer. *Kaohsiung J. Med. Sci.* **2018**, *34*, 423–427. [CrossRef]
15. Manson, J.E.; Cook, N.R.; Lee, I.M.; Christen, W.; Bassuk, S.S.; Mora, S.; Gibson, H.; Gordon, D.; Copeland, T.; D'Agostino, D.; et al. Vitamin D Supplements and Prevention of Cancer and Cardiovascular Disease. *N. Engl. J. Med.* **2019**, *380*, 33–44. [CrossRef]
16. Abbas, S.; Chang-Claude, J.; Linseisen, J. Plasma 25-hydroxyvitamin D and premenopausal breast cancer risk in a German case-control study. *Int. J. Cancer* **2009**, *124*, 250–255. [CrossRef]
17. Brown, R.B. Vitamin D, cancer, and dysregulated phosphate metabolism. *Endocrine* **2019**, *65*, 238–243. [CrossRef]
18. Scaranti, M.; Júnior Gde, C.; Hoff, A.O. Vitamin D and cancer: Does it really matter? *Curr. Opin. Oncol.* **2016**, *28*, 205–209. [CrossRef]
19. Alipour, S.; Hadji, M.; Hosseini, L.; Omranipour, R.; Saberi, A.; Seifollahi, A.; Bayani, L.; Shirzad, N. Levels of serum 25-hydroxyvitamin d in benign and malignant breast masses. *Asian Pac. J. Cancer Prev.* **2014**, *15*, 129–132. [CrossRef]
20. Ward, E.M.; DeSantis, C.E.; Lin, C.C.; Kramer, J.L.; Jemal, A.; Kohler, B.; Brawley, O.W.; Gansler, T. Cancer statistics: Breast cancer in situ. *CA Cancer J. Clin.* **2015**, *65*, 481–495. [CrossRef]
21. Dossus, L.; Benusiglio, P.R. Lobular breast cancer: Incidence and genetic and non-genetic risk factors. *Breast Cancer Res.* **2015**, *17*, 37. [CrossRef] [PubMed]
22. Peppone, L.J.; Rickles, A.S.; Janelsins, M.C.; Insalaco, M.R.; Skinner, K.A. The association between breast cancer prognostic indicators and serum 25-OH vitamin D levels. *Ann. Surg. Oncol.* **2012**, *19*, 2590–2599. [CrossRef] [PubMed]
23. Voutsadakis, I.A. Vitamin D baseline levels at diagnosis of breast cancer: A systematic review and meta-analysis. *Hematol. Oncol. Stem Cell Ther.* **2021**, *14*, 16–26. [CrossRef]
24. Peila, R.; Xue, X.; Cauley, J.A.; Chlebowski, R.; Manson, J.E.; Nassir, R.; Saquib, N.; Shadyab, A.H.; Zhang, Z.; Wassertheil-Smoller, S.; et al. A Randomized Trial of Calcium Plus Vitamin D Supplementation and Risk of Ductal Carcinoma In Situ of the Breast. *JNCI Cancer Spectr.* **2021**, *5*, pkab072. [CrossRef]
25. Gissel, T.; Rejnmark, L.; Mosekilde, L.; Vestergaard, P. Intake of vitamin D and risk of breast cancer—A me-ta-analysis. *J. Steroid Biochem. Mol. Biol.* **2008**, *111*, 195–199. [CrossRef] [PubMed]
26. Peters, J.M.; Gonzalez, F.J. The Evolution of Carcinogenesis. *Toxicol. Sci.* **2018**, *165*, 272–276. [CrossRef]
27. Samuel, S.; Sitrin, M.D. Vitamin D's role in cell proliferation and differentiation. *Nutr. Rev.* **2008**, *66*, S116–S124. [CrossRef]
28. Verma, A.; Schwartz, Z.; Boyan, B.D. 24R,25-dihydroxyvitamin D3 modulates tumorigenicity in breast cancer in an estrogen receptor-dependent manner. *Steroids* **2019**, *150*, 108447. [CrossRef]

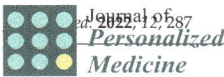

Article

Adjuvant Radiotherapy Is Associated with an Increase in the Survival of Old (Aged over 80 Years) and Very Old (Aged over 90 Years) Women with Breast Cancer Receiving Breast-Conserving Surgery

Chung-Chien Huang [1,2], Chia-Lun Chang [3,4], Mingyang Sun [5], Ming-Feng Chiang [6], Shao-Yin Sum [7], Jiaqiang Zhang [5] and Szu-Yuan Wu [7,8,9,10,11,12,13,14,*]

1. International Ph.D. Program in Biotech and Healthcare Management, School of Health Care Administration, College of Management, Taipei Medical University, Taipei 110, Taiwan; cc-test@tmu.edu.tw
2. Department of Medical Quality, Taipei Municipal Wan Fang Hospital, Taipei Medical University, Taipei 110, Taiwan
3. Department of Hemato-Oncology, Wan Fang Hospital, Taipei Medical University, Taipei 110, Taiwan; richardch9@hotmail.com
4. Department of Internal Medicine, School of Medicine, College of Medicine, Taipei Medical University, Taipei 110, Taiwan
5. Department of Anesthesiology and Perioperative Medicine, Henan Provincial People's Hospital, People's Hospital of Zhengzhou University, Zhengzhou 450052, China; mingyangsun1986@163.com (M.S.); jiaqiang197628@163.com (J.Z.)
6. Division of Gastroenterology and Hepatology, Department of Internal Medicine, Lo-Hsu Medical Foundation, Lotung Poh-Ai Hospital, Yilan 265, Taiwan; chiangmingf@gmail.com
7. Department of General Surgery, Lo-Hsu Medical Foundation, Lotung Poh-Ai Hospital, Yilan 265, Taiwan; b91401126@ntu.edu.tw
8. Department of Food Nutrition and Health Biotechnology, College of Medical and Health Science, Asia University, Taichung 413, Taiwan
9. Big Data Center, Lo-Hsu Medical Foundation, Lotung Poh-Ai Hospital, Yilan 265, Taiwan
10. Graduate Institute of Business Administration, College of Management, Fu Jen Catholic University, Taipei 242062, Taiwan
11. Division of Radiation Oncology, Lo-Hsu Medical Foundation, Lotung Poh-Ai Hospital, Yilan 265, Taiwan
12. Department of Healthcare Administration, College of Medical and Health Science, Asia University, Taichung 413, Taiwan
13. Cancer Center, Lo-Hsu Medical Foundation, Lotung Poh-Ai Hospital, Yilan 265, Taiwan
14. Centers for Regional Anesthesia and Pain Medicine, Taipei Municipal Wan Fang Hospital, Taipei Medical University, Taipei 110, Taiwan
* Correspondence: szuyuanwu5399@gmail.com

Abstract: This study is the first to examine the effect of adjuvant whole-breast radiotherapy (WBRT) on oncologic outcomes such as all-cause death, locoregional recurrence (LRR), and distant metastasis (DM) in old (aged ≥80 years) and very old (aged ≥90 years) women with breast invasive ductal carcinoma (IDC) receiving breast-conserving surgery. After propensity score matching, adjuvant WBRT was associated with decreases in all-cause death, LRR, and DM in old and very old women with IDC compared with no use of adjuvant WBRT. **Background**: To date, no data on the effect of adjuvant whole-breast radiotherapy (WBRT) on oncologic outcomes, such as all-cause death, locoregional recurrence (LRR), and distant metastasis (DM), are available for old (aged ≥80 years) and very old (≥90 years) women with breast invasive ductal carcinoma (IDC) receiving breast-conserving conservative surgery (BCS). **Patients and Methods**: We enrolled old (≥80 years old) and very old (≥90 years old) women with breast IDC who had received BCS followed by adjuvant WBRT or no adjuvant WBRT. We grouped them based on adjuvant WBRT status and compared their overall survival (OS), LRR, and DM outcomes. To reduce the effects of potential confounders when comparing all-cause mortality between the groups, propensity score matching was performed. **Results**: Overall, 752 older women with IDC received BCS followed by adjuvant WBRT, and 752 with IDC received BCS with no adjuvant WBRT. In multivariable Cox regression analysis, the adjusted hazard ratio (aHR) and 95% confidence interval (95% CI) of all-cause death for adjuvant WBRT

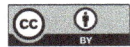

compared with no adjuvant WBRT in older women with IDC receiving BCS was 0.56 (0.44–0.70). The aHRs (95% CIs) of LRR and DM for adjuvant WBRT were 0.29 (0.19–0.45) and 0.45 (0.32–0.62), respectively, compared with no adjuvant WBRT. **Conclusions**: Adjuvant WBRT was associated with decreases in all-cause death, LRR, and DM in old (aged ≥80 years) and very old (aged ≥90 years) women with IDC compared with no adjuvant WBRT.

Keywords: breast cancer; old age; breast-conserving surgery; radiotherapy; survival

1. Introduction

Standard treatments based on cancer treatment guidelines such as the National Comprehensive Cancer Network (NCCN) guidelines are not suitable for every older patient, because many randomized controlled trials (RCTs) for breast cancer therapy do not enroll patients ≥65 years old [1]. Determining optimal treatments for older cancer patients is challenging, especially for those aged 80 years or more. Although trials have enrolled patients ≥70 years old, the sample size of those ≥80 years old is small, and trials including those ≥90 years old are scant [2,3]. However, cancer is commonly a disease of the old, and the median age at diagnosis for all sites is 65 years [4]. Older patients (≥80 years) constitute a substantial percentage of those with breast cancer [5]. Approximately one in four patients with breast cancer are aged more than 65 years, and approximately 10% of the total breast cancer population is 80 years or older [5]. This age group often presents challenges in terms of treatment because of comorbidities and frailty [6].

It is difficult to evaluate long-time overall survival and disease-free survival for elderly breast cancer patients in RCTs, due to their short life-expectancy. Additionally, there is also the cost of treatment to consider in elderly patients with short life-expectancies. Therefore, all comorbidities should be considered in these kinds of elderly patient studies, and be well-matched through propensity score matching (PSM). Most patients should have Charlson comorbidity index (CCI) score of 0–1 with relative health, which might be an association with longer life-expectancy. The selection of relatively healthy, suitable elderly breast cancer patients for the consideration of further adjuvant radiotherapy (RT) would be worthwhile.

Adjuvant RT is applied to eradicate any tumor deposits remaining following surgery [7]. This reduces the risk of locoregional recurrence (LRR) and improves breast cancer-specific survival and overall survival (OS) [7]. For most women treated with breast-conserving surgery (BCS), adjuvant whole-breast RT (WBRT), rather than surgery alone, is recommended according to the NCCN guidelines and the results of RCTs [1,7]. Studies with grade 2B evidence (weak recommendation) have suggested that the omission of RT might be considered in women ≥65 years old with node-negative, hormone receptor-positive, human epidermal growth factor receptor 2 (HER2)-negative primary tumors up to 3 cm, for whom endocrine therapy is planned [8–12]; alternatively, administering RT to these women is also reasonable depending on their values and preferences, and the biologic features of the tumor. For example, women in this subset who wish to minimize their risk of LRR and accept the toxicities associated with RT may reasonably opt for RT. To date, no study with a sufficient sample size and long-term follow-up for older (≥80 years old) women with breast cancer has been conducted; this is especially true for 90-year-old women and above. A head-to-head PSM study mimicking an RCT might be necessary, especially for old (≥80 years) and very old (≥90 years) women.

The radiation oncologist should discuss the advantages and disadvantages of RT with older women with breast cancer receiving BCS prior to making a decision on its omission. For example, in the real world, compliance with endocrine therapy is a critical aspect of treatment, particularly for those with RT omission. A head-to-head study with a sufficiently large sample size and long follow-up is required to estimate the oncologic outcomes of adjuvant WBRT for older women with breast cancer undergoing BCS. We conducted this PSM study to examine the effects of adjuvant WBRT on oncologic outcomes such as OS,

LRR, and distant metastasis (DM) in old (aged ≥80 years) and very old (aged ≥90 years) women, who have scarcely been enrolled in RCTs; these findings would help determine the value of adjuvant WBRT in these patients.

2. Patients and Methods

2.1. Study Population

In this cohort study, data were retrieved from the Taiwan Cancer Registry Database (TCRD). We enrolled old (age ≥80 years) and very old (≥90 years) women with breast invasive ductal carcinoma (IDC) who had received BCS between 1 January 2008 and 31 December 2018. The index date was the date of BCS, and the follow-up duration was from the index date to 31 December 2019. The TCRD of the Collaboration Center of Health Information Application contains detailed cancer-related information of patients, including clinical stage, pathologic stage, chemotherapy regimen, chemotherapy dose, molecular status, drug use, hormone receptor status, HER2 status, radiation modality and dose, and surgical procedure [13–16]. The study protocols were reviewed and approved by the Institutional Review Board of Tzu-Chi Medical Foundation (IRB109-015-B).

2.2. Inclusion and Exclusion Criteria

The diagnoses of the enrolled women with breast IDC were confirmed after their pathological data were reviewed, and women with newly diagnosed IDC were confirmed to have no other cancers or DMs. Women with IDC were included if they were 80 years or older and had clinical stage IA-IIIC (American Joint Committee on Cancer [AJCC], 8th edition) without metastasis. Women with IDC were excluded if they had a history of cancer before the IDC diagnosis date, unknown pathologic types, missing sex data, unclear staging, or non-IDC histology. In addition, women having unclear differentiation of the tumor grade, missing data on hormone receptor status, or unknown HER2 status were excluded. Other adjuvant treatments such as chemotherapy, hormone therapy, or HER2 inhibitors did not constitute exclusion criteria based on the NCCN guidelines [17]. We also excluded women with unclear data on surgical procedures such as BCS or TM, ill-defined nodal surgery, or unclear Charlson comorbidity index (CCI) scores. Hormone receptor-positivity was defined as ≥1% of tumor cells demonstrating positive nuclear staining through immunohistochemistry [18].

After applying the inclusion and exclusion criteria, we divided the population into two groups based on their adjuvant WBRT status to compare all-cause mortality: Group 1 (older women with IDC who received BCS followed by adjuvant WBRT) and Group 2 (older women with IDC who received BCS and no adjuvant WBRT). We also excluded women in Group 1 receiving nonstandard adjuvant WBRT (contrast with standard adjuvant radiotherapy consisting of irradiation to the whole breast with a minimum of 50 Gy). Contemporary RT techniques (i.e., three-dimensional RT and intensity-modulated RT) were included, and the conventional two-dimensional RT technique was excluded. The incidence of comorbidities was scored using the CCI [19,20]. Only comorbidities observed within 6 months before the index date were included; they were classified according to International Classification of Diseases, 10th Revision, Clinical Modification codes (ICD-10-CM codes) at the first admission or based on more than two repetitions of a code recorded at outpatient department visits.

2.3. Study Covariates and Propensity Score Matching

To reduce the effects of potential confounders when comparing all-cause mortality between the adjuvant WBRT and nonadjuvant WBRT groups, PSM was performed. A greedy method was used to match the cohorts at a 1:1 ratio by age, tumor differentiation, AJCC clinical stage, AJCC pathologic stage, pT, pN, neoadjuvant chemotherapy, adjuvant chemotherapy, hormone receptor status, HER2 status, nodal surgical type, CCI score, hypertension, ischemic heart disease, cerebrovascular disease, chronic obstructive pulmonary disease (COPD), diabetes, hospital level (medical center or not), hospital region, and income with a propensity score within a caliper of 0.2 [21]. Moreover, we separated covariates such as hypertension, ischemic heart disease, cerebrovascular disease, COPD, and diabetes [22] from CCI scores and considered these covariates independently in PSM for more precise matching to control for confounders of all-cause death.

2.4. Statistics

Multivariable Cox regression analysis was performed to calculate hazard ratios (HRs) to determine the potential independent predictors of all-cause death, LRR, and DM. PSM was applied to control for potential predictors in the analysis (Table 1), and all-cause death was the primary endpoint in the two groups. LRR and DM were secondary endpoints and were estimated using proportional subdistribution hazard regression to overcome the competing risk of death in the analysis of time-to-event data [23,24].

Table 1. Demographic information of patients aged ≥80 years undergoing breast conservative surgery.

Variables		Raw Population						Propensity Score-Matched Population				
		Total N = 3703		Adjuvant WBRT N = 2776		Non-WBRT N = 927		Adjuvant WBRT N = 752		Non-WBRT N = 752		
		n	(%)	n	(%)	n	(%)	p Value	n	(%)	n	(%)	p Value
Age	Mean (SD)	84.8	(6.1)	84.4	(4.9)	85.9	(7.2)	<0.0001	85.3	(6.0)	85.9	(6.3)	0.9674
	Median (IQR, Q1–Q3)	84	(81–88)	84	(81–88)	84	(82–89)		84	(82–89)	84	(82–90)	
	80–84	1815	(49.0)	1598	(57.6)	217	(23.4)	<0.0001	215	(28.6)	215	(28.6)	1.0000
	85–89	1285	(34.7)	879	(31.7)	406	(43.8)		238	(31.6)	238	(31.6)	
	90+	603	(16.3)	299	(10.8)	304	(32.8)		299	(39.8)	299	(39.8)	
Differentiation	I	851	(23.0)	631	(22.7)	220	(23.7)	0.3441	171	(22.7)	182	(24.2)	0.3075
	II	2071	(55.9)	1544	(55.6)	527	(56.9)		406	(54.0)	418	(55.6)	
	III	781	(21.1)	601	(21.6)	180	(19.4)		175	(23.3)	152	(20.2)	
AJCC Clinical stage	I	2033	(54.9)	1568	(56.5)	465	(50.2)	0.0012	402	(53.5)	398	(52.9)	0.9532
	II	1547	(41.8)	1112	(40.1)	435	(46.9)		329	(43.8)	332	(44.1)	
	III	123	(3.3)	96	(3.5)	27	(2.9)		21	(2.8)	22	(2.9)	
AJCC Pathologic stage	0	41	(1.1)	33	(1.2)	8	(0.9)	0.0029	4	(0.5)	4	(0.5)	1.0000
	I	1894	(51.1)	1449	(52.2)	445	(48.0)		375	(49.9)	375	(49.9)	
	II	1531	(41.3)	1103	(39.7)	428	(46.2)		331	(44.0)	331	(44.0)	
	III	237	(6.4)	191	(6.9)	46	(5.0)		42	(5.6)	42	(5.6)	
pT	0	58	(1.6)	47	(1.7)	11	(1.2)	<0.0001	5	(0.7)	6	(0.8)	0.5977
	1	2214	(59.8)	1710	(61.6)	504	(54.4)		429	(57.0)	424	(56.4)	
	2	1356	(36.6)	975	(35.1)	381	(41.1)		301	(40.0)	301	(40.0)	
	3	45	(1.2)	24	(0.9)	21	(2.3)		8	(1.1)	14	(1.9)	
	4	30	(0.8)	20	(0.7)	10	(1.1)		9	(1.2)	7	(0.9)	
pT	0–1	2272	(61.4)	1757	(63.3)	515	(55.6)	<0.0001	434	(57.7)	430	(57.2)	0.6625
	2–4	1431	(38.6)	1019	(36.7)	412	(44.4)		318	(42.3)	322	(42.8)	
pN	0	2890	(78.0)	2122	(76.4)	768	(82.8)	0.0004	618	(82.2)	608	(80.9)	0.8552
	1	613	(16.6)	488	(17.6)	125	(13.5)		103	(13.7)	113	(15.0)	
	2	140	(3.8)	114	(4.1)	26	(2.8)		22	(2.9)	23	(3.1)	
	3	60	(1.6)	52	(1.9)	8	(0.9)		9	(1.2)	8	(1.1)	
pN	0	2890	(78.0)	2122	(76.4)	768	(82.8)	<0.0001	618	(82.2)	608	(80.9)	0.4111
	1+	813	(22.0)	654	(23.6)	159	(17.2)		134	(17.8)	144	(19.1)	
Neoadjuvant Chemotherapy		115	(3.1)	107	(3.9)	8	(0.9)	<0.0001	8	(1.1)	7	(0.9)	0.7389
Adjuvant chemotherapy		1270	(34.3)	1126	(40.6)	144	(15.5)	<0.0001	162	(21.5)	142	(18.9)	0.0588
Hormone receptor positive		1871	(50.5)	1394	(50.2)	477	(51.5)	0.5132	368	(48.9)	372	(49.5)	0.8168
HER2 positive		231	(6.2)	189	(6.8)	42	(4.5)	0.0130	41	(5.5)	40	(5.3)	0.9081
Nodal surgery	ALND	2259	(61.0)	1688	(60.8)	571	(61.6)	0.6301	432	(57.4)	424	(56.4)	0.3608
	SLNB	1444	(39.0)	1088	(39.2)	356	(38.4)		320	(42.6)	328	(43.6)	
CCI Scores	0	1513	(40.9)	1178	(42.4)	335	(36.1)	<0.0001	279	(37.1)	283	(37.6)	0.9752
	1	1133	(30.6)	863	(31.1)	270	(29.1)		226	(30.1)	224	(29.8)	
	2+	1057	(28.5)	735	(26.5)	322	(34.7)		247	(32.8)	245	(32.6)	
Hypertension		2430	(65.6)	1765	(63.6)	665	(71.7)	<0.0001	543	(72.2)	530	(70.5)	0.4460
Ischemic heart diseases		925	(25.0)	582	(21.0)	343	(37.0)	<0.0001	260	(34.6)	258	(34.3)	0.9811

Table 1. Cont.

		Raw Population						Propensity Score-Matched Population				
		Total N = 3703		Adjuvant WBRT N = 2776		Non-WBRT N = 927			Adjuvant WBRT N = 752		Non-WBRT N = 752	
Variables		n	(%)	n	(%)	n	(%)	p Value	n	(%)	n	(%)	p Value
Cerebrovascular diseases		377	(10.2)	229	(8.2)	148	(17.0)	<0.0001	125	(16.6)	117	(15.6)	0.2624
COPD		552	(14.9)	301	(10.8)	251	(27.1)	<0.0001	211	(28.1)	211	(128.1)	1.0000
Diabetes		1180	(31.9)	862	(31.1)	318	(34.3)	0.0658	268	(35.6)	254	(33.8)	0.4423
Hospital level	Medical center	1973	(53.3)	1394	(50.2)	579	(62.5)	<0.0001	446	(59.3)	461	(61.3)	0.3258
	Non-Medical centers	1730	(46.7)	1382	(49.8)	348	(37.5)		306	(40.7)	291	(38.7)	
Hospital area	North	2017	(54.5)	1563	(56.3)	454	(49.0)	<0.0001	384	(51.1)	374	(49.7)	0.5139
	Center	761	(20.6)	489	(17.6)	272	(29.3)		196	(26.1)	211	(28.1)	
	South/East	925	(25.0)	724	(26.1)	201	(21.7)		172	(22.9)	167	(22.2)	
Income	<NTD 18,000	1331	(35.9)	987	(35.6)	344	(37.1)	0.0599	279	(37.1)	281	(37.4)	0.9108
	NTD 18,000–24,000	1240	(33.5)	928	(33.4)	312	(33.7)		240	(31.9)	248	(33.0)	
	NTD 24,000–36,000	350	(9.5)	283	(10.2)	67	(7.2)		55	(7.3)	56	(7.4)	
	NTD 36,000+	782	(21.1)	578	(20.8)	204	(22.0)		178	(23.7)	167	(22.2)	
Follow-up time, months	Mean (SD)	68.8	(29.1)	70.7	(28.7)	63.1	(29.3)		70.3	(29.2)	64.4	(28.8)	
Death		606	(16.4)	336	(12.1)	270	(29.1)	<0.0001	123	(16.4)	182	(24.2)	<0.0001
Locoregional recurrence		245	(6.6)	144	(5.2)	101	(10.9)	<0.0001	28	(3.7)	88	(11.7)	<0.0001
Distant metastasis		331	(8.9)	214	(7.7)	117	(12.6)	<0.0001	54	(7.2)	108	(14.4)	<0.0001

SD—standard deviation; IQR—interquartile range; WBRT—whole breast radiotherapy; AJCC—American Joint Committee on Cancer; HER2—human epidermal growth factor receptor 2; SLNB—sentinel lymph node biopsy; ALND—axillary lymph node dissection; CCI—Charlson comorbidity index; RT—radiotherapy; T—tumor; N—nodal; pT—pathologic tumor stage; pN—pathologic nodal stage; COPD—chronic obstructive pulmonary disease.

The cumulative incidence of death was estimated using the Kaplan–Meier method, and differences in OS, LRR-free survival, and DM-free survival between older women receiving BCS followed by adjuvant WBRT and those without adjuvant WBRT were determined using a log-rank test. We performed all analyses using SAS version 9.3 (SAS Institute, Cary, NC, USA). p values < 0.05 were considered statistically significant in the two-tailed Wald test. Risk of all-cause death was calculated, and subgroup analyses by age and cancer were conducted using a log-rank test.

3. Results

3.1. Study Cohort

After PSM, 1504 older women with balanced covariates were included (Table 1). Among them, 752 received BCS followed by adjuvant WBRT (Group 1) and 752 with IDC received BCS without adjuvant WBRT (Group 2). After PSM, the results revealed that the covariates between the groups were homogenous. The median follow-up durations after the index date were 70.3 and 64.4 months for Group 1 and Group 2, respectively.

3.2. Impact of Adjuvant WBRT on Oncologic Outcomes of Old and Very Old Women

In multivariable Cox regression analysis, the adjusted HR (aHR) and 95% confidence interval (95% CI) of all-cause death for adjuvant WBRT compared with no adjuvant WBRT was 0.56 (0.44–0.70). The aHRs (95% CIs) of LRR and DM for adjuvant WBRT were 0.29 (0.19–0.45) and 0.45 (0.32–0.62), respectively, compared with no adjuvant WBRT. The aHRs (95% CIs) of all-cause death for old age (85–89 years) and very old age (≥90 years) were 1.85 (1.28–2.69) and 1.67 (1.47–3.46), respectively, compared with the age of 80–84 years. Other confounders were not significantly different for all-cause death, LRR, and DM between the two groups because of the well-matched PSM design without residual imbalance [25,26].

3.3. Age Stratification in Multivariable Cox Regression Analysis

Because age remained an independent prognostic factor of all-cause death even after PSM, residual imbalance existed in the confounder of age for all-cause death (Table 2). We performed multivariable analysis of OS that was stratified by the ages of 80–89 years and ≥90 years (Table 3). The aHRs (95% CIs) of all-cause mortality for adjuvant WBRT compared with no adjuvant WBRT in old (80–89 years) and very old (≥90 years) women receiving BCS were 0.60 (0.40–0.91) and 0.64 (0.48–0.87), respectively (Table 3). In addition, the aHR (95% CI) of all-cause death for the age of 85–89 was 1.48 (1.07–2.27), compared with the age of 80–84 years, and that for the age of ≥95 years was 1.50 (1.10–2.04) compared with the age of 90–94 years.

Table 2. Multivariate analysis for overall survival, local recurrence, and distant metastasis after propensity score-matching patients aged ≥80 years undergoing breast conservative surgery.

		All-Cause Death			Locoregional Recurrence			Distant Metastasis		
		aHR *	(95% CI)	p Value	aHR *	(95% CI)	p Value	aHR *	(95% CI)	p Value
Adjuvant WBRT	No	1		<0.0001	1		<0.0001	1		<0.0001
	Yes	0.56	(0.44–0.70)		0.29	(0.19–0.45)		0.45	(0.32–0.62)	
Age	80–84	1		<0.0001	1		0.6874	1		0.1827
	85–89	1.85	(1.28–2.69)		0.94	(0.61–1.45)		1.05	(0.71–1.56)	
	90+	1.67	(1.47–3.46)		0.77	(0.42–1.41)		0.66	(0.36–1.18)	
Differentiation	I	1		0.6671	1		0.3917	1		0.3724
	II	1.17	(0.90–1.88)		1.09	(0.76–1.71)		1.28	(0.79–1.40)	
	III	1.94	(0.97–2.19)		1.64	(0.77–2.75)		1.59	(0.69–2.46)	
AJCC clinical stage	I	1		0.4779	1		0.5677	1		0.3347
	II	1.08	(0.91–1.76)		1.18	(0.73–1.91)		1.14	(0.78–1.67)	
	III	1.12	(0.87–1.81)		1.75	(0.61–5.03)		1.59	(0.75–5.39)	
pT	pT0–1	1		0.7845	1		0.8537	1		0.7764
	pT2–4	1.06	(0.73–1.27)		1.05	(0.65–1.67)		1.06	(0.73–1.52)	
pN	pN0	1		0.0676	1		0.3442	1		0.3685
	pN1+	1.30	(0.98–1.73)		1.25	(0.79–2.00)		1.20	(0.81–1.77)	
Adjuvant chemotherapy	Yes	0.83	(0.43–1.12)	0.1168	0.93	(0.57–1.51)	0.7727	1.18	(0.78–1.80)	04319
Hormone receptor positive	Yes	0.88	(0.61–1.09)	0.2451	0.80	(0.55–1.18)	0.2617	0.84	(0.60–1.18)	0.3169
HER2 positive	Yes	1.06	(0.72–1.31)	0.2206	1.04	(0.75–1.18)	0.3494	1.14	(0.76–1.21)	0.4070
Nodal surgery	ALND	1		0.2361	1		0.2561	1		0.4612
	SLNB	0.77	(0.49–1.22)		1.16	(0.74–1.84)		1.05	(0.71–1.55)	
CCI Scores	0	1		0.4551	1		0.2721	1		0.0318
	1	1.09	(0.82–1.34)		0.90	(0.57–1.42)		0.94	(0.65–1.35)	
	2+	1.23	(0.81–1.79)		0.69	(0.43–1.09)		0.58	(0.38–0.89)	
Hospital level	Medical center	1		0.3925	1		0.1240	1		0.9823
	Non-Medical centers	1.11	(0.88–1.41)		0.73	(0.49–1.09)		1.00	(0.71–1.42)	

* All of the covariates listed in Table 2 were adjusted. WBRT—whole breast radiotherapy; aHR—adjusted hazard ratio; CI—confidence interval; AJCC—American Joint Committee on Cancer; HER2—human epidermal growth factor receptor 2; SLNB—sentinel lymph node biopsy; ALND—axillary lymph node dissection; CCI—Charlson comorbidity index; pT—pathologic tumor stage; pN—pathologic nodal stage.

Table 3. Multivariate analysis of overall survival of propensity score-matched patients undergoing breast conservative surgery, stratified by old (80 years or over) and very old (90 years or over).

		Age 80–89			Age ≥90		
		aHR *	(95% CI)	p Value	aHR *	(95% CI)	p Value
Adjuvant RT	No	1		0.0156	1		0.0040
	Yes	0.60	(0.40–0.91)		0.64	(0.48–0.87)	
Age	80–84	1		0.0382	–		
	85–89	1.48	(1.07–2.27)		–		
	90–94	–			1		0.0095
	95+	–			1.50	(1.10–2.04)	
Differentiation	I	1		0.2286	1		0.3581
	II	1.01	(0.58–1.76)		1.08	(0.84–1.94)	
	III	1.90	(0.93–2.50)		1.88	(0.90–2.32)	
AJCC clinical stage	I	1		0.4135	1		0.3453
	II	1.13	(0.88–1.54)		1.19	(0.83–1.70)	
	III	1.75	(0.78–2.02)		1.66	(0.70–2.48)	
pT	pT0–1	1		0.7816	1		0.8476
	pT2–4	1.07	(0.66–1.75)		1.04	(0.73–1.47)	
pN	pN0	1		0.1494	1		0.5985
	pN1+	1.36	(0.86–1.96)		1.11	(0.75–1.66)	
Adjuvant chemotherapy		0.64	(0.52–1.22)	0.2338	0.65	(0.52–1.91)	0.2533
HR positive		0.92	(0.60–1.39)	0.6880	0.92	(0.67–1.26)	0.6025
HER2 positive		1.12	(0.77–1.41)	0.5702	1.31	(0.87–1.96)	0.4925
Nodal surgery	ALND	1		0.8517	1		0.0102
	SLNB/+ALND	0.94	(0.57–1.57)		0.77	(0.52–1.15)	
CCI Scores	0	1		0.7365	1		0.8771
	1	1.11	(0.83–1.41)		1.07	(0.84–1.90)	
	2+	1.53	(0.86–2.10)		1.31	(0.85–2.42)	
Hospital level	Medical centers	1		0.8969	1		0.4276
	Non-medical centers	1.03	(0.68–1.57)		1.13	(0.84–1.52)	

* All of the covariates listed in Table 2 were adjusted. WBRT—whole breast radiotherapy; aHR—adjusted hazard ratio; CI—confidence interval; AJCC—American Joint Committee on Cancer; HER2—human epidermal growth factor receptor 2; SLNB—sentinel lymph node biopsy; ALND—axillary lymph node dissection; CCI—Charlson comorbidity index; RT—radiotherapy; pT—pathologic tumor stage; pN—pathologic nodal stage.

3.4. Survival Curves with or without Adjuvant WBRT

Figures 1–3 present Kaplan–Meier curves that illustrate the overall, LRR-free, and DM-free survival curves of the groups. The 5-year OS probability was 90.11% and 83.92% in the adjuvant WBRT and nonadjuvant WBRT groups, respectively (Figure 1A) (log-rank test, $p < 0.0001$). Additionally, 5-year LRR-free survival was 97.81% and 87.32% in the adjuvant WBRT group and nonadjuvant WBRT group, respectively (Figure 2A; log-rank test, $p < 0.0001$). Moreover, 5-year DM-free survival was 95.74% and 85.61% in the adjuvant WBRT group and nonadjuvant WBRT group, respectively (Figure 3A; log-rank test, $p < 0.0001$).

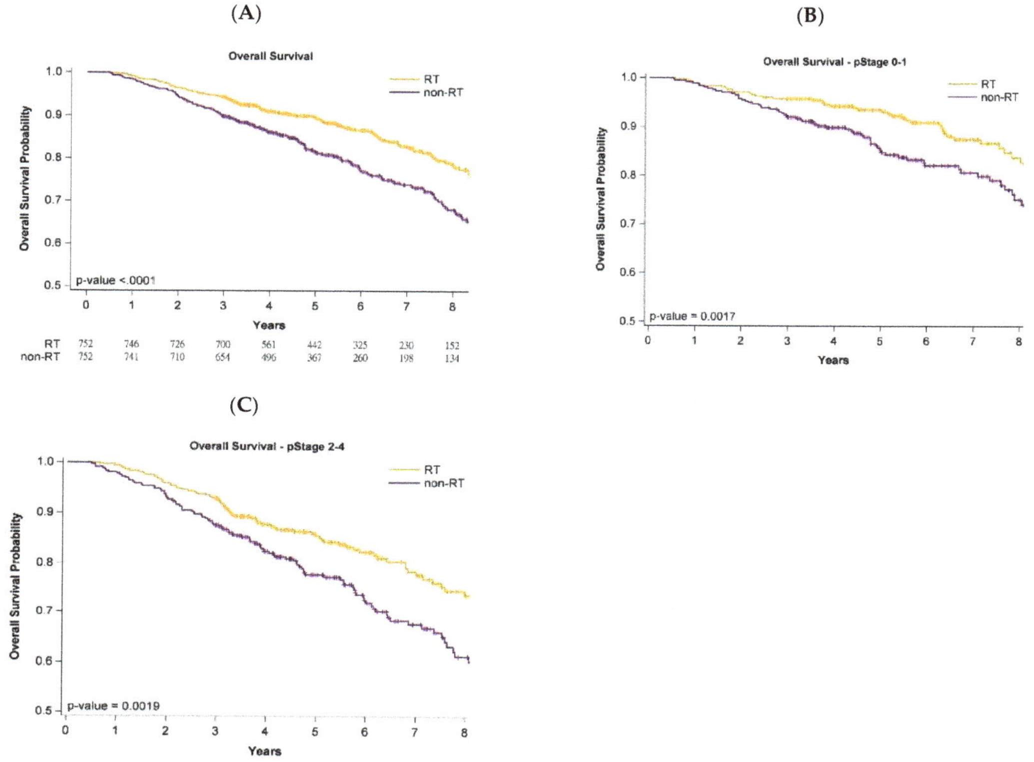

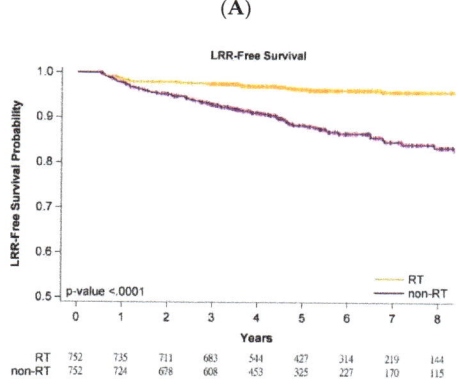

Figure 1. KM curves for overall survival after propensity score matching in patients aged ≥80 years undergoing breast conservative surgery. (**A**)—All stages; (**B**)—Stage 0–1; (**C**)—Stage 2–4.

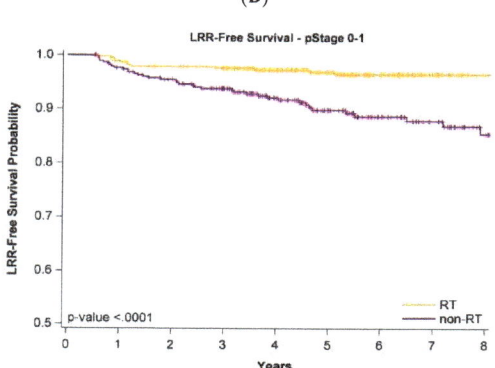

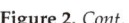

Figure 2. *Cont.*

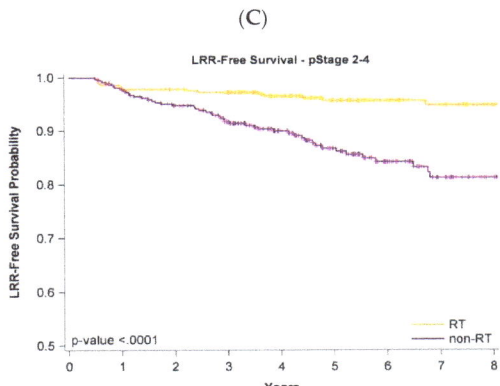

Figure 2. KM survival curves for local recurrence after propensity score matching in patients aged ≥80 years undergoing breast conservative surgery. (**A**)—All stages; (**B**)—Stage 0–1; (**C**)—Stage 2–4.

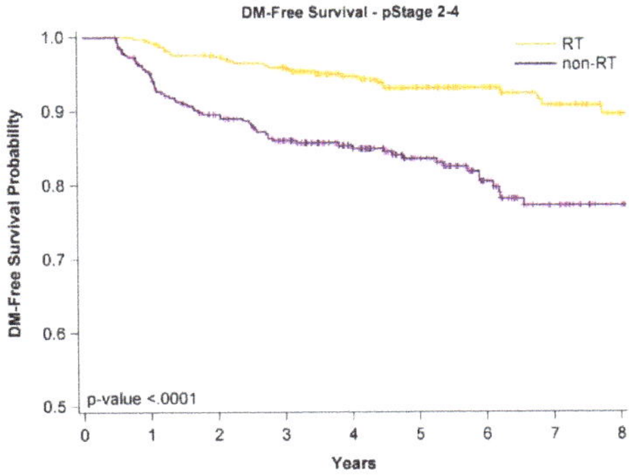

Figure 3. KM survival curves for distant metastasis after propensity score matching in patients aged ≥80 years undergoing breast conservative surgery. (**A**)—All stages; (**B**)—Stage 0–1; (**C**)—Stage 2–4.

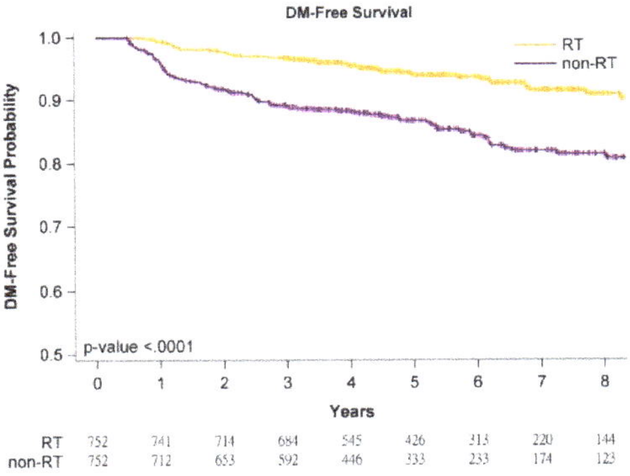

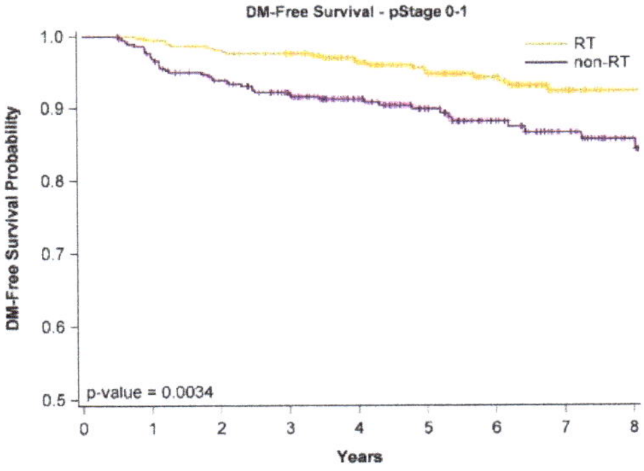

3.5. Survival Curves of Cancer Stages and Age Stratification

Analysis of the impact of stage (early stage (stage 0-I) or advanced stage (stage II-III)) on oncologic outcomes (OS, LRR, and DM) was conducted with stratification by pathologic stages. The OS, LRR-free, and DM-free survival curves of the adjuvant WBRT group remained significantly superior to those of the nonadjuvant WBRT group regardless of stage (Figures 1B,C, 2B,C and 3B,C). Age stratification by 80–89 and $\geq$90 years was also performed. The OS, LRR-free, and DM-free survival curves of the adjuvant WBRT group were significantly superior to those of the non-adjuvant WBRT group in both stratifications (Supplementary Figures S1 and S2).

4. Discussion

4.1. No Solution Regarding Adjuvant WBRT for Older Women with Breast Cancer

Breast cancer is the most common cancer in women, and one in ten patients affected are aged $\geq$80 years [5]. However, this age group is generally excluded from clinical trials, and data to inform their care are sparse [7]. Additionally, no RCT with women aged $\geq$90 years with breast cancer has been conducted. In practice, treatment for older patients with breast cancer involves shared decision-making between physicians and patients based on expected survival lifespan, comorbidities, or prognostic factors of tumor recurrence [8–12]. Nevertheless, few patients in the $\geq$80 years age group receive RT as part of their treatment, especially those aged $\geq$90 years [5,8–12,27]. Studies on the omission of RT in older women with a low recurrence of hormone receptor-positive or HER2-negative breast cancer (as a better prognosis) have been conducted, but studies including women aged $\geq$80 years are scant [8–12]. Breast cancer biologic subtypes of women aged $\geq$80 years exhibit similarities with those of younger postmenopausal women; thus, treatments should be consistent [6]. Possible problems are the expected survival and comorbidities contributing to the incidence of LRR- and DM-related mortality [22–24]. Nonetheless, if older patients with IDC receiving BCS have consistent comorbidities, molecular types (similar hormone receptor status and HER2), the same cancer stages, and similar treatment protocols relative to younger patients, whether adjuvant WBRT should be omitted is unclear.

4.2. Value of PSM in This Population

As shown in Table 1, all potential cofounders of all-cause death for women with breast cancer were matched and controlled through PSM. The cofounders—age, differentiation, AJCC clinical stage, AJCC pathologic stage, pT, pN, neoadjuvant chemotherapy, adjuvant chemotherapy, hormone receptor status, HER2 status, nodal surgical type, CCI score, hospital level (medical center or not), hospital region, and income, all mentioned in previous studies—were matched to balance covariates between the two groups [13–15,28–31]. Because the most common causes of death in older patients are hypertension, ischemic heart disease, cerebrovascular disease, COPD, and diabetes [22], we separated the covariates from the CCI scores and included these covariates in PSM independently for more precise matching to control the confounders of all-cause mortality. PSM allows the design of an observational (non-randomized) study that mimics some of the characteristics of an RCT [32]. After PSM design, we believe the balanced covariates mimic an RCT [32] in our study without selection bias for adjuvant WBRT and no adjuvant WBRT in older women receiving BCS. Before PSM, the trends of selection of no adjuvant WBRT (raw population in Table 1) were compatible with those in previous studies, in which women with node-negative, hormone receptor-positive, HER2-negative cancer or small tumor sizes preferred no adjuvant RT [8–12]. Our findings indicate that women with favorable prognostic factors of OS would not receive adjuvant WBRT (Table 1). Conducting an RCT with patients $\geq$80 years old is difficult. Therefore, a PSM study with balanced conditions is appropriate for evaluating the value of adjuvant WBRT for older women.

4.3. Conditions Different from Previous Studies

Adjuvant WBRT can be omitted in older (≥65 years) women with hormone receptor-positive breast cancer, especially for clinically node-negative, small, or HER2-negative breast cancer [8–12]. Moreover, omission of RT in patients with hormone receptor-positive, node-negative, small breast cancer is supported by a meta-analysis that included postmenopausal women, all of whom received systemic therapy (the majority received tamoxifen) [3]. However, most women had T1, node-negative tumors and were aged ≥65 years, with 39% aged ≥70 years [3]. Only approximately 10% of patients were ≥80 years old in the aforementioned studies [3,8–12]. Comorbidities were not considered in the previous studies with unexpected survival lifespans [3,8–12], and the survival benefit of adjuvant WBRT could not be determined in the aforementioned reports. In the current study, all the enrolled women were ≥80 years old, and approximately 40% were ≥90 years old (Table 1). All comorbidities were considered in our study and were well-matched through PSM. In addition, molecular type, cancer stage, and treatment protocols were controlled for through PSM. Therefore, our study is the first head-to-head PSM study mimicking an RCT with consistent conditions to estimate the oncologic outcomes after adjuvant WBRT in old (aged 80–89 years) and very old (aged ≥90 years) women with IDC receiving BCS.

4.4. Cancer Stage and Age Stratification

Because some reports have indicated that adjuvant RT can be omitted in older women with early-stage breast cancer receiving mastectomy [2,10], we estimated the effects of adjuvant WBRT by using the log-rank test for the PSM population stratified by early or advanced pathologic stage. The results indicated receiving that adjuvant WBRT was significantly superior to not receiving adjuvant WBRT for OS, LRR-free survival, and DM-free survival, even in the earliest stages (stage 0-I) (Figures 1B, 2B and 3B). Previous studies reporting no significant survival difference between adjuvant RT and no adjuvant RT for breast cancer in older women might be attributed to small sample size, short follow-up time, or unknown comorbidities [2,10]. The most common cause of death in these older women is comorbidities [22], but no data on comorbidities have been included in reports [2,10]. Another key concern is that those aged ≥80 years were not the main population, and that those aged ≥90 years were few in the aforementioned studies [2,10]. We used the log-rank test for investigating the effect of adjuvant WBRT or no adjuvant WBRT on oncologic outcomes for different age groups (80–89 years and ≥90 years) in the PSM population (Supplementary Figures S1 and S2). No study of patients aged ≥90 years with breast cancer has been conducted. Our study is the first to demonstrate the benefits of adjuvant RT for women 90 years or older with IDC receiving BCS.

4.5. Limitations

This study has limitations. First, because all the women with IDC were enrolled from an Asian population, the corresponding ethnic susceptibility compared with non-Asian populations remains unclear; hence, our results should be cautiously extrapolated to non-Asian populations. However, no evidence suggests differences in oncologic outcomes between Asian and non-Asian women with breast IDC receiving BCS. Second, the diagnoses of all comorbid conditions were based on ICD-10-CM codes. However, the combination of the TCRD and the National Health Insurance Research Database (NHIRD) in Taiwan appears to be a valid resource for population research on cardiovascular diseases, stroke, or chronic comorbidities [33–35]. The Taiwan Cancer Registry Administration randomly reviews charts and interviews patients to verify the accuracy of diagnoses, and hospitals with outlier chargers or practices may be audited and heavily penalized if malpractice or discrepancies are identified. Accordingly, to obtain crucial information on population specificity and disease occurrence, a large-scale RCT comparing carefully selected patients undergoing suitable treatments is essential. However, as mentioned, enrolling patients ≥80 or even ≥90 years of age in an RCT is difficult. Despite its limitations, a major strength of this study is the use of a nationwide population-based registry with detailed baseline and treatment information. Lifelong follow-up was possible through the linkage of the registry with the national Cause of Death database. Considering the magnitude and statistical significance of the observed effects in the current study, the limitations are unlikely to affect our conclusions.

5. Conclusions

Compared with no adjuvant WBRT, adjuvant WBRT may be associated with decreased all-cause of death, LRR, and DM for older women with breast IDC receiving BCS regardless of stage (early vs. advanced) and age (80–89 vs. ≥90 years). We suggest adjuvant WBRT for old or very old women with IDC receiving BCS, even if the cancer stage is early or the patient is 90 years or older.

Supplementary Materials: The following are available online at https://www.mdpi.com/article/10.3390/jpm12020287/s1, Figure S1: Overall survival, LRR-free survival, and DM-free survival curves for propensity score matched patients aged 80–89 years receiving breast conservative surgery, Figure S2: Overall survival, LRR-free survival, DM-free survival curves for propensity score matched patients aged 90 years or over receiving breast conservative surgery.

Author Contributions: Conception and design, C.-C.H. and S.-Y.W.; collection and assembly of data, C.-C.H., M.S., S.-Y.S., S.-Y.W., C.-L.C. and J.Z.; data analysis and interpretation, C.-C.H., M.S., M.-F.C., C.-L.C. and J.Z.; administrative support, S.-Y.W.; manuscript writing: C.-C.H., C.-L.C., J.Z., S.-Y.S., M.-F.C. and S.-Y.W. All authors have read and agreed to the published version of the manuscript.

Funding: Lo-Hsu Medical Foundation, LotungPoh-Ai Hospital, supports Szu-Yuan Wu's work (Funding Number: 10908, 10909, 11001, 11002, 11003, 11006, and 11013).

Institutional Review Board Statement: The study protocols were reviewed and approved by the Institutional Review Board of Tzu-Chi Medical Foundation (IRB109-015-B).

Informed Consent Statement: Informed consent was waived because the data sets are covered under the Personal Information Protection Act. We used data from the National Health Insurance Research Database and Taiwan Cancer Registry database. The authors confirm that, for approved reasons, some access restrictions apply to the data underlying the findings. The data used in this study cannot be made available in the article, the supplemental files, or in a public repository due to the Personal Information Protection Act executed by Taiwan's government, starting from 2012. Requests for data can be sent as a formal proposal to obtain approval from the ethics review committee of the appropriate governmental department in Taiwan. Specifically, contact information for requesting data appear at http://nhird.nhri.org.tw/en/Data_Subsets.html#S3 and http://nhis.nhri.org.tw/point.html.

Data Availability Statement: The data sets supporting the study conclusions are included in this manuscript and its supplementary files.

Acknowledgments: Lo-Hsu Medical Foundation, LotungPoh-Ai Hospital, supports Szu-Yuan Wu's work (Funding Number: 10908, 10909, 11001, 11002, 11003, 11006, and 11013).

Conflicts of Interest: The authors have no potential conflicts of interest to declare. The data sets supporting the study conclusions are included in the manuscript.

Abbreviations

WBRT, whole-breast radiotherapy; LRR, locoregional recurrence; DM, distant metastasis; IDC, invasive ductal carcinoma; BCS, breast-conserving surgery; OS, overall survival; aHR, adjusted hazard ratio; HR, hazard ratio; CI, confidence interval; AJCC, American Joint Committee on Cancer; TCRD, Taiwan Cancer Registry Database; SD, standard deviation; HER2, human epidermal growth factor receptor 2; SLNB, sentinel lymph node biopsy; ALND, axillary lymph node dissection; CCI, Charlson comorbidity index; ICD-10-CM, International Classification of Diseases, 10th Revision, Clinical Modification; NCCN, National Comprehensive Cancer Network; RT, radiotherapy; T, tumor; N, nodal; pT, pathologic tumor stage; pN, pathologic nodal stage; NHIRD, National Health Insurance Research Database; RCT, randomized controlled trial; PSM, propensity scores matching.

References

1. Mohler, J.; Bahnson, R.R.; Boston, B.; Busby, J.E.; D'Amico, A.; Eastham, J.A.; Enke, C.A.; George, D.; Horwitz, E.M.; Huben, R.P. NCCN Clinical Practice Guidelines in Oncology: Prostate Cancer. Available online: https://www.nccn.org/professionals/physician_gls/pdf/prostate.pdf (accessed on 17 February 2021).
2. Kunkler, I.H.; Williams, L.J.; Jack, W.J.; Cameron, D.A.; Dixon, J.M.; on behalf of the PRIME II investigators. Breast-conserving surgery with or without irradiation in women aged 65 years or older with early breast cancer (PRIME II): A randomised controlled trial. *Lancet Oncol.* **2015**, *16*, 266–273. [CrossRef]
3. van de Water, W.; Bastiaannet, E.; Scholten, A.N.; Kiderlen, M.; de Craen, A.J.; Westendorp, R.G.; van de Velde, C.J.; Liefers, G.J. Breast-conserving surgery with or without radiotherapy in older breast patients with early stage breast cancer: A systematic review and meta-analysis. *Ann. Surg. Oncol.* **2014**, *21*, 786–794. [CrossRef] [PubMed]
4. Siegel, R.L.; Miller, K.D.; Fuchs, H.E.; Jemal, A. Cancer Statistics, 2021. *CA Cancer J. Clin.* **2021**, *71*, 7–33. [CrossRef]
5. Miller, K.D.; Siegel, R.L.; Lin, C.C.; Mariotto, A.B.; Kramer, J.L.; Rowland, J.H.; Stein, K.D.; Alteri, R.; Jemal, A. Cancer treatment and survivorship statistics, 2016. *CA Cancer J. Clin.* **2016**, *66*, 271–289. [CrossRef]
6. Bertolo, A.; Rosso, C.; Voutsadakis, I.A. Breast Cancer in Patients 80 Years-Old and Older. *Eur. J. Breast Health* **2020**, *16*, 208–212. [CrossRef]
7. Early Breast Cancer Trialists' Collaborative, G.; Darby, S.; McGale, P.; Correa, C.; Taylor, C.; Arriagada, R.; Clarke, M.; Cutter, D.; Davies, C.; Ewertz, M.; et al. Effect of radiotherapy after breast-conserving surgery on 10-year recurrence and 15-year breast cancer death: Meta-analysis of individual patient data for 10,801 women in 17 randomised trials. *Lancet* **2011**, *378*, 1707–1716. [CrossRef]
8. Fisher, B.; Bryant, J.; Dignam, J.J.; Wickerham, D.L.; Mamounas, E.P.; Fisher, E.R.; Margolese, R.G.; Nesbitt, L.; Paik, S.; Pisansky, T.M.; et al. Tamoxifen, radiation therapy, or both for prevention of ipsilateral breast tumor recurrence after lumpectomy in women with invasive breast cancers of one centimeter or less. *J. Clin. Oncol. Off. J. Am. Soc. Clin. Oncol.* **2002**, *20*, 4141–4149. [CrossRef] [PubMed]
9. Potter, R.; Gnant, M.; Kwasny, W.; Tausch, C.; Handl-Zeller, L.; Pakisch, B.; Taucher, S.; Hammer, J.; Luschin-Ebengreuth, G.; Schmid, M.; et al. Lumpectomy plus tamoxifen or anastrozole with or without whole breast irradiation in women with favorable early breast cancer. *Int. J. Radiat Oncol. Biol. Phys.* **2007**, *68*, 334–340. [CrossRef] [PubMed]
10. Hughes, K.S.; Schnaper, L.A.; Bellon, J.R.; Cirrincione, C.T.; Berry, D.A.; McCormick, B.; Muss, H.B.; Smith, B.L.; Hudis, C.A.; Winer, E.P.; et al. Lumpectomy plus tamoxifen with or without irradiation in women age 70 years or older with early breast cancer: Long-term follow-up of CALGB 9343. *J. Clin. Oncol. Off. J. Am. Soc. Clin. Oncol.* **2013**, *31*, 2382–2387. [CrossRef] [PubMed]
11. Tinterri, C.; Gatzemeier, W.; Zanini, V.; Regolo, L.; Pedrazzoli, C.; Rondini, E.; Amanti, C.; Gentile, G.; Taffurelli, M.; Fenaroli, P.; et al. Conservative surgery with and without radiotherapy in elderly patients with early-stage breast cancer: A prospective randomised multicentre trial. *Breast* **2009**, *18*, 373–377. [CrossRef]
12. Ford, H.T.; Coombes, R.C.; Gazet, J.C.; Gray, R.; McConkey, C.C.; Sutcliffe, R.; Quilliam, J.; Lowndes, S. Long-term follow-up of a randomised trial designed to determine the need for irradiation following conservative surgery for the treatment of invasive breast cancer. *Ann. Oncol.* **2006**, *17*, 401–408. [CrossRef] [PubMed]
13. Zhang, J.; Lu, C.Y.; Chen, C.H.; Chen, H.M.; Wu, S.Y. Effect of pathologic stages on postmastectomy radiation therapy in breast cancer receiving neoadjuvant chemotherapy and total mastectomy: A Cancer Database Analysis. *Breast* **2020**, *54*, 70–78. [CrossRef] [PubMed]
14. Zhang, J.; Lu, C.Y.; Qin, L.; Chen, H.M.; Wu, S.Y. Breast-conserving surgery with or without irradiation in women with invasive ductal carcinoma of the breast receiving preoperative systemic therapy: A cohort study. *Breast* **2020**, *54*, 139–147. [CrossRef] [PubMed]
15. Zhang, J.; Lu, C.Y.; Chen, H.M.; Wu, S.Y. Neoadjuvant Chemotherapy or Endocrine Therapy for Invasive Ductal Carcinoma of the Breast with High Hormone Receptor Positivity and Human Epidermal Growth Factor Receptor 2 Negativity. *JAMA Netw. Open* **2021**, *4*, e211785. [CrossRef]
16. Liu, W.C.; Liu, H.E.; Kao, Y.W.; Qin, L.; Lin, K.C.; Fang, C.Y.; Tsai, L.L.; Shia, B.C.; Wu, S.Y. Definitive radiotherapy or surgery for early oral squamous cell carcinoma in old and very old patients: A propensity-score-matched, nationwide, population-based cohort study. *Radiother Oncol.* **2020**, *151*, 214–221. [CrossRef]
17. NCCN Clinical Practice Guidelines in Oncology. Available online: http://www.nccn.org/professionals/physician_gls/f_guidelines.asp (accessed on 20 December 2021).
18. Hammond, M.E.; Hayes, D.F.; Dowsett, M.; Allred, D.C.; Hagerty, K.L.; Badve, S.; Fitzgibbons, P.L.; Francis, G.; Goldstein, N.S.; Hayes, M.; et al. American Society of Clinical Oncology/College of American Pathologists guideline recommendations for immunohistochemical testing of estrogen and progesterone receptors in breast cancer. *J. Clin. Oncol. Off. J. Am. Soc. Clin. Oncol.* **2010**, *28*, 2784–2795. [CrossRef]
19. Charlson, M.; Szatrowski, T.P.; Peterson, J.; Gold, J. Validation of a combined comorbidity index. *J. Clin. Epidemiol.* **1994**, *47*, 1245–1251. [CrossRef]
20. Chen, J.H.; Yen, Y.C.; Yang, H.C.; Liu, S.H.; Yuan, S.P.; Wu, L.L.; Lee, F.P.; Lin, K.C.; Lai, M.T.; Wu, C.C.; et al. Curative-Intent Aggressive Treatment Improves Survival in Elderly Patients with Locally Advanced Head and Neck Squamous Cell Carcinoma and High Comorbidity Index. *Medicine* **2016**, *95*, e3268. [CrossRef]

21. Austin, P.C. Optimal caliper widths for propensity-score matching when estimating differences in means and differences in proportions in observational studies. *Pharm. Stat.* **2011**, *10*, 150–161. [CrossRef]
22. Gorina, Y.; Hoyert, D.; Lentzner, H.; Goulding, M. Trends in Causes of Death among Older Persons in the United States. Available online: https://www.cdc.gov/nchs/data/ahcd/agingtrends/06olderpersons.pdf (accessed on 30 October 2005).
23. Berry, S.D.; Ngo, L.; Samelson, E.J.; Kiel, D.P. Competing risk of death: An important consideration in studies of older adults. *J. Am. Geriatr. Soc.* **2010**, *58*, 783–787. [CrossRef]
24. Lau, B.; Cole, S.R.; Gange, S.J. Competing risk regression models for epidemiologic data. *Am. J. Epidemiol.* **2009**, *170*, 244–256. [CrossRef]
25. Nguyen, T.L.; Collins, G.S.; Spence, J.; Daures, J.P.; Devereaux, P.J.; Landais, P.; Le Manach, Y. Double-adjustment in propensity score matching analysis: Choosing a threshold for considering residual imbalance. *BMC Med. Res. Methodol.* **2017**, *17*, 78. [CrossRef]
26. Zhang, Z.; Kim, H.J.; Lonjon, G.; Zhu, Y.; written on behalf of AME Big-Data Clinical Trial Collaborative Group. Balance diagnostics after propensity score matching. *Ann. Transl. Med.* **2019**, *7*, 16. [CrossRef] [PubMed]
27. Kuzan, T.Y.; Koca, E.; Dizdar, O.; Arslan, C.; Eren, T.; Yalcin, S.; Kucukoztas, N.; Aksoy, S.; Rahatli, S.; Dede, D.S.; et al. Breast cancer in octogenarian women: Clinical characteristics and outcome. *J. BUON* **2013**, *18*, 328–334. [PubMed]
28. Zhang, J.; Chang, C.L.; Lu, C.Y.; Chen, H.M.; Wu, S.Y. Paravertebral block in regional anesthesia with propofol sedation reduces locoregional recurrence in patients with breast cancer receiving breast conservative surgery compared with volatile inhalational without propofol in general anesthesia. *Biomed. Pharmacother.* **2021**, *142*, 111991. [CrossRef] [PubMed]
29. Zhang, J.; Lu, C.Y.; Chen, H.M.; Wu, S.Y. Pathologic response rates for breast cancer stages as a predictor of outcomes in patients receiving neoadjuvant chemotherapy followed by breast-conserving surgery. *Surg. Oncol.* **2020**, *36*, 91–98. [CrossRef]
30. Zhang, J.; Sun, M.; Chang, E.; Lu, C.Y.; Chen, H.M.; Wu, S.Y. Pathologic response as predictor of recurrence, metastasis, and survival in breast cancer patients receiving neoadjuvant chemotherapy and total mastectomy. *Am. J. Cancer Res.* **2020**, *10*, 3415–3427. [CrossRef]
31. Zhang, J.Q.; Lu, C.Y.; Qin, L.; Chen, H.M.; Wu, S.Y. Outcome of post-mastectomy radiotherapy after primary systemic treatment in patients with different clinical tumor and nodal stages of breast cancer: A cohort study. *Am. J. Cancer Res.* **2020**, *10*, 2185–2198.
32. Austin, P.C. An Introduction to Propensity Score Methods for Reducing the Effects of Confounding in Observational Studies. *Multivariate Behav. Res.* **2011**, *46*, 399–424. [CrossRef]
33. Cheng, C.L.; Lee, C.H.; Chen, P.S.; Li, Y.H.; Lin, S.J.; Yang, Y.H. Validation of acute myocardial infarction cases in the national health insurance research database in taiwan. *J. Epidemiol.* **2014**, *24*, 500–507. [CrossRef]
34. Cheng, C.L.; Kao, Y.H.; Lin, S.J.; Lee, C.H.; Lai, M.L. Validation of the National Health Insurance Research Database with ischemic stroke cases in Taiwan. *Pharmacoepidemiol. Drug Saf.* **2011**, *20*, 236–242. [CrossRef] [PubMed]
35. Lin, C.C.; Lai, M.S.; Syu, C.Y.; Chang, S.C.; Tseng, F.Y. Accuracy of diabetes diagnosis in health insurance claims data in Taiwan. *J. Formos. Med. Assoc.* **2005**, *104*, 157–163. [PubMed]

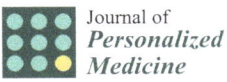

Article

Let-7a-5p, miR-100-5p, miR-101-3p, and miR-199a-3p Hyperexpression as Potential Predictive Biomarkers in Early Breast Cancer Patients

Paola Fuso [1,2,†], Mariantonietta Di Salvatore [2,3,*,†], Concetta Santonocito [2,4], Donatella Guarino [2,4], Chiara Autilio [5], Antonino Mulè [1,2,6], Damiano Arciuolo [1,2,6], Antonina Rinninella [7], Flavio Mignone [7], Matteo Ramundo [2,3], Brunella Di Stefano [2,3], Armando Orlandi [2,3], Ettore Capoluongo [2,8], Nicola Nicolotti [2,9], Gianluca Franceschini [2,10], Alejandro Martin Sanchez [2,10], Giampaolo Tortora [2,3], Giovanni Scambia [1,2], Carlo Barone [2] and Alessandra Cassano [2,3]

Citation: Fuso, P.; Di Salvatore, M.; Santonocito, C.; Guarino, D.; Autilio, C.; Mulè, A.; Arciuolo, D.; Rinninella, A.; Mignone, F.; Ramundo, M.; et al. Let-7a-5p, miR-100-5p, miR-101-3p, and miR-199a-3p Hyperexpression as Potential Predictive Biomarkers in Early Breast Cancer Patients. *J. Pers. Med.* **2021**, *11*, 816. https://doi.org/10.3390/jpm11080816

Academic Editor: Raghu Sinha

Received: 16 May 2021
Accepted: 14 August 2021
Published: 20 August 2021

Publisher's Note: MDPI stays neutral with regard to jurisdictional claims in published maps and institutional affiliations.

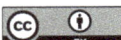

Copyright: © 2021 by the authors. Licensee MDPI, Basel, Switzerland. This article is an open access article distributed under the terms and conditions of the Creative Commons Attribution (CC BY) license (https://creativecommons.org/licenses/by/4.0/).

1. Department of Woman and Child Health and Public Health, Fondazione Policlinico Universitario Agostino Gemelli IRCCS, Largo A. Gemelli 8, 00168 Rome, Italy; paola.fuso@policlinicogemelli.it (P.F.); antonino.mule@policlinicogemelli.it (A.M.); damiano.arciuolo@policlinicogemelli.it (D.A.); giovanni.scambia@policlinicogemelli.it (G.S.)
2. Faculty of Medicine and Surgery, Università Cattolica Del Sacro Cuore, Largo F. Vito 8, 00168 Rome, Italy; concetta.santonocito@policlinicogemelli.it (C.S.); donatella.guarino@policlinicogemelli.it (D.G.); m.ramundo@piafondazionepanico.it (M.R.); brunella.distefano@guest.policlinicogemelli.it (B.D.S.); armando.orlandi@policlinicogemelli.it (A.O.); ettore.capoluongo@unicatt.it (E.C.); nicola.nicolotti@policlinicogemelli.it (N.N.); gianluca.franceschini@policlinicogemelli.it (G.F.); martin.sanchez@policlinicogemelli.it (A.M.S.); giampaolo.tortora@policlinicogemelli.it (G.T.); carlo.barone@unicatt.it (C.B.); alessandra.cassano@policlinicogemelli.it (A.C.)
3. Comprehensive Cancer Center, Medical Oncology Unit, Fondazione Policlinico Universitario "A. Gemelli" IRCCS, Largo A. Gemelli 8, 00168 Rome, Italy
4. Laboratory of Clinical Molecular Biology, Department of Biochemistry and Clinical Biochemistry, Fondazione Policlinico Universitario Agostino Gemelli IRCCS, Largo A. Gemelli 8, 00168 Rome, Italy
5. Department of Biochemistry and Molecular Biology, Faculty of Biology and Research Institute, Universidad Complutense, Av. Sèneca, 2, 28040 Madrid, Spain; cautilio@ucm.es
6. Department of Pathologic Anatomy, Fondazione Policlinico Universitario Agostino Gemelli IRCCS, Largo A. Gemelli 8, 00168 Rome, Italy
7. Department of Science and Innovation Technology, University of Piemonte Orientale, V.le Teresa Michel 11, 15121 Alessandria, Italy; 20001886@studentiunipo.it (A.R.); flavio.mignone@unipo.it (F.M.)
8. Biotecnologie Avanzate, Università Federico II-CEINGE, Corso Umberto I 40, 80138 Naples, Italy
9. Medical Management, Fondazione Policlinico Universitario Agostino Gemelli IRCCS, Largo A. Gemelli 8, 00168 Rome, Italy
10. Multidisciplinary Breast Center, Dipartimento Scienze della Salute della Donna e del Bambino e di Sanità Pubblica, Fondazione Policlinico Universitario Agostino Gemelli IRCCS, Largo A. Gemelli 8, 00168 Rome, Italy
* Correspondence: mariantonietta.disalvatore@policlinicogemelli.it; Tel.: +39-0630-156-212
† Equally contributed to the work.

Abstract: Background: The aim of this study is to identify miRNAs able to predict the outcomes in breast cancer patients after neoadjuvant chemotherapy (NAC). Patients and methods: We retrospectively analyzed 24 patients receiving NAC and not reaching pathologic complete response (pCR). miRNAs were analyzed using an Illumina Next-Generation-Sequencing (NGS) system. Results: Event-free survival (EFS) and overall survival (OS) were significantly higher in patients with up-regulation of let-7a-5p (EFS $p = 0.006$; OS $p = 0.0001$), mirR-100-5p (EFS s $p = 0.01$; OS $p = 0.03$), miR-101-3p (EFS $p = 0.05$; OS $p = 0.01$), and miR-199a-3p (EFS $p = 0.02$; OS $p = 0.01$) in post-NAC samples, independently from breast cancer subtypes. At multivariate analysis, only let-7a-5p was significantly associated with EFS ($p = 0.009$) and OS ($p = 0.0008$). Conclusion: Up-regulation of the above miRNAs could represent biomarkers in breast cancer.

Keywords: subtypes breast cancer; miRNAs; breast cancer treatment; chemotherapy; integrated therapies; next-generation-sequencing; target therapy; precision medicine; personalized medicine

1. Introduction

Breast cancer is a heterogeneous disease and many molecular changes occur during the course of the disease; this is the main cause of treatment failure. This characteristic of breast cancer is reflected on the basis of gene expression pattern classification. It falls under five distinct molecular subtypes including luminal A, luminal B, receptor tyrosine-protein kinase erbB-2 (HER2)-enriched, basal-like, and normal-like subtype. Luminal A breast cancer is hormone-receptor positive (estrogen-receptor (ER) and/or progesterone-receptor (PR) positive), HER2-negative, has low levels of the protein Ki-67, and is low-grade. Luminal B breast cancer is hormone-receptor positive (ER and/or PR positive) and either HER2-positive or HER2-negative with high levels of Ki-67. HER2-enriched breast cancer is hormone-receptor negative (ER and PR negative) and HER2-positive. Triple negative breast cancer (TN) is defined as the absence of estrogen receptor, progesterone receptor, and HER2 expression accounting for approximately 15–20% of all breast cancer patients. The majority of TN patients (up to 70%) overlap with the basal-like gene expression subtype.

Tumor evolution is a unique process for each patient and is influenced by intrinsic genetic variability and external factors such as cancer therapy. Neoadjuvant setting is an ideal scenario to understand tumor evolution at a single patient level, because make it possible to identify molecular changes occurring in tumors due to treatment by comparing pre and post-chemotherapy samples [1–3].

Finding the patients most likely to benefit from NAC is a crucial need and increasing experimental and clinical studies are centered on identifying the predictors of long-term benefit. Several surrogate endpoints have been examined in the neoadjuvant setting such as the pCR, which has been identified as a primary endpoint in numerous clinical trials despite the controversies on its power of predicting the outcome [3,4].

It is noteworthy that not all patients with residual disease after NAC relapse, and the prognostic impact of pCR varies among breast cancer-intrinsic subtypes, whereas patients with luminal A-like breast cancer show a low pCR rate, their overall prognosis is favorable, and patients with TN breast cancer show a high pCR rate but may have a poorer outcome; moreover, if all intrinsic subtypes are considered, the prognostic information of pCR is reduced [5–9].

Several studies have been performed to discover molecular breast cancer biomarkers in order to predict response to neoadjuvant therapy.

miRNAs are involved in pathway regulation (one miRNA can target many genes and a single gene can be modulated by several miRNAs), and finally, miRNAs show tissue and cell-specific expression profiles, and their role in the pathophysiology of the disease is supported extensively in the literature [10].

Each miRNA can regulate the expression of several genes; thus, each one can simultaneously modulate multiple cellular signaling pathways. Depending on their modulation (amplification/deletion) and on target gene function (tumor suppressor/oncogene), miRNA can play alternatively an oncosuppressor or oncogene function. MiRNAs expression in tumors can be altered due to epigenetic, genetic, and transcriptional alterations [11,12].

Several studies have demonstrated that many miRNAs are aberrantly expressed in breast cancer, according to breast cancer molecular subtypes and thus potentially play a role of biomarkers for cancer diagnosis and for response to therapy [13].

We hypothesized that miRNA are differently expressed at different steps of the disease, and it could be possible to identify a set of miRNA associated with disease progression or response to therapy and to attribute to them a predictive and prognostic value.

The aim of the present exploratory study was to identify a set of miRNAs able to predict the prognosis of patients who underwent NAC not achieving pCR.

2. Materials and Methods

2.1. Patients' Characteristics and Tumor Specimen Collection

All procedures performed in studies involving human participants were in accordance with the ethical standards of the institutional and/or national research committee and with the 1964 Helsinki declaration and its later amendments or comparable ethical standards. This study has the approval of the Ethics Committee of Fondazione Poli-clinico A. Gemelli IRCCS of Rome (Italy) (N protocol 27736/16), and all patients gave written informed consent. We analyzed our database that contains clinical and pathological data on ≈200 cases that underwent neoadjuvant treatment from July 1997 to April 2014 at Fondazione Policlinico A. Gemelli. Patients had measurable breast tumors. Patients were staged according to the American Joint Committee on Cancer (AJCC) Eighth edition [14]. A TRU-CUT biopsy was obtained from each patient. Classification of intrinsic subtypes was defined according to 16th St. Gallen and ESMO guidelines. Histological type, tumor grade, Ki67, ER, PR, and HER2 status were evaluated in the pre-NAC biopsy and in post-surgical neoplastic specimens. Treatment of HER2-negative breast cancer patients consisted of a combination of anthracyclines, taxanes, and cyclophosphamide, while patients with HER2-positive tumors received taxanes and carboplatin combined with trastuzumab, the latter continued after surgery to complete one year of treatment. Patients with ER and/or PR positive tumors received adjuvant endocrine treatment for at least 5 years. Adjuvant radiotherapy was offered according to the national guidelines [15]. The pCR was defined as the absence of any residual invasive cancer on resected breast specimen and on all sampled ipsilateral lymph nodes (ypT0/is ypN0) [16,17] (Table 1).

Table 1. Baseline patients' characteristics (N 200).

Characteristics	N	%
Demographic and clinical		
Age		
Mean (SD) (years)	49.4 ± 10.4	
≤40	69	34.5
>40	131	65.5
ER status		
Positive	130	65.0
Negative	55	27.5
Unknown	15	7.5
PR status		
Positive	128	64.0
Negative	58	29.0
Unknown	14	7.0
HER2 status		
Positive	58	29.0
Negative	127	63.5
Unknown	15	7.5
Subtype		
Luminal A	46	23.0
Luminal B/HER2-negative	48	24.0
Luminal B/HER2-positive	37	18.5
HER2-positive (non-luminal)	21	10.5

Table 1. *Cont.*

Characteristics	N	%
Triple negative	33	16.5
Unknown	15	7.5
Ki 67		
≤20%	59	29.5
>20%	120	60.0
Unknown	21	10.5
Grade		
1	0	0.0
2	51	25.5
3	84	42.0
Unknown	65	32.5
2 Histologic type		
Lobular	18	9.0
Ductal	150	75.0
Other	28	14.0
Unknown	4	2.0
3 Tumor characteristics before treatment		
cT stage		
cTx	1	0.5
cT1	11	5.5
cT2	71	35.5
cT3	55	27.5
cT4	48	24.0
Unknown	14	7.0
cN stage		
cN0	33	16.5
cN1	106	53.0
cN2	36	18.0
cN3	9	4.5
Unknown	16	8.0
Clinical AJCC stage		
0	0	0.0
I	1	0.5
II	76	38.0
III	105	52.5
IV	1	0.5
Unknown	17	8.5
Treatment		
Neoadjuvant		
TAC	138	69.0
TCH	54	27.0
Other	8	4.0

Table 1. Cont.

Characteristics	N	%
Adjuvant hormone		
Yes	130	65.0
No	54	27.0
Unknown	16	8.0
Tumor pathology after neoadjuvant treatment		
yT stage		
yT0/is	42	21.0
yT1	75	37.5
yT2	37	18.5
yT3	13	6.5
yT4	7	3.5
Unknown	26	13.0
yN stage		
yN0	83	41.5
yN1	62	31.0
yN2	18	9.0
yN3	12	6.0
Unknown	25	12.5
Pathologic yAJCC stage		
0	34	17.0
I	46	23.0
II	55	27.5
III	37	18.5
IV	1	0.5
Unknown	27	13.0
Treatment outcomes		
Response to neoadjuvant treatment		
Complete response (R0)	44	22.0
Microscopic residual disease (R1)	53	26.5
Macroscopic residual disease (R2)	101	50.5
Unknown	2	1.0
Events within 3 years		
Distant relapse	37	18.5
Local recurrence	11	5.5
Death	12	6.0
Unknown	18	9.0
Median follow-up, months	80	

Abbreviations: TAC, taxanes, anthracyclines, and cyclophosphamide-based regimen; TCH, taxanes, carboplatin, and trastuzumab-based regimen; ER, estrogen receptor; PR, progesterone receptor; HER2, human epidermal growth factor receptor; pCR, pathologic complete response; SD standard deviation.

From the entire database, we selected twenty-four patients homogeneously distributed according to clinical and pathological characteristics not achieving pCR to which the maximum amount of paraffin-embedding samples of both pre- and post-treatment specimen were available (Tables 2 and 3). In particular, we analyzed pre- and post-NAC samples of the three main molecular subtypes, respectively HER2-positive luminal, HER2-positive non-luminal, and TN subtypes, respectively. For each subtype, we selected four patients with good prognosis and four with poor prognosis.

Table 2. Clinicopathological characteristics of breast cancer selected patients (N 1–12).

Patients	1	2	3	4	5	6	7	8	9	10	11	12
Age	42	54	46	40	54	46	45	53	41	68	35	72
Hystological type	IC	DIC	DIC	DIC	IC	DIC	IC	DIC	IC	DIC	DIC	IC
Grade	3		3	3		3	2	3			2	
cKi67	65	40	80	80	45	16	60	30	80	80	45	15
Receptor subtype	B2	B2	B2	B2	B2	B2	B2	B2	TN	TN	TN	TN
cTMN	cT1N1	cT2N1	cT4N1	cT3N1	cT3N1	cT4N1	cT2N1	cT2N1	cT2N1	cT2N2	cT2N1	cT2cN1
Preoperative staging	IIA	IIB	IIIB	IIIA	IIIA	IIIB	IIB	IIB	IIB	IIIA	IIB	IIB
Pathological response	R1	R2	R2	R2	R2	R2	R2	R1	R1	R2	R2	R2
yKi67			70	80			70	45			60	3
ypTNM	ypT1N0	ypT1N1	ypT2N1	ypT1N1	ypT2N1	ypT2N0	ypT1N0	ypT1N0	ypT1N0	ypT1N1	ypT1N1	ypT1N1
ySTADIO	IA	IIA	IIB	IIA	IIB	IA	IA	IA	IA	IIA	IIA	IIA
NAC	TCH	TCH	TCH	TCH	TCH	TCH	TCH	TCH	TAC	TAC	TAC	TC
Type of surgery	Q + L	M + L	M + L	Q + L	M + L	M + L	Q + L	M + L	M + L	M + L	Q + L	M + L
ADJUVANT CHT	H	H	H	H	H	H	H	H	0	0	0	0
ET	X	X	X	X	X	X	X	X				
RT	X			X			X				X	

Table 3. Clinicopathological characteristics of breast cancer selected patients (N 13–24).

Patients	13	14	15	16	17	18	19	20	21	22	23	24
Age	60	52	57	38	67	44	47	40	36	55	57	57
Hystological type	DIC	DIC	IC	DIC	DIC	IC	DIC	DIC	DIC	DIC	DIC	DIC
Grade	3	3	3	3		3	3	3	3	3	3	3
cKi67	45	45	90	80	35		35	60	35	40	15	45
Receptor subtype	TN	TN	TN	TN	H	H	H	H	H	H	H	H
cTMN	cT2N1	cT1N2	cT2N1	cT2N0	cT2N1	cT2N1	cT4N1	cT4N1	cT3N1	cT3N2	cT4N0	cT2N0
Preoperative staging	IIB	IIIA	IIB	IIA	IIB	IIB	IIIB	IIIB	IIIA	IIIA	IIIB	IIA
Pathological response	R2	R1	R2	R2	R1	R2	R1	R2	R2	R1	R1	R1
yKi67	85	6	80	70		70	4		2	40	45	
ypTNM	ypT2N0	ypT1N0	ypT1N1	ypT1N0	ypT1N1	ypT3N0	ypT1N0	ypT1N1	ypT2N1	ypT1N0	ypT1N0	ypT1N0
Pathological staging	IIA	IA	IIA	IA	IIA	IIIA	IA	IIA	IIB	IA	IA	IA
NAC	TAC	TAC	TAC	AC-T	TCH	TCH	TCH	TCH	TCH	TCH	TCH	TCH
Type of surgery	M + L	Q + L	M + L	M + L	M + L	M + L	M + L	M + L	M + L	M + L	M + L	M + L
ADJUVANT CHT			CMF	AC	H	H	H	H	H	H	H	H
ET												
RT		X					X		X		X	X

2.2. Purification of miRNA from Paraffin-Embedding Tissue Sections

Standard formalin-fixation and paraffin-embedding (FFPE) procedures always resulted in significant fragmentation and crosslinking of nucleic acid. For each of the two samples (pre- and post-NAC) for each patient, the starting material for RNA purification was made by up to 4 sections of paraffin-embedding tissue with a thickness of 5 μm combined in one preparation. After microdissection, the total RNA was extracted using miRNeasy FFPE Kit (Qiagen) following the protocol of the manufacturer. The concentration and purity of the total RNA was isolated from tissues and was determined by measuring the absorbance in a spectrophotometer (Nanodrop). The QIAseq miRNA Library Kit (Qiagen) was used for miRNA libraries. In an unbiased rapid reaction, adapters were ligated sequentially to the 3' and 5' ends of the miRNAs. Subsequently, universal cDNA synthesis with UMI (Unique Molecular Index) assignment, cDNA cleanup, library amplification, and library cleanup were performed following the manufacturer's recommendation. The integrity and size distribution of the total RNA from the tissue was confirmed using an automated analysis system (Agilent 2100 Bioan-alyzer). Successively, the miRNA sequencing libraries was sequenced using MiSeq® Il-lumina NGS system: the molarity of each sample (in nM) was calculated using the following equation: $(X\ ng/\mu L)(106)/(112450) = Y\ nM$. Individual libraries were diluted to 4 nM using nuclease-free water and then combined in equimolar amounts.

2.3. MiRNA Discovery

2.3.1. Analysis Procedure

The QIAseq miRNA-NGS data analysis software (Qiagen) was used. The results were confirmed manually by aligning the fastqs with the sequences corresponding to all human miRNAs. The miRNA sequences were extracted from the miRBase database [18].

The miRNAs were selected based on the number of reads, and those that differed between pre-NAC and post-NAC were taken into consideration.

2.3.2. MiRNA Target Prediction

To know the potential target site, a computational approach was applied for their validation [19]. The miRNA targets were predicted by the instrument MiRDB [20]. This is an online database for miRNA target prediction and functional annotations with a focus on mature miRNAs. It provides a web interface for target prediction generated by an SVM machine learning algorithm. All gene targets were converted by the Human Gene ID Converter tool into their corresponding NCBI entrez gene ID. Some NCBI-gene ID were searched manually on the HUGO Gene Nomenclature Committee (HGNC) database. Perl language scripts have been made to list the NCBI entrez gene ID for each of the miRNAs to be analyzed. For the mapping of the genes, the KEGG Mapper—Search & Color Pathway tool was used. Only the pathways related to the disease were selected and where the mapped genes were more numerous. The pathways related to the disease were selected in consultation with the bibliographic articles in Pubmed-NCBI.

2.4. Statistical Analysis

The primary endpoint was event-free survival (EFS). The secondary endpoint was overall survival (OS). EFS was considered as the time from diagnosis to any relevant event (progression of disease that precludes surgery, local or distant recurrence, or death due to any cause) and was censored at the last follow-up visit. OS was estimated as the interval from diagnosis to death from any cause, and it was censored at the last follow-up visit for the patients still alive. The Kaplan–Meier method was applied for survival probabilities estimation. For univariate analysis, we used the Fisher exact test. Variables (IHC-based molecular subtypes, histological type, tumor grade, Ki67% value, tumor size, clinical lymph node status, cTNM stage, surgery) were included in the multivariate analysis if the univariate p-value was <0.05. Multivariate analysis was done using the Cox proportional hazard model. A two-sided p-value < 0.05 was considered statistically significant. Analyses were performed using SPSS statistical package version 13.0.

3. Results

3.1. Patients Charachteristics

Within the entire database, we selected 24 early breast cancer patients, who had undergone neoadjuvant chemotherapy at the IRCCS Fondazione Policlinico A. Gemelli, homogeneously stratified according to clinical and pathological characteristics, and not achieving pCR. In particular, we analyzed pre- and post-NAC samples of eight patients for the following subtypes: HER2-positive luminal, HER2-positive non-luminal, and TN subtypes. Median age at time of study entry was 50.2 years (range, 35 to 72 years). Median follow-up was 80 months, median EFS was 40.7 months, and median OS was 63.3 months.

3.2. Clinicopathological Variables and Outcome

We analyzed the correlation between IHC-based molecular subtypes (luminal B/HER2-positive, HER2-positive/non-luminal and TN breast cancer), histological type (ductal invasive breast cancer and others), tumor grade, Ki67% value, tumor size, clinical lymph node status, cTNM stage, surgery, and clinical outcome. Variables showing p-values < 0.05 in univariate analyses were used for multivariate logistic regression. However, none of the selected variables were statistically significant at univariate analysis.

3.3. miRNAs and Outcome

Thanks to the computational algorithms and bioinformatics database, we identified 27 miRNAs that were significantly hypo- or hyper-expressed in pre- versus post-NAC samples: hsa-let-7a-5p, hsa-let-7f-5p, hsa-miR-100-5p, hsa-miR-101-3p, hsa-miR-103a-3p, hsa-miR-10a-5p, hsa-miR-10b-5p, hsa-miR-125a-5p, hsa-miR-125b-5p, hsa-miR-126-3p, hsa-miR-143-3p, hsa-miR-191-5p, hsa-miR-196a-5p, hsa-miR-199a-3p, hsa-miR-205-5p, hsa-miR-26a-5p, hsa-miR-26b-5p, hsa-miR-29a-3p, hsa-miR-29c-3p, hsa-miR-30a-5p, hsa-miR-30d-5p, hsa-miR-30e-5p, hsa-miR-510-3p, hsa-miR-92a-3p, hsa-miR-93-5p, hsa-miR-99a-5p, hsa-miR-99b-5p. In Scheme 1, we show the modulation of expression of miRNAs for each subtypes. In Table 4 we presented miRNAs predictive target genes.

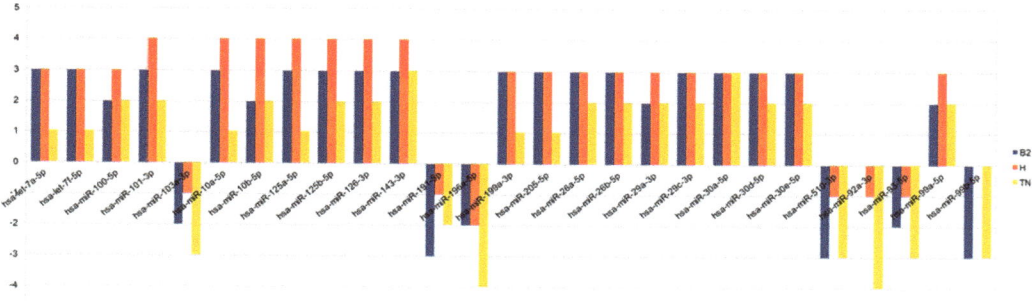

Scheme 1. The chart summarizes—for each miRNA and for each subtype—the number of samples that show the same over/under-expression pattern. Bars above the 0 represent overexpression, while bars below represent under-expression.

Table 4. miRNAs predictive target genes.

miRNAs	Gene Target Predicted
Let 7a-5p	SMARCAD1 FAM178A LIN28B GATM LRIG3 GNPTAB BZW1 ZNF322 ADAMTS8 C8orf58 ADRB2 DNA2 IGDCC3 TTLL4 NME6 TMPRSS2 HIC2 MAPK6 DMD SCN4B ZFYVE26 FZD3 LIMD2 SMIM3 TMEM2 PCGF3 COL3A1 ZBTB5 ACVR1C EIF4G2 CLP1 SLC25A27 NPHP3 PRTG B3GNT7 COIL CCNJ IGF2BP3 FOXP2 TRIM71 PARD6B FRAS1 MAP4K3 HAND1 UTRN GNG5 NAP1L1 UHRF2 LRIG2 ACER2 RICTOR PRPF38B NR6A1 BEGAIN NHLRC3 IFI44L E2F5 BACH1 PAPPA STK40 SLC5A9 PDP2 RDX THRSP FIGN ZBP1 IGF1R ERCC6 C5orf51 PBX3 RNF20 TGFBR1 C15orf41 ADAMTS15 TSEN34 C14orf28 FIGNL2 ZNF275 CPEB1 ARHGAP28 EDN1 C15orf39 USP38 E2F6 FNDC3A ARG2 SPRYD4 IGDCC4 HIP1 SLC10A7 KCTD21 NDST2 DDI2 TRIM41 SLC20A1 DPP6 PLXNC1 LIPT2 CPA4 FBXL12 PALD1 EEA1 HMGA1 RAB11FIP4 STX3 CEP135 GDF6 TRIM67 SLC5A6 OSBPL3 PLEKHG6 TMEM110 DDX26B PLAGL2 PGRMC1 CLDN12 HMGA2 TOR1AIP2 CLASP2 DDX19A KMT2D RPUSD3 ZNF583 AKAP6 SMAP2 RGS16 TAF9B ESR2 CHD4 MFSD4 PPP1R15B TARBP2 CRTAM ATP8B4 FRMD4B HIF1AN RPUSD2 PARS2 CEP120 USP32 GCNT4 GALNT1 SMC1A NRAS PRRX1 MXD1 TMOD2 RANBP2 KLHL31 FNIP1 ULK2 YOD1 ZSWIM5 FAM104A RALB GLRX APBB3 SLC17A9 DCLRE1B USP24 GALC SERF2 PXT1 CCL7 RRM2 TMEM167A RFX5 TMPPE C9orf40 PPAPDC1B PLEKHA8 SCD AHCTF1 RSPO2 PBX1 ZNF318 ZBTB8B ZNF512B GPR26 SLC2A12 ZNF362 AP1S1 SIGLEC14 RASGRP1 DLST TGFBR3 NGF MTUS1 ZNF10 MED8 GAB2 ESPL1 AMT CRY2 NYNRIN ABCG4 KIAA0930 IQCB1 KLHL23 KLHDC8B COL24A1 GAS7 XKR8 NAA30 ADRB3 ARRDC4 CBX5 CADM2 DDX19B OPA3 RIOK3 TET3 FGD6 SEMA3F GXYLT1 LBR COL4A6 BIN3 CDC34 CLDN1 SNX16 RAB3GAP2 FZD4 MAPK8 PPAPDC2 NNT SDR42E1 RNF5 LOC101930255 LOC102723960 PDPR SEMA4F SLC25A18 GFM2 CASP3 BZW2 CCR7 AGPAT6 THAP9 GRPEL2 MEIS3 CGNL1 ZNF644 SKIL NXT2 TXNDC8 PARP16 LGR4 ARHGEF38 RDH10 PIGA ZNF710 WDR37 AFF2 COL5A2 POLLDOK3 COL1A2 MARS2 MDM4 GAN LRRC17 RFX6 DNAJA2 AMER3 MIB1 IKBKAP MYO1F MGAT4A SEMA4C NKD1 KATNBL1 AGBL1 ABT1 TBC1D13 GGA3 SOX13 FAM210A SESTD1 NRARP NME4 PITPNM3 ANKRD46 KCTD17 SLC52A3 MBTPS2 MAP3K1 DIP2A ABHD14B CCDC141 CBL LOR ABCB9 ASPH USP12 RMI2 ELOVL4 SLC25A24 MTDH MICAL3 TNFRSF1B ZCCHC3 SOCS1 PRKAA2 CHRD ARHGEF15 ZNF516 DCAF15 TOLD3 DLGAP4 FMO4 MAB21L3 E2F2 FASLG PEX11B PLA2G3 TIA1 SOWAHA PLXND1 CYP4F2 DCNA BCC5 DUSP22 DAPK1 ZNF879 ELF4 BRWD3 CLDN16 CDKN1A SCN11A KLHL13 MAP4K4 CERCAM ITGB3 CYP46A1 RNMT SLAMF6 GSG1L MC2R ENTPD7 AMOT RUFY3 B3GNT1 KLK10 SCN8A SNX30 EDEM3 FAS KLF9 ATG10 FRMD5 CD86 MMS22L OGG1 AEN LMX1A CCNF ZNF273 CECR6 SUB1 CYB561D1 PRSS22 TBKBP1 DMRT2 DDN SERPINB9 SNAI3 PLA2G15 DAGLA INTS2 FAXC DPP3 C19orf47 GREB1 ERGIC1 LIMK2 ANKRD49 C2 HOOK1 SLC25A40 PARM1 SLC11A2 DPF2 MDFI ABCC10 SMARCC1 IGF2BP1 SPATA2 FAM84B MFSD8 CDC25A C20orf112 SLC6A1 SMCR8 MIER1 IGF2BP2 UBXN2B DZIP1L IRS2 ERCC4 PAG1 CELF3 NEK3 BTBD9 MBD2 ENTHD2 SLC25A12 TMED5 KIAA1429 HDLBP ARPP19 HOXD1 ZBTB39 RAD18 ODF2L CPM TSPAN18 LAMP2 STAT2 CD59 TPK1 RBMS2 DCX ZNF566 IMPG2 MASP1 PNKD NOVA1 SREBF2 SLC25A32 ZC3H3 SPRYD7 SYNPO2L EEF2K LIPH
miR-100-5p	KBTBD8 S3ST2 ZZEF1 MTOR MBNL1 TRIB2 SMARCA5 TTC39A ZADH2 RAVER2 PPP3CA AP1AR FGFR3 HS3ST3B1 NOX4 BAZ2A ZNF845 AGO2 PCSK9 NR6A1 TAOK1 FZD8 MTMR3 EPDR1 ETFDH FZD5 CTDSPL
miR-101-3p	MPPE1 MOB4 CACNB2 TNPO1 STC1 ABHD17C FLRT3 MYCN TSHZ3 LCOR C3orf58 SOCS5 ZFP36L2 FZD6 REV3L FZD4 RORA TMEM65 ZNF654 FGA RFX3 TGFBR1 ZNF532 CDYL DR1 CPEB3 RANBP9 FOS SCN2A SLC12A2 NLK CDH11 FAT3 ADAMTS17 KBTBD8 FAM214A ATXN1L EZH2 PRKCE PRPF4B USP47 ZFHX4 RASD2 DIP2B INO80D STAG2 UBE2D1 RAP2C ZNF746 MFSD6 UBE2A SMARCA1 ADAMTSL2 ANKRD44 SEL1L MTMR2 ZNF451 SLC1A1 ARID1A EED SMARCD1 ZMAT3 PAPOLG BCL9 EYA1 RAB5A ETV5 SH2B3 EMP2 ICK CBFA2T2 SGK1 SULT4A1 ZEB1 NEK7 ZBTB34 BEAN1 ENY2 ATXN1 ZNF385B HTRA3 PPFIA1 SUB1 TMEM194B MKL2 HSPE1-MOB4 GLCCI1 TET2 PIEZO1 NPNT CTTNBP2 UBE2D2 ING3 TNKS2 BDP1 ZSWIM6 COL10A1 ERBB2IP AJAP1 SHISA6 KIF2A CHAC2 ANKRD11 SSBP2 ASPN CAV3 KIAA1804 KLF3 FBXW7 ETNK1 ANKRD17 GPR85 EXOC5 PCDH8 SLC39A10 MBNL1 UBN2 UNC79 SIX4 SEPT11 EMP1 DUSP1 ZNF207 PLXNA2 FAM46A CAPN2 NR1D2 BTBD3 MTCL1 ZFAND3 ABHD17B CERS2 CEP350 MAGI1 DAG1 GLTSCR1 DIP2C PIP5K1C DISC1 MORN4 MGAT4A ARNTL2 GAB1 NRK IFFO2 PCGF5 PTGS2 MAK PDE4D ARHGEF3 FBN2 B3GALNT2 SCN8A ARAP2 STAMBP STAU2 KLHDC1 LIN7C ZNF518A PHF20L1 POMP RAB39B ZNF217 SLC38A2 LMNB1 UTS2B LRP2 RAB1A AP3D1 ADAMTS3 GSK3B SLC19A2 PPP1R2 DENND1B PPARGC1B RIN2 FBXO30 SLC7A11 MYRIP TCEB1 SYNCRIP DDIT4 ABCC5 FAM83B IMPA1 AP3S1 TGFBR3 DNMT3A FAM114A1 CDK8 CERS6 BICD2 DCBLD2 TAL1 NUPL2 TRPC4 MARK1 NDFIP1 PANK3 DLG5 HELZ CCNJ INPP5F TRIM24 KIAA1244 KCNH7 N4BP2 LRRN1 IKZF2 CPEB2 ADRB1 KAT7 CEP63 TDG RAP1B NOVA1 PPFIA2 SYT4 AEBP2 RSF1 ZDHHC21 PIKFYVE PNISR PABPC5 MED13 SLC39A6 DOT1L SLC2A13 ATP8A1 LRCH1 CAMKK1 SASH1 CLDN11 EVI5 TULP4 PURG DCAF5 KCNA1 ST7 RBM25 DMXL2 PPM1L LHFP ABLIM3 IL1R1 ACAD9 CAMTA1 CIR1 GJA1 ENPP2 ZBTB21 GID4 FKTN MED14OS ZNF557 CYB561D2 RAC1 TFB2M TNRC18 CTNND2 EDEM3 KCTD6 ASAP1 FAM179B PRKAA1 C8orf76 HNRNPA0 PPTC7 RAB4A RAPH1 GCNT3 KLF6 METAP1 TMEM161B TIA1 ZIK1 CDH5 GFRA1 TBRG1 MMGT1 DSC1 ERO1LB SLC30A7 GLRA2 LRCH2 NDST3 CDK5R1 PMPCB POGZ RNF219 KDM3B FAM78A H2AFV UGGT1 SPATA2 MAP3K13 MAML3 MPHOSPH9 AKT3 FA2H PRKD3 MRGBP CEBPA KIAA1586

Table 4. *Cont.*

miRNAs	Gene Target Predicted
miR-101-3p	ASCC3 RAB27A BEGAIN ZNF510 RFPL4B CCDC68 TLK2 TAGAP FUCA2 ZNF549 RAB15 OTUD4 CCSER1 ZBED4 RASGRP3 GRIN2A ANXA10 WWC3 HNRNPF KAT6B HAS2 DCUN1D1 CTCF CCDC88A FAM73A MTSS1L BBX FAM60A RNF19A RCN2 PKD2 ATRX POLR3K MAP3K9 N4BP1 DNM1L MRPL42 KHDRBS2 STX6 CSNK1G3 NOTCH1 GABRB2 SPOP GLIPR1L1 KIF5B C9orf72 DENND2C SACM1L LRRC4 MAP3K2 SPG11 DCAF7 ARHGEF10 KLF2 ZCCHC2 KPNB1 KIAA1432 CRLS1 BTLA NSD1 MAPK1 TMEM167A PDS5B OGT KDM6B GCNT1 C11orf70 ANKZF1 RNF38 ROBO2 SGMS2 EPT1 SLMO2 HIVEP3 FAR1 CAPS2 TMEM231 TKTL1 TMEM68 ZNF469 SGPL1 RXRB WDR72 DESI2 NACA2 MTMR4 LGI2 CREBRF XPO5 PTCH1 NACA GABBR2 PRR11 CTDSPL DCLRE1B DDX3X MAB21L3 MLEC FAM103A1 GNB1 SPATS2L PRRC2C UBR7 FYTTD1 CD86 RIPK1 CNIH3 NAIP MON2 ATRNL1 KIAA1462 BCL2L11 RANBP1 FMNL3 PHTF2 TMF1 LANCL3 ZNF33A TIMM17A PLEKHG1 PBX3 MTX3 UNKL TEX2 RANBP6 AGAP1 ZNF235 CCDC126 FAM169A PTBP3 CADM2 KCNE1 FAM216B OTUD3 MAP10 FLRT2 PIK3C2B PCK1 PYGO1 TMEM201 C7orf73 C1orf52 SPRED1 B3GNT3 NDUFB5 TKTL2 ATP11B NEGR1 CADM1 TMED5 SMARCA4 SMN2 IKZF4 ZNF24 XKR6 PLA2R1 CDKN1A NAV1 PYGO2 NAA15 FRYL PCDH20 KIAA1377 PACRG NF1 SUPT7L C2orf88 RRM1 SMN1 FAM53B INPP4B IPO5 SRPK2 BBS7 STAR GDE1 FBXW11 JDP2 CRISPLD1 MAD2L1 SLTM DPY19L2 TBC1D12 ADH5 VSX1 LONRF1 COTL1 RBBP7 JAK2 SOAT1 NEK4 UBE2F MNX1 AGFG1 PTPRJ KTI12 PHACTR2 C16orf72 ARHGAP32 POGK IQGAP3 FAM122C USP38 CCNT2 DTD2 TMEM170B STMN1 PITPNB PCDH7 ZIC1 LRAT PDP1 CISD2 FOXN2 ZNF260 EPB41L5 DENR SLC25A4 ZC3H7A GRSF1 TMEM132D RHOT1 C10orf12 JAKMIP2 AP1S3 CASP3 BAZ2A
miR-199-3a	ETNK1 CELSR2 ADAMTSL3 KLHL3 ACVR2A LRP2 BCAR3 SERPINE2 NOVA1 MAP3K4 FAM110C KIAA0319L RB1 ZHX1 KDM5A PSD2 LIN28B LLGL2 ITGA3 CHMP5 TUBGCP3 FAM60A NLK CD2AP NID2 UTP20 PAK4 C9orf40 KDM6A CDK7 C2orf49 KATNBL1 CDK17 PPP2R2A APLP2 MCFD2 CDNF PRPF40A CXADR PPP2R5E G3BP2 FUBP1 NEDD4 SLC24A2 RASEF SDC2 PDGFRA SCD SUMO3 ITPK1 ARHGEF3 ESRP1 ATAD1 MAP3K5 APLF ASTN1 EMC1 GGNBP2 CYB5R4 PAWR NXPH1 PIP5K1B ATRX NUFIP2 KTN1 RNGTT MDGA2 GORAB PNRC1 VGLL2 FAM199X DEPDC1B GNPTAB NFIA DNHD1 RAPH1 TPPP WDR7 ARL15 ADAM10 NLRP1 CBLB RAPGEF4 SEMA3A COL12A1 TACC2 KLF13 SPIRE1 FAM115C ANKRD44 MS4A7 LRRC1 PTPN3 AEBP2 COL4A5 CBLL1 CISD2 CCDC85C FN1 ATP6V1A NRBP2 PTPRZ1 SP1 ATL1 DNMT3A NET1 FOS PROSER1 RFX3 WFDC8 MFSD6 TAOK1 ZBTB18 PTPRC C20orf194 ITGA6 RPS6KA6 LPAR4 LCOR MAPRE1 CD151 FXR1 PLCB1 MPP7 YWHAE EPG5 SMARCC2 EPB41L5 SLC25A46 C21orf91 SMIM8 GPBP1L1 KIDINS220 GPM6A VPS33A PON2 TMED5 HNF1B WAPAL DCBLD2 CNIH2 C9orf170 RALGPS2 LAMP3 BEND7 FAM129A ITGB8 ANKRD61 CETN3 KCMF1 FAM76B PDE4B HYPK SLC39A10 NAA25 NTRK2 KDM3A GLT8D2 WDR47 MBNL1 MTOR SOWAHC RGS4 FGL2 ALX4 YWHAG STARD9 ENOX2 MAP3K1 GALNT7 YWHAZ CREBRF TENM1 TAB2 EML4 RP1 FMN1 CHKA PVRL2 VAMP3 ZCCHC17 TEAD1 SYNJ1 SLC16A12 PCDH7 ABHD4 DUSP5 KCND2 SECISBP2L DIMT1 PPP1R9A ATP6V1C2 MEIS1 ARG2 CHAD SORL1 RNF216 ELAVL2 CAPRIN1 FCGR3A LONRF3 ADD3 RRM2B CNOT7 SRR IL1RL1 ECM2 MVB12B ADRB1 CLDN8 FCGR3B CCSAP CA5B VLDLR UBQLN1 EFCAB14 TMEM62 PTPRU ABCA1 CABLES1 SH3GLB1 ERO1L ANK2 TMEM218 KIAA0907 ASAP2 ACOX1 SYPL1 BRWD3 DPAGT1 PIK3CB NF1 ZNF614 SLC39A9 SLC5A7 HRNR CYP1B1 ZC3H14 LOC101929844 PCDHB12 HECTD2 PLEKHH1 UCK2 HNMT CDC42BPB RFX7 CCSER1 KCTD7 CITED2 CFL2 RHOT1 UBXN2B HGF KIAA0141 FBXW11 GPR160 KCNH2 TRMT61B GNA12 GRHL1 SLC44A5 PHF6 KLF12 CYP24A1 CDK5R1 MAP3K2 ATP1B4 CCDC88C ADAM22 C10orf2 TXLNG CEP85L KAZN PRKCB BAG4 FAM46D CALCRL PRC1 KIAA1244 SEC16B FKBP14 CDC14A CTNNA2 NAP1L1 UNC45A DDIT4 PAQR3

Up-regulation of let-7a-5p, miR-100-5p, miR-101-3p, and miR-199a-3p in post-NAC specimens was significantly correlated with better EFS and OS compared to those with normal or lower expression, independent from breast cancer subtypes.

At subgroup analysis, the overexpression of mentioned miRNAs in post-NAC samples was linked with an improvement in EFS and OS only in HER2-positive non-luminal subtypes (Table 5). Furthermore, when we stratified patients according to a sort of miRNA signature (let-7a-5p, mirR-100-5p, miR-101-3p, miR-199a-3p), we found that patients who concurrently overexpress all four miRNAs experimented a significantly better prognosis in terms of EFS and OS (Table 5; Figures 1–5). However, at multivariate analysis, EFS ($p = 0.009$) and OS ($p = 0.0008$) showed a statistically association exclusively with up-regulation of let-7a-5p.

Table 5. Prognostic impact of miRNA expression profile on EFS and OS in all populations and in HER2 non-luminal subtypes.

	EFS (Months)	p Value	Hazard Ratio (CI 95%)	OS (Months)	p-Value	Hazard Ratio (CI 95%)
Let-7a-5p in all populations	58 vs. 28	0.006	0.38 (0.08–0.66)	65 vs. 35	0.0001	0.27 (0.03–0.33)
Let-7a-5p in HER2 non-luminal subtypes	61 vs. 36	0.05	0.58 (0.29–6.28)	71 vs. 44	0.05	0.31 (0.02–1.0)
miR-100-5p in all populations	56 vs. 17	0.01	0.39 (0.11–0.75)	56 vs. 39	0.03	0.45 (0.15–0.94)
miR-100-5p in HER2 non-luminal subtypes	61 vs. 20	0.004	0.21 (0.01–0.30)	70 vs. 35	0.004	0.19 (0.00–0.30)
miR-101-3p in all populations	56 vs. 20	0.05	0.48 (0.16–1.03)	58 vs. 35	0.01	0.38 (0.10–0.75)
miR-101-3p in HER2 non-luminal subtypes	61 vs. 24	0.02	0.28 (0.01–0.77)	71 vs. 40	0.02	0.27 (0.01–0.77)
miR-199a-3p in all populations	61 vs. 20	0.02	0.41 (0.14–0.85)	69 vs. 46	0.01	0.39 (0.13–0.80)
miR199a-3p in HER2 non-luminal subtypes	61 vs. 20	0.02	0.27 (0.00–0.70)	70 vs. 45	0.04	0.29 (0.01–0.96)
Signature in all populations	64 vs. 20	0.004	0.31 (0.4–0.66)	71 vs. 46	0.005	0.31 (0.11–0.68)

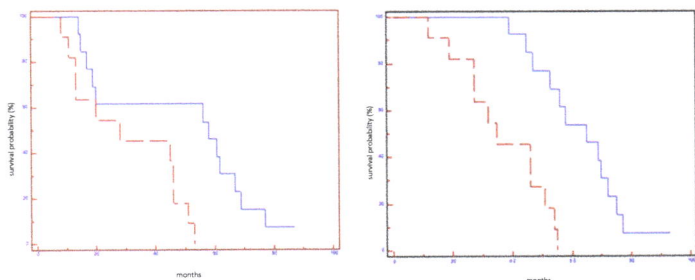

Figure 1. Prognostic impact of Let7a-5p on EFS (on the left) and on OS (on the right) in all population: blue line refers to patients with overexpression of Let7a; red line refers to patients without overexpression of Let7a-5p.

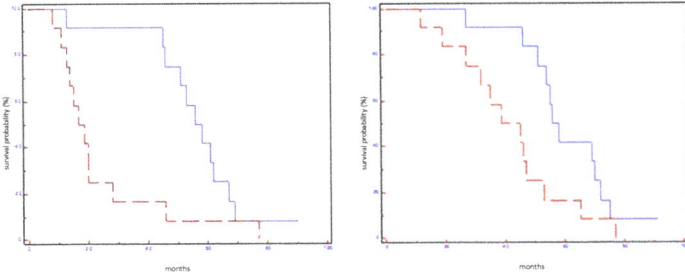

Figure 2. Prognostic impact of miR100-5p on EFS (on the left) and on OS (on the right) in all population: blue line refers to patients with overexpression of miR100-5p; red line refers to patients without overexpression of miR100-5p.

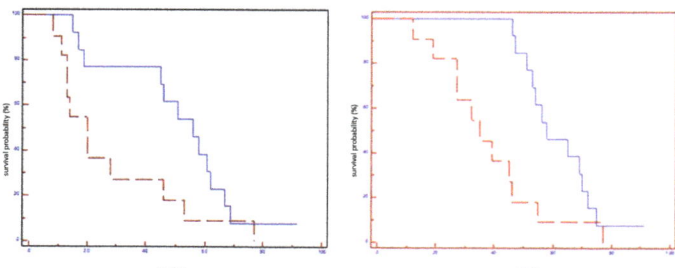

Figure 3. Prognostic impact of miR101-3p on EFS (on the left) and on OS (on the right) in all population: blue line refers to patients with overexpression of miR101-5p; red line refers to patients without overexpression of miR101-5p.

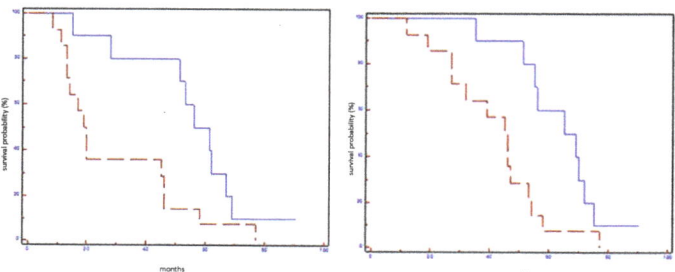

Figure 4. Prognostic impact of miR199a-3p on EFS (on the left) and on OS (on the right) in all population: blue line refers to patients with overexpression of miR199a-3p; red line refers to patients without overexpression of miR199a-3p.

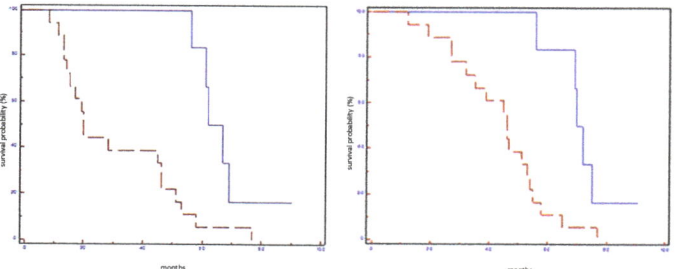

Figure 5. Prognostic impact of miRNA signature on EFS (on the left) and OS (on the right) in all population: blue line refers to patients with overexpression of miRNA signature; red line refers to patients without overexpression of miRNA signature.

4. Discussion

Recent suggestions have revealed that the miRNAs can modulate the expression of oncogenes or tumor suppressor genes. Based on this evidence, miRNAs appear as hopeful biomarkers of breast cancer [21].

Bertoli et al. analyzed the role of several miRNAs in breast cancer and showed that some of them could be useful for diagnostic tools (i.e., miR-9, miR-10b, and miR-17-5p); other miRNAs (i.e., miR-148a and miR-335) may have a prognostic role, while still others (i.e., miR-30c, miR-187, and miR-339-5p) may be predictive of treatment response [22].

In our study, we investigated the potential role of miRNAs as predictors of outcome in early breast cancer patients. We found a significantly differential miRNA expression among some breast cancer subtypes in pre-NAC and post-NAC paraffin-embedding tissue: in particular, we found that the up-regulation of let-7a-5p, miR-100-5p, miR-101-3p, and miR199a-3p in post-NAC samples was significantly associated with better prognosis in terms of EFS and OS, but at multivariate analysis, only overexpression of let-7 was correlated with survival.

Although miR100, miR101, and miR199 did not maintain a statistically significant correlation with survival outcome in multivariate analysis, there is a strong biological rationale supporting their role in breast cancer prognosis and, in our opinion, they deserve further studies.

Interestingly, all these miRNAs have shown to be normally down-regulated in breast cancer and have a role in cancer pathogenesis affecting cell cycle, proliferation, and metastasis diffusion.

Let-7 employs its antiproliferative activities and its tumor-suppressor role by controlling key checkpoints of several mitogenic pathways and by suppressing different oncogenes, including HMGA2, RAS, and MYC [23,24]. Let-7 expression levels have a role as a prognostic marker in several cancers, and the loss of its expression is a marker for less differentiated cancers [25,26]. It is newsworthy that HMGA2 and H-RAS oncogenes are targeted by an induced expression of let-7 in breast cancer cells, and in a murine model of breast cancer, exogenous let-7 delivery represses mammosphere formation, cell proliferation, and the undifferentiated cell population by downregulating both H-RAS and HMGA2 oncogenes [27]. Barh demonstrated that in silico analysis, apart from repressing HMGA2, RAS, and MYC, let-7 may also target CYP19A1, ESR1, and ESR2, thereby potentially blocking estrogen signaling in ER-positive breast cancers [28]. Moreover, Kim et al. affirmed that let-7a inhibits breast cancer cell migration and invasion through the down-regulation of C-C chemokine receptor type 7 expression (CCR7) [29]. Other authors described a new role of let-7a in regulating energy metabolism in neoplastic cells [30]. To underline the role of Let-7 restoration to prevent tumor progression, our study found that the overexpression of let-7 family members in post-NAC samples is associated with a better prognosis in patients with no pCR. From the therapeutic viewpoint, let-7 is an attractive molecule for preventing tumorigenesis and angiogenesis; thus, it could be a potential therapeutic target in several cancers that lose let-7.

miR-100, miR-99a, and miR-99b belong to the miR-100 family. The miRNA-100 controls several genes playing an important modulatory role. mTOR, PI3K, AKT1, IGF1-R, HS3ST2, HOXA1, RAP1B, and FGFR3 are some of the multiple targets of miR-100. Modulating these important genes, miRNA 100 could block proliferation by promoting cell cycle arrest and apoptosis in tumor cells. Furthermore, recent findings suggest that in breast cancer, the miR-100 may act as a pro-differentiating agent for cancer stem cell modulating Wnt/β-catenin pathway and Polo-like kinase 1 gene. It was found that miR100 overexpression has the capability to inhibit the Wnt pathway. Recent evidence showed that miRNA-100 downregulates Polo-like kinase 1 in basal-like cancer, blocking the maintenance and expansion of breast cancer stem cells (BrCSCs), inducing BrCSC differentiation, thus favoring the transition from undifferentiated tumors into well-differentiated ones [31,32]. Petrelli et al. analyzed 123 early node-negative breast cancer tumor specimens: patients were categorized on the basis of the miR-100 expression status. Patients with low miR-100 levels experienced worst distant metastasis-free survival [32]. According to the literature, the miR-100 family could convert an aggressive tumor into a well differentiated, biologically favorable, phenotype. In support of this potential role, miRNA-100 family members are understudied as targets for differentiation therapy: this therapeutic strategy aims to induce the transformation of aggressive cancer cells into well-differentiated ones, which are more sensitive to therapy [31,32].

miR-101 is known to be involved in many important cancer processes such as inhibition of proliferation, chemoresistance, angiogenesis, invasion, and metastasis [33]. According to this hypothesis, several reports showed that the loss of miR-101 is frequent and is associated to a worse outcome in many types of tumors [34–39]. Several studies demonstrated that EZH2, a mammalian histone methyltransferase, is emerging as one of the most important targets of miR-101: loss of miR-101 function induces the overexpression of EZH2, which is related to cancer evolution [40,41]. A meta-analysis showed that the down-regulation of miR-101 expression is correlated with a poor prognosis [13]. Liu at al. revealed that a high expression of miR-101 inhibits TNBC progression and increases chemotherapeutic drug-induced apoptosis in TNBC by directly targeting myeloid cell leukemia 1 (MCL-1) [42]. Other authors demonstrated that miR-101 is hypo-expressed in different breast cancer subtypes and stimulates cellular proliferation and invasiveness by targeting Stathmin1 (Stmn1) [43]. According to these findings, our study showed that higher levels of miR-101-3p were correlated with a better EFS and OS, independently from breast cancer subtypes in patients not achieving pCR. Therefore, it is possible to say that miR-101 could be a potential therapeutic target and a novel prognostic factor.

The role in breast cancer progression is unclear regarding miR-199a/b-3p. Some studies showed a loss of miR-199a/b-3p expression in aggressive breast cancer [44]; other evidence demonstrated the ability of miR-199a/b-3p to inhibit proliferation, migration, and multi-drug resistance. miR-199a/b-3p seems to be down-expressed in many types of cancer [45–52]. According to Shou-Qing Li et al., PAK4 could be a possible target of miR-199a/b-3p with an oncosuppresive role: in human breast cell lines, ectopic expression of miR-199a/b-3p blocks the PAK4/MEK/ERK pathway to inhibit breast cancer progression by inducing G1 phase arrest [52]. Xuelong et al. have shown that the hyper-expression of miR-199a-3p inhibits mitochondrial transcription factor A (TFAM) expression, enhancing sensitivity to cisplatin in breast cancer cells. Hence, miR-199a/b-3p could represent a good prognostic and predictive biomarker [53]. It was found that the overexpression of miR-199a-3p regulates the activation of the G protein coupled receptor (GPER), which is involved in tumorigenesis, and suppresses cells' proliferation, invasion, and epithelial–mesenchymal transition in TNBC [54].

Taking into consideration all our findings, our hypothesis is that miRNA patterns of expression could help identify, in the group of patients not achieving pCR, a population with better outcome. Moreover, in our opinion, the present study is interesting because it gives further support to the fundamental role of the miRNAs in cancer biology and their potential application as target cancer therapies. Several studies have been conducted in order to modulate cellular miRNA levels as inhibiting the oncogenic miRNAs and as restoring the tumor-suppressive ones, with encouraging results [55–58].

Although larger case series are needed, our findings provide a basis for broader, prospective, and multicenter trials to support the potential role of miRNAs as predictive and prognostic biomarkers not only in early but also in advanced disease. We hope that the identified miRNAs will help in comprehensively understanding their pathway mechanism in breast cancer and improve the therapeutic strategies [59].

5. Conclusions

miRNAs have changed our understanding of cell pathway modulation and opened fields not only for the development of novel cancer target therapies but even for new diagnostic tools. At present, important topics in cancer research are discovering the underlying pathways involved in miRNA expression and secretion and understanding miRNA modulation in different phases of cancer progression. Large cohort studies are still required to analyze and confirm the diagnostic, prognostic, and therapeutic application of miRNA.

Author Contributions: Conceptualization, P.F. and M.D.S.; methodology, P.F., M.D.S., G.T., G.S., C.B. and A.C.; Writing—review and editing, all authors; supervision, P.F., M.D.S., G.T., G.S., G.F., C.B. and A.C. All authors have read and agreed to the published version of the manuscript.

Funding: This research received no external funding.

Institutional Review Board Statement: The study was conducted according to the guidelines of the Declaration of Helsinki, and approved by the Ethics Committee of FONDAZIONE POLICLINICO GEMELLI (protocol code 27736/16 and date of approval (20 October 2016).

Informed Consent Statement: Informed consent was obtained from all subjects involved in the study.

Conflicts of Interest: The authors declare no conflict of interest.

References

1. Mauri, D.; Pavlidis, N.; Ioannidis, J.P. Neoadjuvant versus adjuvant systemic treatment in breast cancer: A meta-analysis. *J. Natl. Cancer Inst.* **2005**, *97*, 188–194. [CrossRef]
2. van der Hage, J.A.; van de Velde, C.J.; Julien, J.P.; Tubiana-Hulin, M.; Vandervelden, C.; Duchateau, L. Preoperative chemotherapy in primary operable breast cancer: Results from the European Organization for Research and Treatment of Cancer trial 10902. *J. Clin. Oncol.* **2001**, *19*, 4224. [CrossRef]
3. Rastogi, P.; Anderson, S.J.; Bear, H.D.; Geyer, C.E.; Kahlenberg, M.S.; Robidoux, A.; Margolese, R.G.; Hoehn, J.L.; Vogel, V.G.; Dakhil, S.R.; et al. Preoperative chemotherapy: Updates of National Surgical Adjuvant Breast and Bowel Project Protocols B-18 and B-27. *J. Clin. Oncol.* **2008**, *26*, 778–785. [CrossRef]
4. Kuerer, H.M.; Newman, L.A.; Smith, T.L.; Ames, F.C.; Hunt, K.K.; Dhingra, K.; Theriault, R.L.; Singh, G.; Binkley, S.M.; Sneige, N.; et al. Clinical course of breast cancer patients with complete pathologic primary tumor and axillary lymph node response to doxorubicin-based neoadjuvant chemotherapy. *J. Clin. Oncol.* **1999**, *17*, 460–469. [CrossRef]
5. von Minckwitz, G.; Untch, M.; Blohmer, J.U.; Costa, S.D.; Eidtmann, H.; Fasching, P.A.; Gerber, B.; Eiermann, W.; Hilfrich, J.; Huober, J.; et al. Definition and impact of pathologic complete response on prognosis after neoadjuvant chemotherapy in various intrinsic breast cancer subtypes. *J. Clin. Oncol.* **2012**, *30*, 1796–1804. [CrossRef]
6. von Minckwitz, G.; Untch, M.; Nüesch, E.; Loibl, S.; Kaufmann, M.; Kümmel, S.; Fasching, P.A.; Eiermann, W.; Blohmer, J.U.; Costa, S.D.; et al. Impact of treatment characteristics on response of different breast cancer phenotypes: Pooled analysis of the German neo-adjuvant chemotherapy trials. *Breast Cancer Res. Treat.* **2011**, *125*, 145–156. [CrossRef] [PubMed]
7. Gampenrieder, S.P.; Rinnerthaler, G.; Greil, R. Neoadjuvant chemotherapy and targeted therapy in breast cancer: Past, present, and future. *J. Oncol.* **2013**, *732047*. [CrossRef] [PubMed]
8. Bear, H.D.; Anderson, S.; Brown, A.; Smith, R.; Mamounas, E.P.; Fisher, B.; Margolese, R.; Theoret, H.; Soran, A.; Wickerham, D.L.; et al. The effect on tumor response of adding sequential preoperative docetaxel to preoperative doxorubicin and cyclophosphamide: Preliminary results from National Surgical Adjuvant Breast and Bowel Project Protocol B-27. *J. Clin. Oncol.* **2003**, *21*, 4165–4174. [CrossRef]
9. Sataloff, D.M.; Mason, B.A.; Prestipino, A.J.; Seinige, U.L.; Lieber, C.P.; Baloch, Z. Pathologic response to induction chemotherapy in locally advanced carcinoma of the breast: A determinant of outcome. *J. Am. Coll. Surg.* **1995**, *180*, 297–306.
10. Berezikov, E. Evolution of microRNA diversity and regulation in animals. *Nat. Rev. Genet.* **2011**, *12*, 846–860. [CrossRef]
11. Weber, B.; Stresemann, C.; Brueckner, B.; Lyko, F. Methylation of human microRNA genes in normal and neoplastic cells. *Cell Cycle* **2007**, *6*, 1001–1005. [CrossRef]
12. Calin, G.A.; Sevignani, C.; Dumitru, C.D.; Hyslop, T.; Noch, E.; Yendamuri, S.; Shimizu, M.; Rattan, S.; Bullrich, F.; Negrini, M.; et al. Human microRNA genes are frequently located at fragile sites and genomic regions involved in cancers. *Proc. Natl. Acad. Sci. USA* **2004**, *101*, 2999–3004. [CrossRef] [PubMed]
13. Blenkiron, C.; Goldstein, L.D.; Thorne, N.P.; Spiteri, I.; Chin, S.-F.; Dunning, M.J.; Barbosa-Morais, N.L.; Teschendorff, A.E.; Green, A.R.; Ellis, I.O.; et al. MicroRNA expression profiling of human breast cancer identifies new markers of tumor subtype. *Genome Biol.* **2007**, *8*, R214. [CrossRef]
14. Amin, M.B.; Greene, F.L.; Edge, S.; Compton, C.C.; Gershenwald, J.E.; Brookland, R.K.; Meyer, L.; Gress, D.M.; Byrd, D.R.; Winchester, D.P.; et al. *Cancer Staging Manual*, 8th ed.; Springer: New York, NY, USA, 2017.
15. But-Hadzić, J.; Bilban-Jakopin, C.; Hadzić, V. The role of radiation therapy in locally advanced breast cancer. *Breast J.* **2010**, *16*, 183–188. [CrossRef] [PubMed]
16. Green, M.C.; Buzdar, A.U.; Smith, T.; Ibrahim, N.K.; Valero, V.; Rosales, M.F.; Cristofanilli, M.; Booser, D.J.; Pusztai, L.; Rivera, E.; et al. Weekly paclitaxel improves pathologic complete remission in operable breast cancer when compared with paclitaxel once every 3 weeks. *J. Clin. Oncol.* **2005**, *23*, 5983–5992. [CrossRef] [PubMed]
17. Baselga, J.; Bradbury, I.; Eidtmann, H.; Di Cosimo, S.; Aura, C.; De Azambuja, E.; Gomez, H.; Dinh, P.; Fauria, K.; Van Dooren, V.; et al. Abstract S3-3: First results of the NeoALTTO trial (BIG 01-06/EGF106903): A phase III, randomized, open label, neoadjuvant study of lapatinib, trastuzumab, and their combination plus paclitaxel in women with HER2-positive primary breast cancer. *Cancer Res.* **2010**, *70*. [CrossRef]
18. miRBase: The microRNA Database. Available online: http://www.mirbase.org/ (accessed on 1 August 2021).
19. Li, L.; Xu, J.; Yang, D.; Tan, X.; Wang, H. Computational approaches for microRNA studies. *Mamm. Genome* **2010**, *21*, 1–12. [CrossRef]
20. miRDB. Available online: http://www.mirdb.org (accessed on 1 August 2021).
21. Peng, Y.; Croce, C.M. The role of MicroRNAs in human cancer. *Signal. Transduct. Target. Ther.* **2016**, *1*, 15004. [CrossRef]
22. Bertoli, G.; Cava, C.; Castiglioni, I. MicroRNAs: New Biomarkers for Diagnosis, Prognosis, Therapy Prediction and Therapeutic Tools for Breast Cancer. *Theranostics* **2015**, *5*, 1122–1143. [CrossRef]

23. Bussing, I.; Slack, F.J.; Grosshans, H. let-7 microRNAs in development, stem cells and cancer. *Trends Mol. Med.* **2008**, *14*, 400–409. [CrossRef]
24. Worringer, K.A.; Rand, T.A.; Hayashi, Y.; Sami, S.; Takahashi, K.; Tanabe, K.; Narita, M.; Srivastava, D.; Yamanaka, S. The let-7/LIN-41 pathway regulates reprogramming to human induced pluripotent stem cells by controlling expression of prodifferentiation genes. *Cell Stem Cell.* **2014**, *14*, 40–52. [CrossRef] [PubMed]
25. Akao, Y.; Nakagawa, Y.; Naoe, T. Let-7 microrna functions as a potential growth suppressor in human colon cancer cells. *Biol. Pharm. Bull.* **2006**, *29*, 903–906. [CrossRef]
26. Johnson, S.M.; Grosshans, H.; Shingara, J.; Byrom, M.; Jarvis, R.; Cheng, A.; Labourier, E.; Reinert, K.L.; Brown, D.; Slack, F.J. Ras is regulated by the let-7 microrna family. *Cell* **2005**, *120*, 635–647. [CrossRef] [PubMed]
27. Yu, F.; Yao, H.; Zhu, P.; Zhang, X.; Pan, Q.; Gong, C.; Huang, Y.; Hu, X.; Su, F.; Lieberman, J.; et al. Let-7 regulates self renewal and tumorigenicity of breast cancer cells. *Cell* **2007**, *131*, 1109–1123. [CrossRef] [PubMed]
28. Barh, D.; Parida, S.; Parida, B.P. Let-7, mir -125, mir -205, and mir -296 are prospective therapeutic agents in breast cancer molecular medicine. *Gene Ther. Mol. Biol.* **2008**, *12*, 189–206.
29. Seok-Jun, K.; Ji-Young, S.; Kang-Duck, L.; Bae, Y.-K.; Sung, K.W.; Nam, S.J.; Chun, K.H. MicroRNA let-7a suppresses breast cancer cell migration and invasion through downregulation of C-C chemokine receptor type 7. *Breast Cancer Res.* **2012**, *14*, R14. [CrossRef]
30. Serguienk, A.; Grad, I.; Wennerstrøm, A.B.; Meza-Zepeda, L.A.; Thiede, B.; Stratford, E.W.; Myklebost, O.; Munthe, E. Metabolic reprogramming of metastatic breast cancer and melanoma by let-7a microRNA. *Oncotarget* **2015**, *6*, 2451–2465. [CrossRef]
31. Chen, L.; Yanping, G.; Kai, Z.; Chen, J.; Han, S.; Feng, B.; Wang, R.; Chen, L. Multiple Roles of MicroRNA-100 in Human Cancer and its Therapeutic Potential. *Cell Physiol. Biochem.* **2015**, *37*, 2143–2159. [CrossRef]
32. Petrelli, A.; Carollo, R.; Cargnelutti, M.; Iovino, F.; Callari, M.; Cimino, D.; Todaro, M.; Mangiapane, L.R.; Giammona, A.; Cordova, A.; et al. By promoting cell differentiation, miR-100 sensitizes basal-like breast cancer stem cells to hormonal therapy. *Oncotarget* **2015**, *6*, 2315–2330. [CrossRef]
33. Lei, Y.; Li, B.; Tong, S.; Qi, L.; Hu, X.; Cui, Y.; Li, Z.; He, W.; Zu, X.; Wang, Z.; et al. miR-101 suppresses vascular endothelial growth factor C that inhibits migration and invasion and enhances cisplatin chemosensitivity of bladder cancer cells. *PLoS ONE* **2015**, *10*, e0117809. [CrossRef]
34. Ye, Z.; Yin, S.; Su, Z.; Bai, M.; Zhang, H.; Hei, Z.; Cai, S. Downregulation of miR-101 contributes to epithelial-mesenchymal transition in cisplatin resistance of NSCLC cells by targeting ROCK2. *Oncotarget* **2016**, *7*, 37524–37535. [CrossRef] [PubMed]
35. Luo, L.; Zhang, T.; Liu, H.; Lv, T.; Yuan, D.; Yao, Y.; Lv, Y.; Song, Y. MiR-101 and Mcl-1 in non-small cell lung cancer: Expression profile and clinical significance. *Med. Oncol.* **2012**, *29*, 1681–1686. [CrossRef] [PubMed]
36. Li, J.T.; Jia, L.T.; Liu, N.N.; Zhu, X.-S.; Liu, Q.-Q.; Wang, X.-L.; Yu, F.; Liu, Y.-L.; Yang, A.-G.; Gao, C.-F. MiRNA-101 inhibits breast cancer growth and metastasis by targeting CX chemokine receptor 7. *Oncotarget* **2015**, *6*, 30818–30830. [CrossRef] [PubMed]
37. Zheng, F.; Liao, Y.J.; Cai, M.Y.; Liu, T.-H.; Chen, S.-P.; Wu, P.-H.; Wu, L.; Bian, X.-W.; Guan, X.-Y.; Zeng, Y.-X.; et al. Systemic delivery of microRNA-101 potently inhibits hepatocellular carcinoma in vivo by repressing multiple targets. *PLoS Genet.* **2015**, *11*, e1004873. [CrossRef]
38. Slattery, M.L.; Herrick, J.S.; Pellatt, D.F.; Mullany, L.E.; Stevens, J.R.; Wolff, E.; Hoffman, M.D.; Wolff, R.K.; Samowitz, W. Site-specific associations between miRNA expression and survival in colorectal cancer cases. *Oncotarget* **2016**, *7*, 60193–60205. [CrossRef]
39. Varambally, S.; Cao, Q.; Mani, R.S.; Shankar, S.; Wang, X.; Ateeq, B.; Laxman, B.; Cao, X.; Jing, X.; Ramnarayanan, K.; et al. Genomic loss of microRNA-101 leads to overexpression of histone methyltransferase EZH2 in cancer. *Science* **2008**, *322*, 1695–1699. [CrossRef]
40. Zhang, J.G.; Guo, J.F.; Liu, D.L.; Liu, Q.; Wang, J.-J. MicroRNA-101 exerts tumorsuppressive functions in non-small cell lung cancer through directly targeting enhancer of Zeste homolog 2. *J. Thorac. Oncol.* **2011**, *6*, 671–678. [CrossRef]
41. Hu, J.; Wu, C.; Zhao, X.; Liu, C. The prognostic value of decreased miR-101 in various cancers: A meta-analysis of 12 studies. *Onco Targets Ther.* **2017**, *10*, 3709–3718. [CrossRef]
42. Xiaoping, L.; Tang, H.; Chen, J.; Song, C.; Yang, L.; Liu, P.; Wang, N.; Xie, X.; Lin, X.; Xie, X. MicroRNA-101 inhibits cell progression and increases paclitaxel sensitivity by suppressing MCL-1 expression in human triple-negative breast cancer. *Oncotarget* **2015**, *6*, 20070–20083. [CrossRef]
43. Rui, W.; Hong-Bin, W.; Chan, J.H.; Cui, Y.; Han, X.-C.; Hu, Y.; Li, F.-F.; Xia, H.-F. Ma XMiR-101 Is Involved in Human Breast Carcinogenesis by Targeting Stathmin. *PLoS ONE* **2012**, *7*, e46173. [CrossRef]
44. Hou, J.; Lin, L.; Zhou, W.; Wang, Z.; Ding, G.; Dong, Q.; Qin, L.; Wu, X.; Zheng, Y.; Yang, Y.; et al. Identification of miRNomes in human liver and hepatocellular carcinoma reveals miR-199a/b-3p as therapeutic target for hepatocellular carcinoma. *Cancer Cell* **2011**, *19*, 232–243. [CrossRef] [PubMed]
45. Duan, Q.; Wang, X.; Gong, W.; Li, N.; Chen, C.; He, X.; Chen, F.; Yang, L.; Wang, P.; Wang, D.W. ER stress negatively modulates the expression of the miR-199a/214 cluster to regulates tumor survival and progression in human hepatocellular cancer. *PLoS ONE* **2012**, *7*, e31518. [CrossRef] [PubMed]
46. Wang, Z.; Ting, Z.; Li, Y.; Chen, G.; Lu, Y.; Hao, X. microRNA-199a is able to reverse cisplatin resistance in human ovarian cancer cells through the inhibition of mammalian target of rapamycin. *Oncol. Lett.* **2013**, *6*, 789–794. [CrossRef]
47. Tsukigi, M.; Bilim, V.; Yuuki, K.; Ugolkov, A.; Naito, S.; Nagaoka, A.; Kato, T.; Motoyama, T.; Tomita, Y. Re-expression of miR-199a suppresses renal cancer cell proliferation and survival by targeting GSK-3beta. *Cancer Lett.* **2012**, *315*, 189–197. [CrossRef]

48. Duan, Z.; Choy, E.; Harmon, D.; Liu, X.; Susa, M.; Mankin, H.; Hornicek, F. MicroRNA199a-3p is downregulated in human osteosarcoma and regulates cell proliferation and migration. *Mol. Cancer Ther.* **2011**, *10*, 1337–1345. [CrossRef]
49. Tian, Y.; Zhang, Y.Z.; Chen, W. MicroRNA-199a-3p and microRNA-34a regulate apoptosis in human osteosarcoma cells. *Biosci. Rep.* **2014**, *34*, e00132. [CrossRef] [PubMed]
50. Minna, E.; Romeo, P.; De Cecco, L.; Dugo, M.; Cassinelli, G.; Pilotti, S.; Degl'Innocenti, D.; Lanzi, C.; Casalini, P.; Pierotti, M.A.; et al. miR-199a-3p displays tumor suppressor functions in papillary thyroid carcinoma. *Oncotarget* **2014**, *5*, 2513–2528. [CrossRef]
51. Wu, D.; Huang, H.J.; He, C.N.; Wang, K.-Y. MicroRNA-199a-3p regulates endometrial cancer cell proliferation by targeting mammalian target of rapamycin (mTOR). *Int. J. Gynecol. Cancer* **2013**, *23*, 1191–1197. [CrossRef] [PubMed]
52. Li, S.Q.; Wang, Z.H.; Mi, X.G.; Liu, L.; Tan, Y. MiR-199a/b-3p suppresses migration and invasion of breast cancer cells by downregulating PAK4/MEK/ERK signaling pathway. *IUBMB Life* **2015**, *67*, 768–777. [CrossRef]
53. Xuelong, F.; Shangcheng, Z.; Miao, Z.; Deng, X.; Yi, Y.; Huang, T. MiR-199a-3p enhances breast cancer cell sensitivity to cisplatin by downregulating TFAM (TFAM). *Biomed. Pharmacother.* **2017**, *88*, 507–514. [CrossRef]
54. Ruiyan, H.; Junbai, L.; Feng, P.; Zhang, B.; Yao, Y. The activation of GPER inhibits cells proliferation, invasion and EMT of triple-negative breast cancer via CD151/miR-199a-3p bio-axis. *Transl Res.* **2020**, *12*, 32–44.
55. Krützfeldt, J.; Rajewsky, N.; Braich, R.; Rajeev, K.G.; Tuschl, T.; Manoharan, M.; Stoffel, M. Silencing of microRNAs in vivo with 'antagomirs'. *Nature* **2005**, *438*, 685–689. [CrossRef] [PubMed]
56. Weiler, J.; Hunziker, J.; Hall, J. Anti-miRNA oligonucleotides (AMOs): Ammunition to target miRNAs implicated in human disease? *Gene Ther.* **2006**, *13*, 496–502. [CrossRef] [PubMed]
57. Lim, L.P.; Lau, N.C.; Garrett-Engele, P.; Grimson, A.; Schelter, J.M.; Castle, J.; Bartel, D.P.; Linsley, P.S.; Johnson, J.M. Microarray analysis shows that some microRNAs downregulate large numbers of target mRNAs. *Nature* **2005**, *433*, 769–773. [CrossRef] [PubMed]
58. Sun, L.; Yao, Y.; Lin, B.; Lin, L.; Yang, M.; Zhang, W.; Chen, W.; Pan, C.; Liu, Q.; Song, E.; et al. MiR-200b and miR-15b regulate chemotherapy-induced epithelial-mesenchymal transition in human tongue cancer cells by targeting BMI1. *Oncogene* **2012**, *31*, 432–445. [CrossRef] [PubMed]
59. Chan, M.; Liaw, C.S.; Ji, S.M.; Tan, H.H.; Wong, C.Y.; Thike, A.A.; Tan, P.H.; Ho, G.H.; Lee, A.S.-G. Identification of circulating microRNA signatures for breast cancer detection. *Clin Cancer Res.* **2013**. [CrossRef]

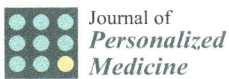

Systematic Review

Ovarian Reserve after Chemotherapy in Breast Cancer: A Systematic Review and Meta-Analysis

Alessia Romito [1], Sonia Bove [1], Ilaria Romito [1,*], Drieda Zace [2], Ivano Raimondo [1], Simona Maria Fragomeni [3], Pierluigi Maria Rinaldi [4,5], Domenico Pagliara [1], Antonella Lai [6], Fabio Marazzi [5], Claudia Marchetti [2,3], Ida Paris [3], Gianluca Franceschini [3,7], Riccardo Masetti [3,7], Giovanni Scambia [1,2], Alessandra Fabi [3] and Giorgia Garganese [1,2]

1. Gynecology and Breast Care Center, Mater Olbia Hospital, 07026 Olbia, Italy; alessia.romito@materolbia.com (A.R.); sonia.bove@materolbia.com (S.B.); ivano.raimondo@materolbia.com (I.R.); domenico.pagliara@materolbia.com (D.P.); giovanni.scambia@policlinicogemelli.it (G.S.); giorgia.garganese@materolbia.com (G.G.)
2. Dipartimento Scienze della Vita e Sanità Pubblica, Università Cattolica del Sacro Cuore, 00168 Roma, Italy; drieda.zace@unicatt.it (D.Z.); claudia.marchetti@policlinicogemelli.it (C.M.)
3. Dipartimento Scienze della Salute della Donna, del Bambino e di Sanità Pubblica, Fondazione Policlinico Universitario Agostino Gemelli IRCCS, 00168 Roma, Italy; simona.fragomeni@policlinicogemelli.it (S.M.F.); ida.paris@policlinicogemelli.it (I.P.); gianluca.franceschini@policlinicogemelli.it (G.F.); riccardo.masetti@policlinicogemelli.it (R.M.); alessandra.fabi@policlinicogemelli.it (A.F.)
4. Radiology and Interventional Radiology Unit, Mater Olbia Hospital, 07026 Olbia, Italy; pierluigi.rinaldi@materolbia.com
5. Dipartimento di Diagnostica per Immagini, Radioterapia Oncologica ed Ematologia, Fondazione Policlinico Universitario Agostino Gemelli IRCCS, 00168 Roma, Italy; fabio.marazzi@unicatt.it
6. Department of Oncology, Mater Olbia Hospital, 07026 Olbia, Italy; antonella.lai@materolbia.com
7. Dipartimento di Medicina e Chirurgia traslazionale, Università Cattolica del Sacro Cuore, 00168 Roma, Italy
* Correspondence: ilaria.romito@materolbia.com; Tel.: +39-392-415-1114

Abstract: Background: Worldwide, breast cancer (BC) is the most common malignancy in the female population. In recent years, its diagnosis in young women has increased, together with a growing desire to become pregnant later in life. Although there is evidence about the detrimental effect of chemotherapy (CT) on the menses cycle, a practical tool to measure ovarian reserve is still missing. Recently, anti-Mullerian hormone (AMH) has been considered a good surrogate for ovarian reserve. The main objective of this paper is to evaluate the effect of CT on AMH value. Methods: A systematic review and meta-analysis were conducted on the PubMed and Scopus electronic databases on articles retrieved from inception until February 2021. Trials evaluating ovarian reserves before and after CT in BC were included. We excluded case reports, case-series with fewer than ten patients, reviews (narrative or systematic), communications and perspectives. Studies in languages other than English or with polycystic ovarian syndrome (PCOS) patients were also excluded. AMH reduction was the main endpoint. Egger's and Begg's tests were used to assess the risk of publication bias. Results: Eighteen trials were included from the 833 examined. A statistically significant decline in serum AMH concentration was found after CT, persisting even after years, with an overall reduction of −1.97 (95% CI: −3.12, −0.82). No significant differences in ovarian reserve loss were found in the BRCA1/2 mutation carriers compared to wild-type patients. Conclusions: Although this study has some limitations, including publication bias, failure to stratify the results by some important factors and low to medium quality of the studies included, this metanalysis demonstrates that the level of AMH markedly falls after CT in BC patients, corresponding to a reduction in ovarian reserve. These findings should be routinely discussed during oncofertility counseling and used to guide fertility preservation choices in young women before starting treatment.

Keywords: breast cancer; AMH; ovarian reserve; chemotherapy; pregnancy desire

1. Introduction

Breast cancer (BC) is the most common cancer in the female population, with an estimated 2.3 million new cases worldwide in 2020 [1].

While the death rate has dropped by 40% since 1989, an increase in BC among young women has been reported, with around 10% of new cases diagnosed in patients younger than 40 years old [2].

Physicians should carry out counseling on fertility issues and fertility preservation in patients who have not completed childbearing before starting treatment [3].

Recent evidence has shown that age and the use of cyclophosphamide-based chemotherapy are the main factors influencing ovarian failure. In particular, the risk of chemotherapy-induced amenorrhea (CIA) was 55% [95% CI 50–60%], ranging from 26% to 77% in women younger than 35 years old compared to those older than 40 [4]. However, CIA might not be the best indicator of fertility because resumption of menses can resume even one year after chemotherapy treatment [4]. In the last two decades, there has been increased interest in the role of anti-Mullerian hormone (AMH) as a marker of ovarian reserve. Preantral and antral follicles, which remain in the growing phase for many weeks, independently of FSH or menses fluctuation, release AMH [5]. AMH is superior in terms of accuracy compared to other conventional indicators of ovarian function such as menstruation, estradiol or FSH [6,7]. Recently, a growing body of literature has been published on the effect of chemotherapy on the ovarian reserve in women with BC, assessed by AMH [8–25]. The summarization and synthesis of these results could provide BC patients and healthcare professionals with crucial information on the reproductive health consequences of chemotherapy treatment and the possibility of achieving pregnancy after completion of endocrine therapy.

In this context, this systematic review aims to evaluate the impact of chemotherapy treatment on the ovarian reserve in fertile women with BC through the quantification of AMH.

2. Materials and Methods

The present work has been reported according to the Preferred Reporting Items for Systematic Reviews and Meta-Analyses (PRISMA) statement [26].

2.1. Research Question

To address our objective, we structured a specific research question based on the PI/ECOS framework (Population, Intervention/Exposure, Comparison, Outcome, Setting/Time) as follows:

- Population: Fertile women who have been diagnosed with breast cancer and have gone through chemotherapy treatment
- Intervention: Chemotherapy treatment
- Comparison: Not Applicable
- Outcome: Ovarian reserve measured by AMH
- Setting/Time: All

2.2. Literature Search

The research was conducted on the PubMed and Scopus electronic databases. A search string was first built for PubMed, using MeSH terms, Boolean operators, and free text words. The string was subsequently adapted for use in the other database. The search was restricted to articles published in English, without any further restrictions and was last performed on 17 February 2021 for all databases. Supplementary Material (Table S1) shows the complete search strategy.

The reference lists of included studies were hand-searched for additional articles. Reference lists with trials, previous reviews or meta-analyses were also reviewed.

2.3. Study Selection and Inclusion/Exclusion Criteria

All studies that compared AMH levels at baseline and after chemotherapy in BC patients younger than 50 years old were considered pertinent. Only studies that reported a minimum of one-month follow-up were included in the systematic review. Only peer-reviewed articles reporting primary data, with no time limits, were included. We excluded case reports, case-series (reporting data for fewer than ten patients) reviews (narrative or systematic), communications and perspectives. We also excluded studies in languages other than English or with polycystic ovarian syndrome (PCOS) patients.

All articles retrieved from the search strategy were imported to Rayyan QCRI [27] and duplicates were removed. Two independent reviewers (A.R. and I.R.) selected the identified studies based on the title and abstract. We evaluated the full-text version of the studies if the title or abstract did not clarify the topic.

Discussion by a multidisciplinary team, including breast surgeons (S.B., S.M.F. and D.P.), gynecologists (Iv.R. and C.M.), a radiologist (P.M.R.) and medical oncologists (A.L., F.M. and I.P.) resolved uncertainties about the eligibility of the papers. A statistician experienced in meta-analysis (D.Z.), along with the two reviewers, analyzed data. We discussed the results in a multidisciplinary setting.

Finally, an expert committee (G.F., R.M., G.S., A.F. and G.G.) performed an independent review and gave the final approval.

2.4. Data Extraction

Two researchers (A.R. and I.R.) performed the data extraction process. We used a standardized Excel spreadsheet to extract following data: first author; year of publication; study design; sample size; mean age of patients; type of chemotherapy; follow-up duration; AMH assay; basal AMH; AMH immediately after chemotherapy; and AMH at 6 months, 1 year, 2 years and 3 years of follow-up.

2.5. Data Synthesis and Statistical Analyses

Treatment effect, defined as the difference between basal AMH and the value of AMH immediately, 6 months, 1 year, 2 years and 3 years after treatment, was calculated for each included study. If the AMH was undetectable after chemotherapy, we used the lower detection limit for the specific assay. The variance in the treatment effect, derived from standard deviations or standard errors of paired differences between baseline and the end of follow-up, was calculated. If these statistics were not given, they were calculated, where appropriate data were available [28]. The mean effect size was calculated using the inverse variance method in random-effect models. Forest plots were used for the graphical representation of each study. Heterogeneity was examined using the I^2 test, with $I^2 > 50\%$ considered important [29]. Publication bias was examined using the analyses described by Egger and Begg, where $p < 0.05$ indicated significant publication bias [30,31]. Galbraith's test and sensitivity analysis were conducted to investigate the impact each study had on the overall estimate and its contribution to Q-statistics [32]

An overall analysis of data from all studies was performed (at 1 month, 6 months, 1 year, 2 years and 3 years of follow-up). Subsequently, to account for confounding factors, subgroup analyses were performed based on the patient's age, AMH kits used, BRCA status, chemotherapy regimen and hormone therapy. Statistical analysis was performed using Cochrane Collaboration RevMan 5.1 software (http://www.cochrane.org, accessed on 16 May 2021) and STATA software (StataCorp, 2015, Stata Statistical Software: Release 15; StataCorp LP 4905 Lakeway Drive, College Station, TX, USA).

2.6. Quality Assessment

The methodological quality of the included studies was assessed based on the study design. The Newcastle–Ottawa scale was applied for cohort studies to evaluate the following quality parameters: selection of study groups, comparability of study groups and ascertainment of outcome, giving scores that range from 0 to 9. The Jadad tool was used to assess the methodological quality of randomized controlled trials (RCTs) included in the systematic review. It evaluates the randomization process, blinding, dropouts and withdrawal and assigns up to 5 points. To summarize the overall evidence quality, we grouped the articles into three categories: good methodological quality (studies that met at least 75% of the quality criteria), moderate methodological quality (studies that met between 50% and 74% of the quality criteria) and poor methodological quality (studies that met less than 50% of the quality criteria).

3. Results

Figure 1 shows the number of studies assessed and excluded through the stages of the meta-analysis.

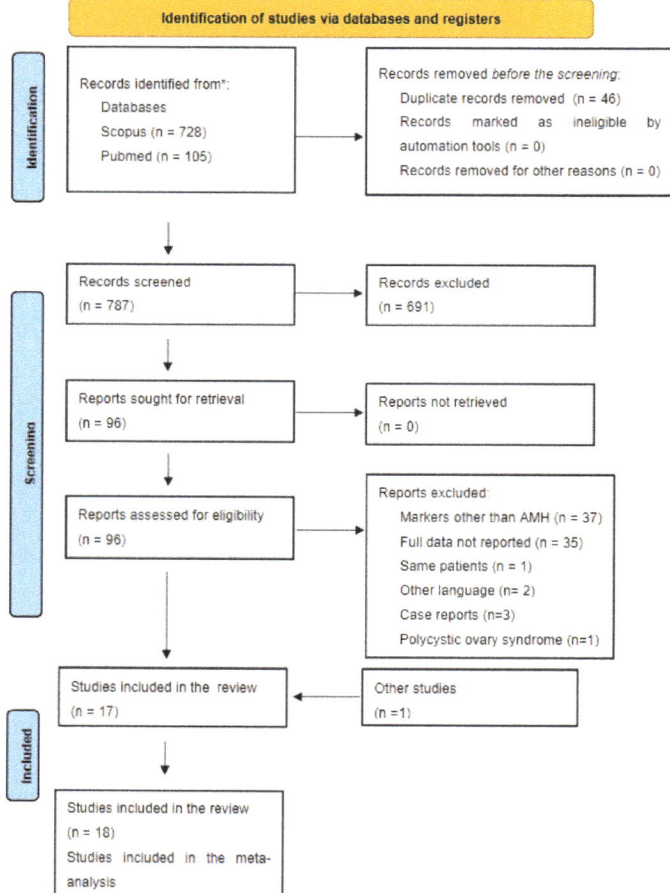

Figure 1. PRISMA flow diagram.

3.1. Bibliographical Search

The defined search strategy retrieved 833 studies from PubMed and Scopus. After the first screening process, 96 articles were deemed pertinent, and their full texts were thoroughly read. Based on this step, 79 articles were excluded for the following reasons: outcome other than AMH, incomplete data and full text in languages other than English. One study was excluded because it reported the same sample of patients as another [33] and three studies were excluded because they included fewer than ten patients [34–37]. One article was additionally added after hand-searching the references of the included studies [8]. A total of 18 studies were deemed eligible for this systematic review and meta-analysis [8–25]. Anderson et al. carried out two studies on the same population but with different follow-up periods; thus, both studies were included [10,11].

3.2. Description of the Included Studies

The main characteristics of the included studies are shown in Supplementary Material (Tables S2 and S3). Nine studies (50%) were carried out in Europe [10,11,15,16,18,21–24], three (16%) were carried out in the USA [17,20,25], four (22%) were carried out in Asia [8,9,12,19], one (6%) was carried out in Africa [14] and one (6%) was carried out in South America [13].

All included studies had a cohort design [8–11,13–15,17–23], except for three RCT [16,24,25] and one case–control study [12]. The study by Trapp et al. was a sub-analysis of the SUCCESS-A study [37]. It compared the disease-free survival (DFS) of patients receiving three cycles of fluorouracil, epirubicin and cyclophosphamide (FEC) followed by three cycles of docetaxel (D) versus three cycles of FEC chemotherapy followed by three cycles of gemcitabine and docetaxel (DG). This study included only premenopausal patients, younger than 40 years old, treated with FEC-D. The RCT of Hadji et al. and Yu et al. randomized patients to receive zoledronic acid versus a placebo after the standard treatment. For both studies, the two aims were combined in the overall analysis [16,25].

The sample size varied from 23 [13] to 250 patients [15], for a total of 1219 women. The mean age varied from 26 [13] to 41 [10,11]. The chemotherapy regimen was variable (cyclophosphamide, FEC, FEC-D, FEC-D plus methotrexate plus fluorouracil (CFM), doxorubicin plus cyclophosphamide (AC) in association with taxanes (AC-T), treatment with aGnRH during or after chemotherapy, and hormone therapy often not reported (in 52%, 32% and 37% of the studies, respectively). Six different AMH kits were used. Elecsys AMH assay was used in four studies [13,18,21,22], AMH Gen II assay was used in six studies [8,12,16,17,19,24], four articles used the Immunotech (IOT) [10,11,14,15], one article used the Diagnostic Systems Laboratories (DSL) [25], one used the ultrasensitive AMH ELISA kit [23] and one used the picoAMH ELISA kit [20]. One study did not specify the AMH kits used [9].

Seven studies reported AMH value immediately after chemotherapy [8,9,14,17,21,24,25], four studies reported it six months after chemotherapy [10,14,16,25], ten studies reported it one year after chemotherapy [10,13,16–20,22,23,25], four studies reported it two years after chemotherapy [11,15,20,24] and three studies reported it three years after chemotherapy [11,18,22].

3.3. Quality Assessment

Five out of fifteen cohort and case–control studies were considered of high quality (satisfied 75% or more of the quality criteria), while two out of three RCT were of medium quality (satisfied between 50% and 74% of the quality criteria) (Supplementary Material: Tables S4 and S5).

3.4. Meta-Analysis

All studies were analyzed, followed by a subgroup analysis for age, AMH kits and BRCA status. The insufficient data did not permit the subgroup analysis for a chemotherapy regimen and endocrine therapy.

3.4.1. Ovarian Reserve after Chemotherapy

An analysis of seven studies including 410 patients revealed a statistically significant decline in serum AMH concentration immediately after chemotherapy, with an overall reduction of -1.97 (95% CI: $-3.12, -0.82$). There was significant heterogeneity in the pooled analysis (p for heterogeneity < 0.00001, $I2 = 99\%$). After six months, there was a slight recovery (Mean Difference (MD): -1.61 (95% CI: $-2.38, -0.84$)) with a pooled population of 190 patients (p for heterogeneity < 0.00001, $I2 = 89\%$). One year after chemotherapy, there was a further reduction (MD: −2.21 (95% CI: −2.95, −1.48)) (*p* for heterogeneity < 0.00001, I2 = 98%) to achieve a steady state after two and three years of follow-up (MD after 2 and 3 years: −2.59 (95% CI: −3.95, −1.24) (*p* for heterogeneity < 0.00001, I2 = 99%) and −2.57 (95% CI: −3.99, −1.15) (*p* for heterogeneity < 0.00001, I2 = 97%), respectively (See Figure 2)). Galbraith's test was conducted, but heterogeneity remained high (more than 80%). Egger's and Begg's tests showed no significant publication bias for studies assessing AMH values immediately after chemotherapy (*p* = 0.5 and *p* = 0.3, respectively) and for those assessing AMH values 1 year after chemotherapy (*p* = 0.4 and *p* = 0.1, respectively).

3.4.2. Subgroup Analysis

Considering the high heterogeneity in the overall analysis, subgroup analysis was performed when data were available based on factors that could contribute to heterogeneity between the included studies.

Subgroup Analysis: Age

The first subgroup analysis was conducted among patients with a median age of more than 40 years old, from ages 35 to 40 years old and from ages 30 to 35 years old, one year after chemotherapy. We included ten studies. Only one study reported results on women younger than 30 years old [13]; thus, a meta-analysis was not performed.

An analysis of three studies including 140 patients older than 40 years revealed a statistically significant decline in serum AMH concentration of −1.01 (95% CI: −1.37, −0.65). Two studies (n° of pts = 134) included patients from 35 to 40 years old, reporting a higher impairment (MD −2.69 (95% CI: −2.87, −2.50). Higher toxicity was shown in younger patients (MD −2.73 (95% CI: −3.77, −1.70) aged between 30 and 35 years) assessed in four studies (N = 307). Heterogeneity was acceptable (I^2 = 53%, I^2 = 0% and I^2 = 85%) (See Figure 3).

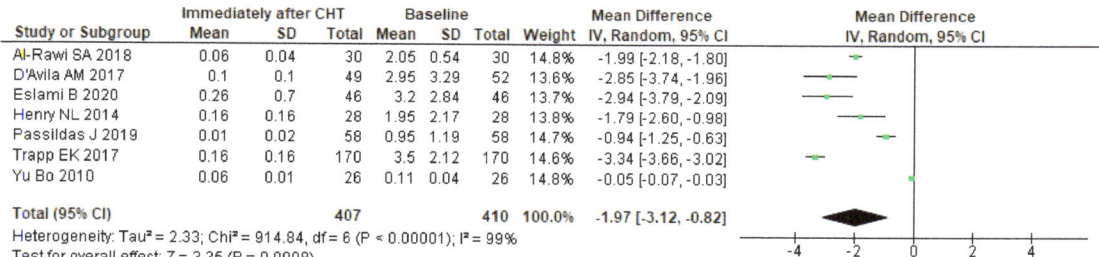

Figure 2. *Cont.*

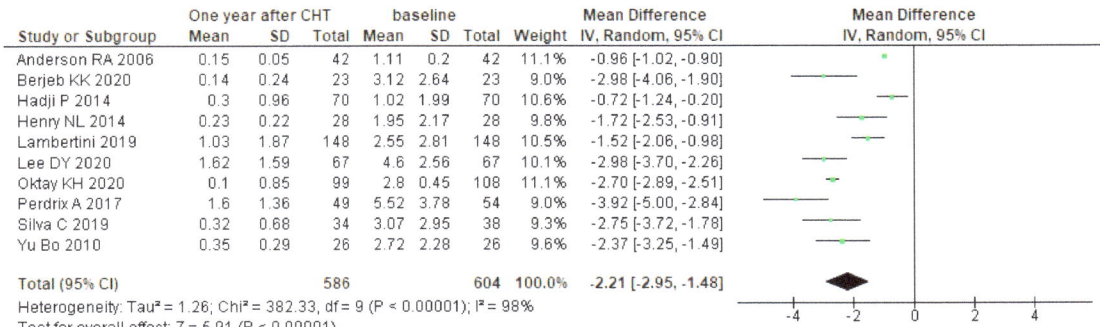

Figure 2. Forest plot for post-operative AMH levels in all BC women. AMH level were assessed (**A**) immediately after chemotherapy, (**B**) 6 months later, (**C**) 1 year later, (**D**) 2 years later and (**E**) 3 years later.

Subgroup Analysis: AMH Assay

We performed a subgroup analysis accordingly with different AMH kits one year after chemotherapy (more data available). A pooled analysis of three studies (N = 225) using Elecsys AMH kits showed a statistically significant decline in serum AMH concentration one year after chemotherapy with an overall reduction of -2.75 (95% CI: -4.28, -1.22) (p for heterogeneity < 0.0001, I^2 = 89%). The level of AMH was higher than that in the analysis of the three studies (n = 165) using AMH Gen II kits, which revealed an overall reduction of -1.79 (95% CI: $-3-17$, -0.41), also with high heterogeneity (p for heterogeneity < 0.00001, I^2 = 92%). Only one study used each of the other four AMH assays (DSL, IOT, pico-AMH and ultrasensitive AMH); therefore, meta-analysis was not performed (See Figure 4).

Study or Subgroup	One year after CHT Mean	SD	Total	Basal Mean	SD	Total	Weight	Mean Difference IV, Random, 95% CI
Anderson RA 2006	0.15	0.05	42	1.11	0.2	42	58.7%	-0.96 [-1.02, -0.90]
Hadji P 2014	0.3	0.96	70	1.02	1.99	70	26.6%	-0.72 [-1.24, -0.20]
Henry NL 2014	0.23	0.22	28	1.95	2.17	28	14.8%	-1.72 [-2.53, -0.91]
Total (95% CI)			**140**			**140**	**100.0%**	**-1.01 [-1.37, -0.65]**

Heterogeneity: Tau² = 0.06; Chi² = 4.22, df = 2 (P = 0.12); I² = 53%
Test for overall effect: Z = 5.52 (P < 0.00001)

(**A**)

Study or Subgroup	One year after CHT Mean	SD	Total	Basal Mean	SD	Total	Weight	Mean Difference IV, Random, 95% CI
Oktay KH 2020	0.1	0.85	99	2.8	0.45	108	95.7%	-2.70 [-2.89, -2.51]
Yu Bo 2010	0.35	0.29	26	2.72	2.28	26	4.3%	-2.37 [-3.25, -1.49]
Total (95% CI)			**125**			**134**	**100.0%**	**-2.69 [-2.87, -2.50]**

Heterogeneity: Tau² = 0.00; Chi² = 0.51, df = 1 (P = 0.47); I² = 0%
Test for overall effect: Z = 28.67 (P < 0.00001)

(**B**)

Study or Subgroup	One year after CHT Mean	SD	Total	Basal Mean	SD	Total	Weight	Mean Difference IV, Random, 95% CI
Lambertini 2019	1.03	1.87	148	2.55	2.81	148	27.6%	-1.52 [-2.06, -0.98]
Lee DY 2020	1.62	1.59	67	4.6	2.56	67	26.1%	-2.98 [-3.70, -2.26]
Perdrix A 2017	1.6	1.36	49	5.52	3.78	54	22.6%	-3.92 [-5.00, -2.84]
Silva C 2019	0.32	0.68	34	3.07	2.95	38	23.7%	-2.75 [-3.72, -1.78]
Total (95% CI)			**298**			**307**	**100.0%**	**-2.73 [-3.77, -1.70]**

Heterogeneity: Tau² = 0.94; Chi² = 20.67, df = 3 (P = 0.0001); I² = 85%
Test for overall effect: Z = 5.16 (P < 0.00001)

(**C**)

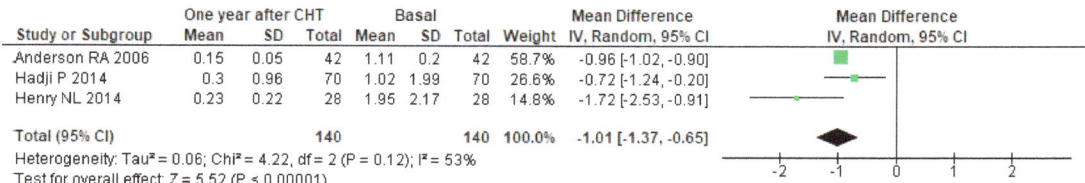

Figure 3. Forest plot for post-operative AMH levels accordingly with age. AMH levels were assessed in women (**A**) older than 40 years, (**B**) between 35 to 40 years, and (**C**) between 30 to 35 years.

Study or Subgroup	One year after CHT Mean	SD	Total	Basal Mean	SD	Total	Weight	Mean Difference IV, Random, 95% CI
Berjeb KK 2020	0.14	0.24	23	3.12	2.64	23	31.9%	-2.98 [-4.06, -1.90]
Lambertini 2019	1.03	1.87	148	2.55	2.81	148	36.2%	-1.52 [-2.06, -0.98]
Perdrix A 2017	1.6	1.36	49	5.52	3.78	54	31.9%	-3.92 [-5.00, -2.84]
Total (95% CI)			**220**			**225**	**100.0%**	**-2.75 [-4.28, -1.22]**

Heterogeneity: Tau² = 1.60; Chi² = 17.76, df = 2 (P = 0.0001); I² = 89%
Test for overall effect: Z = 3.53 (P = 0.0004)

(**A**)

Study or Subgroup	One year after CHT Mean	SD	Total	Basal Mean	SD	Total	Weight	Mean Difference IV, Random, 95% CI
Hadji P 2014	0.3	0.96	70	1.02	1.99	70	34.6%	-0.72 [-1.24, -0.20]
Henry NL 2014	0.23	0.22	28	1.95	2.17	28	32.3%	-1.72 [-2.53, -0.91]
Lee DY 2020	1.62	1.59	67	4.6	2.56	67	33.1%	-2.98 [-3.70, -2.26]
Total (95% CI)			**165**			**165**	**100.0%**	**-1.79 [-3.17, -0.41]**

Heterogeneity: Tau² = 1.37; Chi² = 25.13, df = 2 (P < 0.00001); I² = 92%
Test for overall effect: Z = 2.54 (P = 0.01)

(**B**)

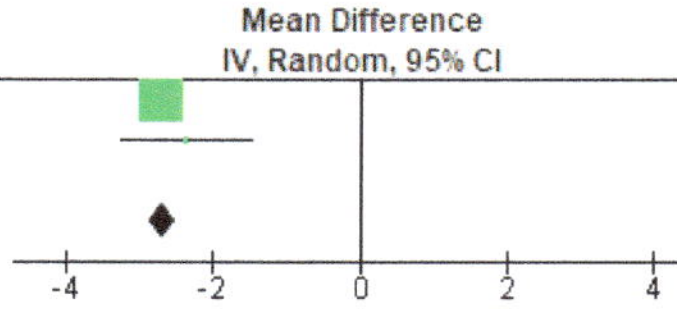

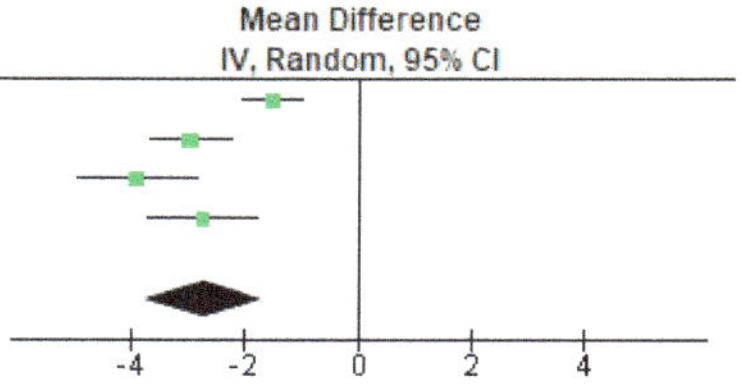

Figure 4. Forest plot for post-operative AMH levels accordingly with AMH assay. AMH levels were assessed with (**A**) ELECSYS kit (**B**) and AMH Gen II Elisa.

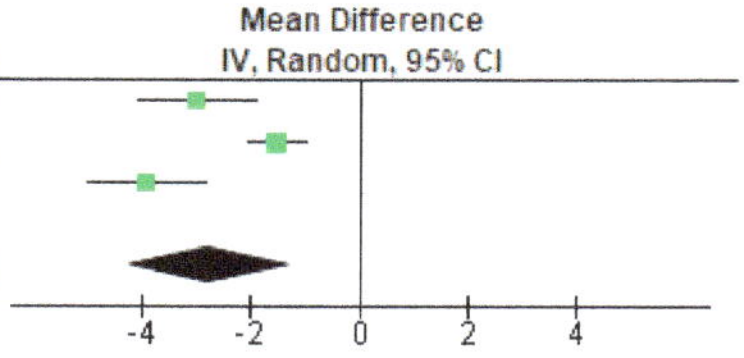

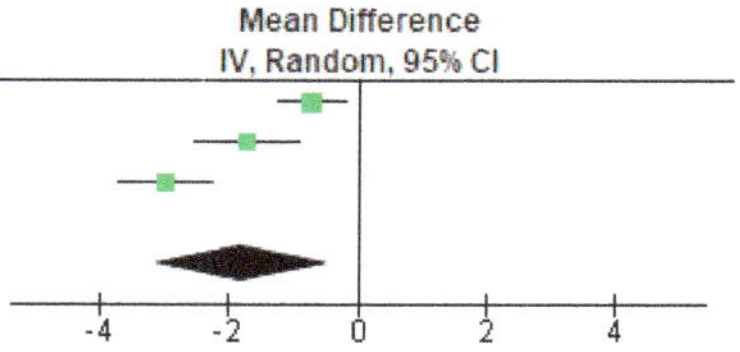

Subgroup Analysis: BRCA Subgroup Analysis

A subgroup analysis was performed accordingly with BRCA status one year after chemotherapy (more data available). An analysis of two studies including 49 patients revealed a decline in serum AMH concentration one year after chemotherapy of −2.50 (95% CI: −2.97, −2.04) for BRCA mutated (m-BRCA) patients (p for heterogeneity < 0.00001, $I^2 = 0$), similar to the reduction for wild-type BRCA (wt-BRCA) (MD: −2.47 (95% CI: −2.68, −2.25) on 172 patients (p for heterogeneity < 0.00001, $I^2 = 0$)) (See Figure 5).

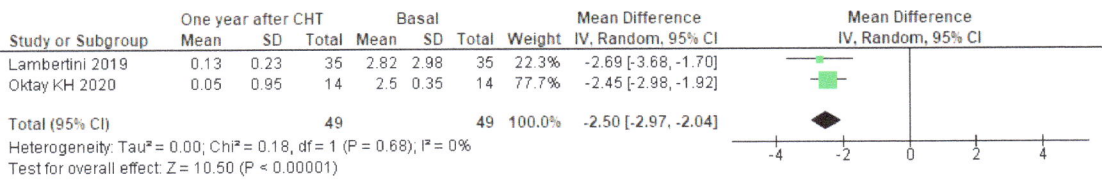

(A)

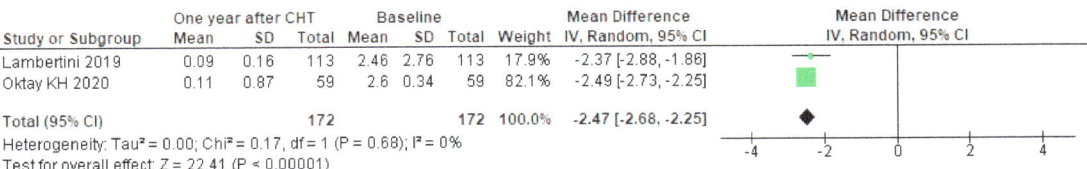

(B)

Figure 5. Forest plot for post-operative AMH levels accordingly with BRCA status. AMH levels were assessed at (**A**) m-BRCA (**B**) and wt-BRCA.

4. Discussion

This paper is the first systematic review and meta-analysis to evaluate the effect of chemotherapy on AMH in BC patients. The overall analysis revealed a marked decline of AMH value after chemotherapy treatment. AMH levels drop significantly soon after chemotherapy, with some recovery 6 months later. However, combining the detrimental effect of older age and the damage caused by chemotherapy, the ovarian reserve was almost completely depleted for women over 35 years old.

Fertile women represent almost 10% of cases with BC diagnosis [2]. In 2018, to improve the quality of life in cancer survivors [38,39], the American Society of Clinical Oncology suggested a discussion of this reproductive issue and offered fertility preservation strategies before starting cancer treatment [40]. Especially for BC, generally undergoing a polychemotherapy regimen, the risk of ovarian reserve loss is very high [41].

Different authors proposed chemotherapy-induced amenorrhea (CIA) as markers of ovarian reserve to assess the effect of chemotherapy. Women older than 40 years of age had between 77% to 100% risk of developing CIA (77–100%) compared with younger people (0–40%) [42–44].

However, amenorrhea is a poor surrogate for fertility because it serves as an instant measure of ovarian function. Above all, resumption of menses could occur after a long time. In addition, pregnancy can also arise during amenorrhea due to sporadic ovulation [45].

In our study, we evaluate chemotherapy-induced gonadotoxicity by AMH levels. In the last 15 years, AMH showed a strong correlation with ovarian reserve, with higher accuracy compared with other markers such as FSH [7].

This metanalysis demonstrated a marked fall in the ovarian reserve after chemotherapy. Although a few months later there was a slight recovery, AMH values remained in the poor responder's threshold. Therefore, BC women, after ovarian stimulation, will probably obtain a low number of oocytes, resulting in poor chances of becoming pregnant [46].

In our paper, AMH recovers following the first chemotherapy decline, dropping again after 6 months, probably due to physiological aging decline [47]. Previously, Andersen et al. have shown that recovery slope and peak depend on age and type of treatment; in fact, while BC patient's recovery was slight [10], in other cancers such as lymphoma, for which median age is younger, recovery was greater and longer [48].

The high statistical heterogenicity found in the overall meta-analysis could be due to the high clinical variability, including different ages, chemotherapy regimens, hormone therapies, AMH assay kits and BRCA mutations [49]. In order to reduce heterogeneity, we could perform a sub-group analysis for some of these items, with an overall decrease in heterogeneity that was significant for age and BRCA status and slighter for AMH assay kit.

Instead, given the lack of data, a subgroup analysis for other items, such as chemotherapy regimens, aGnRH treatments and endocrine therapies, remained unaddressed in this meta-analysis. Furthermore, the differences in the methodological quality of the included studies could contribute to the high statistical heterogeneity.

Regarding age, in our study, we showed a different chemotherapy effect accordingly for each age category. Indeed, a lower reduction was shown for older compared with younger women (M D was -1.01, -2.69 and -2.73 for the >40 years, 35 to 40 years and 30 to 35 years subgroups, respectively). The lower baseline level of AMH in older patients probably explains this effect. In fact, through the years, serum AMH levels gradually decline even in healthy women (5.6% per year) [47].

However, the most important finding from this analysis is the AMH value after chemotherapy. It appears to be very low for women older than 35 years of age (mean AMH values one year after CHT for the age category were 0.24 ± 0.69, 0.15 ± 0.77 and 1.14 ± 1.65 ng/mL for the >40 years, 35 to 40 years and 30 to 35 years subgroups, respectively). For these patients, pre-treatment counseling should be mandatory to inform them about the expected fertility drop. Physicians should inform women with pregnancy desire about fertility preservation strategies that could be implemented before starting BC treatment.

Among the 18 included studies, six different AMH assays were used. To reduce bias, standardizing the methodology might be useful in future research, especially since each test reported different sensitivities, detection limits and inter-variability [50]. Indeed, heterogeneity was slightly reduced in the subgroup that used the best performing kit [51].

We also analyzed the impact of CT on AMH levels among BRCA mutation carriers (m-BRCA). Indeed, several studies focused on their fertility potential, since the baseline ovarian reserve is expected to be reduced because of the lack of DNA double-stranded break repair [52]. However, studies on the reduction of AMH levels in the m-BRCA women compared to wild type before cancer treatments are controversial, with opposite results [53].

Moreover, data on the effects of chemotherapy depending on BRCA status are poor. In our sub-analysis, we identified only two studies. Our results suggest that BRCA mutation do not seem to change the effect of chemotherapy on ovarian reserve (MD: -2.50 (95% CI: -2.97, -2.04) versus -2.47 (95% CI: -2.68, -2.25) in mBRCA and wtBRCA, respectively). Further studies are needed to clarify this issue, as the total population in the meta-analysis was small (mBRCA $n = 172$; wtBRCA $n = 49$).

This systematic review and meta-analysis highlighted several gaps in current knowledge and could potentially help guide future research. Indeed, many sub-analyses that would be clinically very helpful and informative cannot be performed with the available data. Many relevant questions remain unsolved: First, what is the possible role of different chemotherapy regimens? Chemotherapy drugs are already known to impact menses in different ways. Anthracycline has a higher risk of amenorrhea than other drugs, but it is not known whether it directly affects ovarian reserve [4].

Second, what are the effects of GnRHa administered during and after chemotherapy on ovarian reserve? No studies in the literature investigate this topic in patients with BC, although several authors have demonstrated that GnRHa could influence AMH levels in healthy women. This question is particularly relevant for BC women since 2015. Based on evidence from the SOFT and TEXT trials, all high-risk patients younger than 35 years of age undergoing chemotherapy are currently receiving ovarian suppression with GnRHa as a standard [54,55].

Third, how do AMH levels vary during adjuvant endocrine therapy? We already know that tamoxifen could induce amenorrhea. Despite this, the effect on AMH remains unknown. There are no data in the literature, but as 75% of women with BC are suitable for endocrine therapy [56], we should clarify the effect of tamoxifen or aromatase inhibitors on ovarian reserve.

The results of this meta-analysis should be interpreted in the light of some limitations, such as publication bias, having included only peer-reviewed, English-language articles; the failure to stratify the results by factors such as chemotherapy regimen, ovarian suppression administration and endocrine therapy because data were unavailable; in general, the low- to-medium methodological quality of the studies were unrepresentative and carried out on small sample sizes, for which no stratified analysis had been performed to contain possible confounding factors.

However, despite the above limitations, this meta-analysis provides a practical tool for predicting ovarian reserve in BC patients undergoing chemotherapy. These findings should be routinely discussed during oncofertility counseling and used to guide fertility preservation choices or even simply to reduce the emotional stress associated with unexpected reproductive health impairment. Future efforts should be made to improve knowledge with more systematically collected data, precisely oriented toward clinical stratification based on the key risk factors.

Supplementary Materials: The following are available online at https://www.mdpi.com/article/10.3390/jpm11080704/s1, Supplementary Material Table S1: Search strategy; Supplementary Material Table S2: Data extraction 1; Supplementary Material Table S3: Data extraction 2; Supplementary Material Table S4: Quality assessment 1; Supplementary Material Table S5: Quality assessment 2.

Author Contributions: Conceptualization, A.R., I.R.(Ilaria Romito) and G.G.; methodology, A.R. and D.Z.; software, A.R. and D.Z.; validation, S.B., S.M.F., D.P., I.R.(Ilaria Romito), C.M., P.M.R., A.L, F.M., I.P. and G.G.; formal analysis, A.R. and D.Z.; investigation, A.R. and I.R (Ilaria Romito).; resources and data curation, A.R., I.R. (Ilaria Romito) and I.R. (Ivano Raimondo); writing—review and editing, A.R., I.R.(Ivano Raimondo) and G.G.; visualization, S.B., S.M.F., D.P., I.R. (Ivano Raimondo), C.M., P.M.R., A.L., F.M. and I.P.; supervision, G.F., R.M., G.S., A.F. and G.G. All authors have read and agreed to the published version of the manuscript.

Funding: This research received no external funding.

Institutional Review Board Statement: Not applicable.

Informed Consent Statement: Not applicable.

Data Availability Statement: Not applicable.

Conflicts of Interest: The authors declare no conflict of interest.

References

1. Sung, H.; Ferlay, J.; Siegel, R.L.; Laversanne, M.; Soerjomataram, I.; Jemal, A.; Bray, F. Global cancer statistics 2020: GLOBOCAN estimates of incidence and mortality worldwide for 36 cancers in 185 countries. *CA Cancer J. Clin.* **2021**, *71*, 209–249. [CrossRef]
2. Bardia, A.; Hurvitz, S. Targeted Therapy for Premenopausal Women with HR+, HER2− Advanced Breast Cancer: Focus on Special Considerations and Latest Advances. *Clin. Cancer Res.* **2018**, *24*, 5206–5218. [CrossRef] [PubMed]
3. Cardoso, F.; Kyriakides, S.; Ohno, S.; Penault-Llorca, F.; Poortmans, P.; Rubio, I.T.; Zackrisson, S.; Senkus, E. Early breast cancer: ESMO Clinical Practice Guidelines for diagnosis, treatment and follow-up. *Ann. Oncol.* **2019**, *30*, 1194–1220. [CrossRef]
4. Zavos, A.; Valachis, A. Risk of chemotherapy-induced amenorrhea in patients with breast cancer: A systematic review and meta-analysis. *Acta Oncol.* **2016**, *55*, 664–670. [CrossRef] [PubMed]
5. Hansen, K.R.; Hodnett, G.M.; Knowlton, N.; Craig, L.B. Correlation of ovarian reserve tests with histologically determined primordial follicle number. *Fertil. Steril.* **2011**, *95*, 170–175. [CrossRef] [PubMed]

6. Alipour, F.; Rasekhjahromi, A.; Maalhagh, M.; Sobhanian, S.; Hosseinpoor, M. Comparison of Specificity and Sensitivity of AMH and FSH in Diagnosis of Premature Ovarian Failure. *Dis. Markers* **2015**, *2015*, 1–4. [CrossRef]
7. Broekmans, F.J.; Kwee, J.; Hendriks, D.J.; Mol, B.W.; Lambalk, C.B. A systematic review of tests predicting ovarian reserve and IVF outcome. *Hum. Reprod. Updat.* **2006**, *12*, 685–718. [CrossRef]
8. Eslami, B.; Jalaeefar, A.; Moini, A.; Omranipour, R.; Haghighi, M.; Alipour, S. Significant Post-Chemotherapy Decrease of Ovarian Reserve in Iranian Women With Breast Cancer. *Acta Med. Iran.* **2020**, *58*, 400–403. [CrossRef]
9. Al-Rawi, S.A.; Saleh, B.O.; Al-Naqqash, M. Serum anti-müllerian hormone levels in evaluation of chemotherapy effect on ovarian reserve in women with breast cancer. *Saudi Med. J.* **2018**, *39*, 733–735. [CrossRef]
10. Anderson, R.A.; Themmen, A.P.N.; Al-Qahtani, A.; Groome, N.P.; Cameron, D.A. The effects of chemotherapy and long-term gonadotrophin suppression on the ovarian reserve in premenopausal women with breast cancer. *Hum. Reprod.* **2006**, *21*, 2583–2592. [CrossRef]
11. Anderson, R.A.; Cameron, D.A. Pretreatment Serum Anti-Müllerian Hormone Predicts Long-Term Ovarian Function and Bone Mass after Chemotherapy for Early Breast Cancer. *J. Clin. Endocrinol. Metab.* **2011**, *96*, 1336–1343. [CrossRef]
12. Bala, J.; Seth, S.; Dhankhar, R.; Ghalaut, V.S. Chemotherapy: Impact on Anti-Müllerian Hormone Levels in Breast Carcinoma. *J. Clin. Diagn. Res.* **2016**, *10*, BC19–BC21. [CrossRef]
13. Berjeb, K.K.; Debbabi, L.; Braham, M.; Zemni, Z.; Chtourou, S.; Hannachi, H.; Hamdoun, M.; Ayadi, M.; Kacem, K.; Zhioua, F.; et al. Evaluation of ovarian reserve before and after chemotherapy. *J. Gynecol. Obstet. Hum. Reprod.* **2021**, *50*, 102035. [CrossRef]
14. D'Avila, Â.M.; Capp, E.; Corleta, H.V.E. Antral Follicles Count and Anti-Müllerian Hormone Levels after Gonadotoxic Chemotherapy in Patients with Breast Cancer: Cohort Study. *Rev. Bras. Ginecol. Obs. RBGO Gynecol. Obstet.* **2017**, *39*, 162–168. [CrossRef]
15. Dezellus, A.; Barriere, P.; Campone, M.; Lemanski, C.; Vanlemmens, L.; Mignot, L.; Delozier, T.; Levy, C.; Bendavid, C.; Debled, M.; et al. Prospective evaluation of serum anti-Müllerian hormone dynamics in 250 women of reproductive age treated with chemotherapy for breast cancer. *Eur. J. Cancer* **2017**, *79*, 72–80. [CrossRef]
16. Hadji, P.; Kauka, A.; Ziller, M.; Birkholz, K.; Baier, M.; Muth, M.; Kann, P. Effect of adjuvant endocrine therapy on hormonal levels in premenopausal women with breast cancer: The ProBONE II study. *Breast Cancer Res. Treat.* **2014**, *144*, 343–351. [CrossRef]
17. Henry, N.L.; Xia, R.; Schott, A.F.; McConnell, D.; Banerjee, M.; Hayes, D.F. Prediction of Postchemotherapy Ovarian Function Using Markers of Ovarian Reserve. *Oncology* **2013**, *19*, 68–74. [CrossRef] [PubMed]
18. Lambertini, M.; Olympios, N.; LeQuesne, J.; Calbrix, C.; Fontanilles, M.; Loeb, A.; Leheurteur, M.; Demeestere, I.; Di Fiore, F.; Perdrix, A.; et al. Impact of Taxanes, Endocrine Therapy, and Deleterious Germline BRCA Mutations on Anti-müllerian Hormone Levels in Early Breast Cancer Patients Treated With Anthracycline- and Cyclophosphamide-Based Chemotherapy. *Front. Oncol.* **2019**, *9*, 575. [CrossRef] [PubMed]
19. Lee, D.-Y.; Kim, J.-Y.; Yu, J.; Kim, S.W. Prediction of Successful Ovarian Protection Using Gonadotropin-Releasing Hormone Agonists During Chemotherapy in Young Estrogen Receptor-Negative Breast Cancer Patients. *Front. Oncol.* **2020**, *10*, 863. [CrossRef] [PubMed]
20. Oktay, K.H.; Bedoschi, G.; Goldfarb, S.B.; Taylan, E.; Titus, S.; Palomaki, G.E.; Cigler, T.; Robson, M.; Dickler, M.N. Increased chemotherapy-induced ovarian reserve loss in women with germline BRCA mutations due to oocyte deoxyribonucleic acid double strand break repair deficiency. *Fertil. Steril.* **2020**, *113*, 1251–1260.e1. [CrossRef] [PubMed]
21. Passildas, J.; Collard, O.; Savoye, A.-M.; Dohou, J.; Ginzac, A.; Thivat, E.; Durando, X.; Kwiatkowski, F.; Penault-Llorca, F.; Abrial, C.; et al. Impact of Chemotherapy-induced Menopause in Women of Childbearing Age With Non-metastatic Breast Cancer—Preliminary Results From the MENOCOR Study. *Clin. Breast Cancer* **2019**, *19*, e74–e84. [CrossRef]
22. Perdrix, A.; Saint-Ghislain, M.; Degremont, M.; David, M.; Khaznadar, Z.; Loeb, A.; Leheurteur, M.; Di Fiore, F.; Clatot, F. Influence of adjuvant chemotherapy on anti-Müllerian hormone in women below 35 years treated for early breast cancer. *Reprod. Biomed. Online* **2017**, *35*, 468–474. [CrossRef]
23. Silva, C.; Rama, A.C.R.; Soares, S.R.; Moura-Ramos, M.; Santos, T.A. Adverse reproductive health outcomes in a cohort of young women with breast cancer exposed to systemic treatments. *J. Ovarian Res.* **2019**, *12*, 1–10. [CrossRef]
24. Trapp, E.; Steidl, J.; Rack, B.; Kupka, M.; Andergassen, U.; Jückstock, J.; Kurt, A.; Vilsmaier, T.; de Gregorio, A.; Tzschaschel, M.; et al. Anti-Müllerian hormone (AMH) levels in premenopausal breast cancer patients treated with taxane-based adjuvant chemotherapy—A translational research project of the SUCCESS A study. *Breast* **2017**, *35*, 130–135. [CrossRef]
25. Yu, B.; Douglas, N.; Ferin, M.J.; Nakhuda, G.S.; Crew, K.; Lobo, R.A.; Hershman, D.L. Changes in markers of ovarian reserve and endocrine function in young women with breast cancer undergoing adjuvant chemotherapy. *Cancer* **2010**, *116*, 2099–2105. [CrossRef] [PubMed]
26. Page, M.J.; McKenzie, J.E.; Bossuyt, P.M.; Boutron, I.; Hoffmann, T.C.; Mulrow, C.D.; Shamseer, L.; Tetzlaff, J.M.; Akl, E.A.; Brennan, S.E.; et al. The PRISMA 2020 statement: An updated guideline for reporting systematic reviews. *BMJ* **2021**, *372*, n71. [CrossRef]
27. Ouzzani, M.; Hammady, H.; Fedorowicz, Z.; Elmagarmid, A. Rayyan—a web and mobile app for systematic reviews. *Syst. Rev.* **2016**, *5*, 1–10. [CrossRef] [PubMed]
28. Wan, X.; Wang, W.; Liu, J.; Tong, T. Estimating the sample mean and standard deviation from the sample size, median, range and/or interquartile range. *BMC Med. Res. Methodol.* **2014**, *14*, 1–13. [CrossRef]
29. Higgins, J.P.T.; Thompson, S.G.; Deeks, J.J.; Altman, D.G. Measuring inconsistency in meta-analyses. *BMJ* **2003**, *327*, 557–560. [CrossRef]

30. Egger, M.; Smith, G.D.; Schneider, M.; Minder, C. Bias in meta-analysis detected by a simple, graphical test. *BMJ* **1997**, *315*, 629–634. [CrossRef] [PubMed]
31. Begg, C.B.; Mazumdar, M. Operating Characteristics of a Rank Correlation Test for Publication Bias. *Biometrics* **1994**, *50*, 1088–1099. [CrossRef]
32. Galbraith, R.F. A note on graphical presentation of estimated odds ratios from several clinical trials. *Stat. Med.* **1988**, *7*, 889–894. [CrossRef]
33. Anderson, R.; Mansi, J.; Coleman, R.; Adamson, D.; Leonard, R. The utility of anti-Müllerian hormone in the diagnosis and prediction of loss of ovarian function following chemotherapy for early breast cancer. *Eur. J. Cancer* **2017**, *87*, 58–64. [CrossRef]
34. Wakimoto, Y.; Fukui, A.; Wakimoto, G.; Ikezawa, Y.; Matsuoka, M.; Omote, M.; Sugiyama, Y.; Ukita, Y.; Kato, T.; Shibahara, H. Association between spontaneous ovulation and serum anti-Müllerian hormone levels in a premature ovarian insufficiency patient after a multimodal treatment for breast cancer. *J. Obstet. Gynaecol. Res.* **2019**, *45*, 2297–2301. [CrossRef] [PubMed]
35. Mahany, E.B.; Hershman, D.L.; Sauer, M.V.; Choi, J.M. Pregnancy despite ovarian insufficiency in a patient with breast cancer. *Reprod. Med. Biol.* **2013**, *12*, 35–38. [CrossRef] [PubMed]
36. Miyoshi, Y.; Ohta, H.; Namba, N.; Tachibana, M.; Miyamura, T.; Miyashita, E.; Hashii, Y.; Oue, T.; Isobe, A.; Tsutsui, T.; et al. Low Serum Concentrations of Anti-Müllerian Hormone Are Common in 53 Female Childhood Cancer Survivors. *Horm. Res. Paediatr.* **2013**, *79*, 17–21. [CrossRef] [PubMed]
37. Andergassen, U.; Kasprowicz, N.S.; Hepp, P.; Schindlbeck, C.; Harbeck, N.; Kiechle, M.; Sommer, H.; Beckmann, M.W.; Friese, K.; Janni, W.; et al. Participation in the SUCCESS-A Trial Improves Intensity and Quality of Care for Patients with Primary Breast Cancer. *Geburtshilfe Frauenheilkd.* **2013**, *73*, 63–69. [CrossRef]
38. Benedict, C.; Thom, B.; Friedman, D.N.; Pottenger, E.; Raghunathan, N.; Kelvin, J.F. Fertility information needs and concerns post-treatment contribute to lowered quality of life among young adult female cancer survivors. *Support. Care Cancer* **2018**, *26*, 2209–2215. [CrossRef] [PubMed]
39. Gorman, J.R.; Su, H.I.; Mph, S.C.R.; Dominick, S.A.; Malcarne, V. Experiencing reproductive concerns as a female cancer survivor is associated with depression. *Cancer* **2015**, *121*, 935–942. [CrossRef]
40. Oktay, K.; Harvey, B.; Partridge, A.H.; Quinn, G.; Reinecke, J.; Taylor, H.S.; Wallace, W.H.; Wang, E.T.; Loren, A.W. Fertility Preservation in Patients With Cancer: ASCO Clinical Practice Guideline Update. *J. Clin. Oncol.* **2018**, *36*, 1994–2001. [CrossRef]
41. Early Breast Cancer Trialists' Collaborative Group (EBCTCG). Effects of chemotherapy and hormonal therapy for early breast cancer on recurrence and 15-year survival: An overview of the randomised trials. *Lancet* **2005**, *365*, 1687–1717. [CrossRef]
42. Smith, I.E.; Dowsett, M.; Yap, Y.-S.; Walsh, G.; Lonning, P.E.; Santen, R.J.; Hayes, D. Adjuvant Aromatase Inhibitors for Early Breast Cancer After Chemotherapy-Induced Amenorrhoea: Caution and Suggested Guidelines. *J. Clin. Oncol.* **2006**, *24*, 2444–2447. [CrossRef] [PubMed]
43. Davis, A.L.; Klitus, M.; Mintzer, D.M. Chemotherapy-Induced Amenorrhea from Adjuvant Breast Cancer Treatment: The Effect of the Addition of Taxanes. *Clin. Breast Cancer* **2005**, *6*, 421–424. [CrossRef] [PubMed]
44. Walshe, J.M.; Denduluri, N.; Swain, S.M. Amenorrhea in Premenopausal Women After Adjuvant Chemotherapy for Breast Cancer. *J. Clin. Oncol.* **2006**, *24*, 5769–5779. [CrossRef]
45. Van Der Wijden, C.; Manion, C. Lactational amenorrhoea method for family planning. *Cochrane Database Syst. Rev.* **2015**, *12*, CD001329. [CrossRef]
46. Polyzos, N.P.; Drakopoulos, P.; Parra, J.; Pellicer, A.; Santos-Ribeiro, S.; Tournaye, H.; Bosch, E.; Garcia-Velasco, J. Cumulative live birth rates according to the number of oocytes retrieved after the first ovarian stimulation for in vitro fertilization/intracytoplasmic sperm injection: A multicenter multinational analysis including ~15,000 women. *Fertil. Steril.* **2018**, *110*, 661–670.e1. [CrossRef]
47. Api, M. Is ovarian reserve diminished after laparoscopic ovarian drilling? *Gynecol. Endocrinol.* **2009**, *25*, 159–165. [CrossRef]
48. Decanter, C.; Morschhauser, F.; Pigny, P.; Lefebvre, C.; Gallo, C.; Dewailly, D. Anti-Müllerian hormone follow-up in young women treated by chemotherapy for lymphoma: Preliminary results. *Reprod. Biomed. Online* **2010**, *20*, 280–285. [CrossRef]
49. Higgins, J.; Thompson, S.; Deeks, J.; Altman, D. Statistical heterogeneity in systematic reviews of clinical trials: A critical appraisal of guidelines and practice. *J. Heal. Serv. Res. Policy* **2002**, *7*, 51–61. [CrossRef]
50. Su, H.I.; Sammel, M.D.; Homer, M.V.; Bui, K.; Haunschild, C.; Stanczyk, F.Z. Comparability of antimüllerian hormone levels among commercially available immunoassays. *Fertil. Steril.* **2014**, *101*, 1766–1772.e1. [CrossRef] [PubMed]
51. Gassner, D.; Jung, R. First fully automated immunoassay for anti-Müllerian hormone. *Clin. Chem. Lab. Med.* **2014**, *52*, 1143–1152. [CrossRef]
52. Venkitaraman, A.R. Cancer Susceptibility and the Functions of BRCA1 and BRCA2. *Cell* **2002**, *108*, 171–182. [CrossRef]
53. Corrado, G.; Marchetti, C.; Trozzi, R.; Scambia, G.; Fagotti, A. Fertility preservation in patients with BRCA mutations or Lynch syndrome. *Int. J. Gynecol. Cancer* **2021**, *31*, 332–338. [CrossRef] [PubMed]
54. Francis, P.; Regan, M.M.; Fleming, G.F.; Láng, I.; Ciruelos, E.; Bellet, M.; Bonnefoi, H.R.; Climent, M.A.; Da Prada, G.A.; Burstein, H.J.; et al. Adjuvant Ovarian Suppression in Premenopausal Breast Cancer. *N. Engl. J. Med.* **2015**, *372*, 436–446. [CrossRef] [PubMed]

55. Regan, M.M.; Pagani, O.; Fleming, G.F.; Walley, B.A.; Price, K.N.; Rabaglio, M.; Maibach, R.; Ruepp, B.; Coates, A.S.; Goldhirsch, A.; et al. Adjuvant treatment of premenopausal women with endocrine-responsive early breast cancer: Design of the TEXT and SOFT trials. *Breast* **2013**, *22*, 1094–1100. [CrossRef] [PubMed]
56. Kennecke, H.; Yerushalmi, R.; Woods, R.; Cheang, M.C.U.; Voduc, D.; Speers, C.H.; Nielsen, T.O.; Gelmon, K. Metastatic Behavior of Breast Cancer Subtypes. *J. Clin. Oncol.* **2010**, *28*, 3271–3277. [CrossRef] [PubMed]

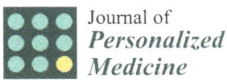

Review

Oligometastatic Breast Cancer: How to Manage It?

Vittoria Barberi [1], Antonella Pietragalla [2], Gianluca Franceschini [3], Fabio Marazzi [4], Ida Paris [5], Francesco Cognetti [1], Riccardo Masetti [3], Giovanni Scambia [2] and Alessandra Fabi [6,*]

[1] Medical Oncology 1, Regina Elena National Cancer Institute, IRCCS, 00144 Rome, Italy; vittoria.barberi@ifo.gov.it (V.B.); francesco.cognetti@ifo.gov.it (F.C.)
[2] Scientific Directorate, Department of Woman and Child Health and Public Health, Fondazione Policlinico Universitario A. Gemelli, IRCCS, 00168 Rome, Italy; antonella.pietragalla@policlinicogemelli.it (A.P.); giovanni.scambia@policlinicogemelli.it (G.S.)
[3] Comprehensive Cancer Center, Multidisciplinary Breast Unit, Fondazione Policlinico Universitario Agostino Gemelli IRCCS, Università Cattolica del Sacro Cuore, 00168 Rome, Italy; gianluca.franceschini@policlinicogemelli.it (G.F.); riccardo.masetti@policlinicogemelli.it (R.M.)
[4] UOC Radiotherapy, Department of Imaging Diagnostic, Fondazione Policlinico Universitario A. Gemelli, IRCCS, 00168 Rome, Italy; fabio.marazzi@policlinicogemelli.it
[5] Department of Woman and Child Health and Public Health, Fondazione Policlinico Universitario A. Gemelli IRCCS, 00168 Rome, Italy; ida.paris@policlinicogemelli.it
[6] Unit of Precision Medicine in Breast Cancer, Scientific Directorate, Department of Woman and Child Health and Public Health, Fondazione Policlinico Universitario A. Gemelli, IRCCS, 00168 Rome, Italy
* Correspondence: alessandra.fabi@policlinicogemelli.it; Tel.: +39-30157337

Abstract: Breast cancer (BC) is the most frequent cancer among women and represents the second leading cause of cancer-specific death. A subset of patients with metastatic breast cancer (MBC) presents limited disease, termed 'oligometastatic' breast cancer (OMBC). The oligometastatic disease can be managed with different treatment strategies to achieve long-term remission and eventually cure. Several approaches are possible to cure the oligometastatic disease: locoregional treatments of the primary tumor and of all the metastatic sites, such as surgery and radiotherapy; systemic treatment, including target-therapy or immunotherapy, according to the biological status of the primary tumor and/or of the metastases; or the combination of these approaches. Encouraging results involve local ablative options, but these trials are limited by being retrospective and affected by selection bias. Systemic therapy, e.g., the use of CDK4/6 inhibitors for hormone receptor-positive (HR+)/HER-2 negative BC, leads to an increase of progression-free survival (PFS) and overall survival (OS) in all the subgroups, with favorable toxicity. Regardless of the lack of substantial data, this subset of patients could be treated with curative intent; the appropriate candidates could be mostly young women, for whom a multidisciplinary aggressive approach appears suitable. We provide a global perspective on the current treatment paradigms of OMBC.

Keywords: oligometastatic breast cancer; locoregional therapy; CDK4/6 inhibitors; multidisciplinary

1. Introduction

Breast cancer is the most frequent cancer among women and represents the second leading cause of cancer-specific death [1]. Metastatic breast cancer (MBC) includes about 6% of cases of de novo disease, and about 20–30% of early-stage cancers recurred at distant sites [2]. The behavior of stage IV breast cancer may differ, depending on the biology of the tumor, the likelihood of spreading to certain sites (e.g., bone in hormone receptor-positive disease), and the disease burden. A subset of patients with MBC presents limited disease, termed 'oligometastatic' breast cancer (OMBC) [3].

The concept of oligometastases represents a condition midway between locoregionally confined cancer and disseminated disease, in which tumor burden is low and the number of affected organs is limited, typically with 1 to 5 secundarisms [4–8].

Even though the incidence of OMBC is not clearly defined (1–10%), it seems that a considerable amount of all new MBC presents as oligometastatic. A tri-institutional retrospective analysis of 2249 patients with stage I–III disease who had first treatment failure showed that 21.9% were characterized by oligometastatic disease [9]. This boundary between oligo- and polymetastatic disease is increasingly recognized because of treatment and survival implications [3].

Given the likelihood of limited spread, it is possible to achieve longer survival, and, in 2–3% of cases, cure, with aggressive metastasis-directed therapy [5,8].

Moreover, OMBC is characterized by its chronicity and evolvement: primary cancer may present synchronous limited metastases, or the primitive tumor over time can develop a few metachronous metastases. We define oligorecurrence as the development of metachronous oligometastases with a controlled primary site [10], whereas oligoprogression represents a condition where a limited number of metastases progress, while all other sites of the disease remain stable, commonly during systemic treatment [11,12]. This distinction is representative of different scenarios and related prognosis, and it has a clinical implication in terms of survival [4].

For example, the patients with oligometastatic disease included in the previously cited study present a significantly longer overall survival (OS) as compared to polymetastatic patients with a follow-up of more than three years.

Prior reviews on oligometastatic disease investigated the effect of local techniques, namely surgical and radiotherapy. Recently, new techniques directed to disease biology provide information about next-generation treatment strategies, leading to a deeper biological understanding of OMBC and related treatment options. We provide a global perspective on the current treatment paradigms of OMBC [3].

2. Options for Treatment of Oligometastatic Breast Cancer

The oligometastatic disease can be managed with different treatment strategies to achieve long-term remission and eventually cure. In Figure 1 a flow chart of treatment options is presented.

Several approaches are possible to cure the metastatic disease: locoregional treatment of the primary tumor and the metastases; systemic treatment, including target-therapy or immunotherapy, according to the biological status of the primary tumor and/or of the metastases; or the combination of these approaches [13].

Locoregional options both of the primitive tumor and of the metastases lead to long-lasting remissions reported in several case series; however, unlike other tumor entities, prospective data are lacking [13].

2.1. Surgery

In oligometastatic cancer, several trials involve surgery [14] (Table 1). The role of surgery in metastatic disease is unknown in terms of prognosis. Retrospective analyses demonstrate that patients who underwent surgery on the primitive tumor show a better prognosis compared to those who received only systemic therapy [15,16].

To corroborate a possible role of local treatments for the prognosis at the beginning of the metastatic disease, there is evidence that a multidisciplinary approach (surgery + radiotherapy, axillary dissection) is better for locoregional control of the disease, despite it being only surgery of the mammary node/mastectomy [17]. However, the findings of these studies are weakened due to selection bias: for example, patients with a less extended metastatic disease and/or who are responsive to medical treatments have more opportunities to undergo surgery on the primitive tumor than those who present a more advanced disease and/or who are less responsive to medical treatments.

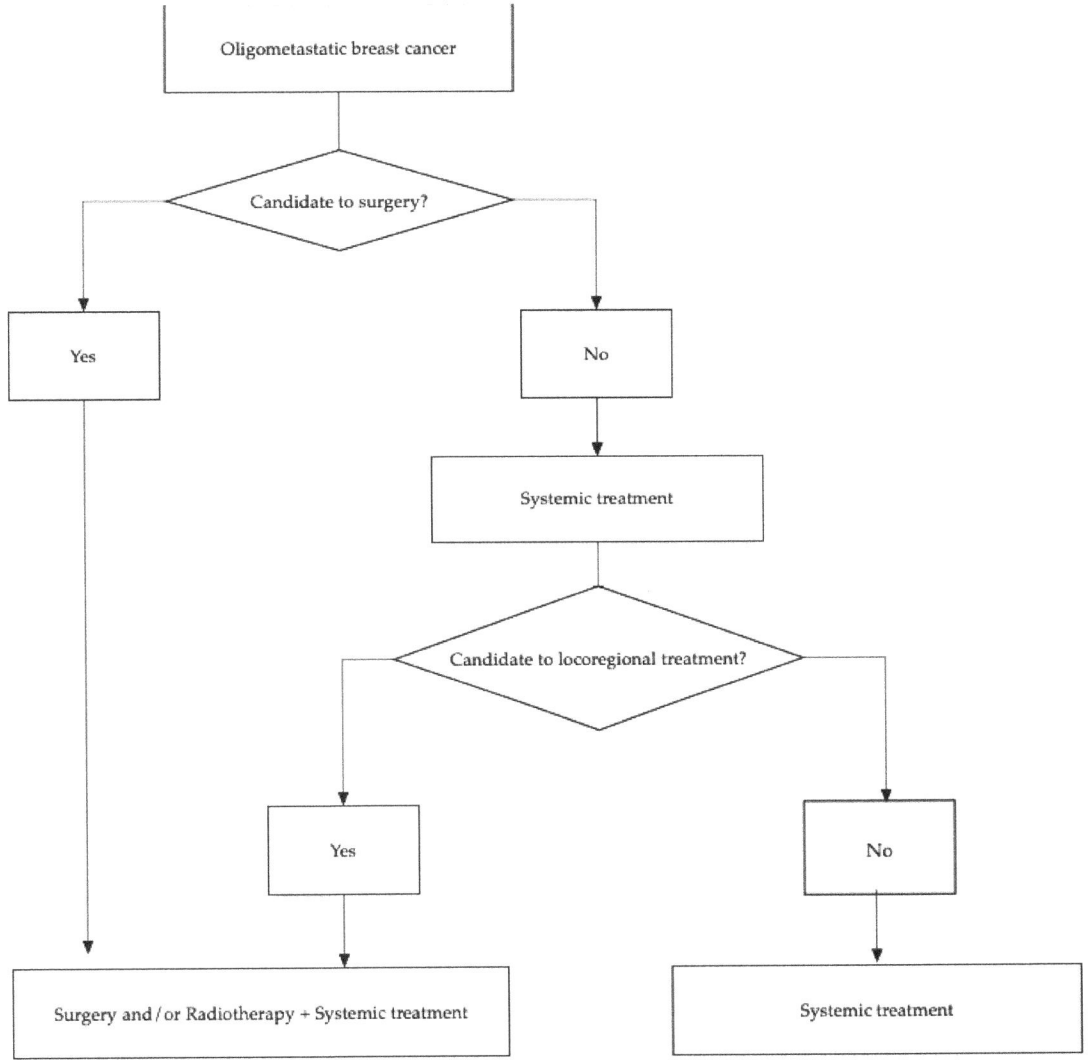

Figure 1. Diagram flow of therapeutic options in oligometastatic breast cancer.

In the literature, three randomized trials evaluated the efficacy of surgery in MBC at the beginning of the disease.

In Tata Memorial Trial [18], among 350 women who enrolled, 173 underwent surgery and medical treatment and 177 received only medical treatment. This trial demonstrates that there are no differences in OS between the two groups. Surgical treatment is related to a better locoregional PFS, but also a worse DPFS (distant progression-free survival).

In the MF0701 [19] study, of 274 women who were enrolled, 138 underwent surgery and systemic treatment, while 136 were administered only systemic treatment. Patients with HR+ could receive hormone therapy. The protocol permitted upfront randomization (before the beginning of medical treatment) and the option of surgery on the primitive tumor during the local progression in the systemic treatment group. This trial showed a significant increase in median survival in those patients who underwent surgery upfront (46 vs. 37 months, HR 0.66 $p < 0.005$). An analysis of the subgroups showed that the survival was superior to locoregional treatment in women with luminal tumors, age < 55 years, and solitary bone metastases.

ECOG-ACRIN E 2108 [20] studied 258 patients with de novo MBC with no progression after 4–8 months of systemic treatment that were randomized to continue systemic treatment or to receive radical locoregional treatment (surgery with free margins and subsequent radiotherapy, if indicated). About 60% presented an HR+/HER-2 negative tumor, 26% HER-2+, 15% were triple negative. In addition, 37% of these patients presented only bone metastases. The survival analysis showed no difference in OS and PSF in the two cohorts in the general population. The subgroup analysis suggests a possible detrimental effect of locoregional treatment in the subgroup of patients with triple-negative BC. Thus, even though we observed an increase of 2.5 times in the risk of locoregional progression in patients who received systemic therapy without locoregional treatment, there is no benefit in terms of quality of life from locoregional treatment.

Moreover, a prospective cohort trial [21] shows that in patients who have responded to first-line treatment, surgery on the primitive tumor does not improve PFS and OS, so that the predominant prognostic role is given by medical treatments, histopathologic features, and tumor burden. Conclusively, in patients with de novo MBC, the surgery approach has a palliative role (e.g., ulcerative lesions). In the absence of results of the effectiveness in OS, this procedure is considered in selected cases and after discussion with the patient.

There are three other randomized trials, one of which has finished the accrual, and it could furnish other elements to the argument.

In clinical practice, surgery is reserved for vertebral metastases with medullary compression, pathological fractures, pleural or pericardial effusion, and single visceral metastasis (e.g., liver, lung, brain).

In this regard, the resection of liver metastases in MBC is little explored, although in other tumors such as colorectal cancer it is widely recognized [6].

Different case series [6,22–36] show different survival rates (22–61 months) for liver metastases resection. A monocentric experience with 51 patients reported a 16% increase of 10-year OS rate [26]; 8.9% of these patients never presented any recurrence after surgery. However, this result is affected by a selection bias of the sample: the resection, but also the indolent course of the disease, the specific genetic profile of the tumor, and the ability of subclones to metastasize to a certain organ likely play a crucial prognostic role. Therefore, these reports need confirmation with prospective randomized trials [37].

A prospective data collection of 41 patients, who underwent liver metastases resection, revealed that positive resection margins and a short disease-free interval until the detection of liver metastases may lead to poor long-term survival [38]. Comparable results can be assumed for pulmonary lesions metastasectomy [39,40]: a short disease-free interval, the presence of several metastases, incomplete resection of them, and a non-luminal subtype are considered negative prognostic factors [41].

In summary: in OMBC, surgery on the metastases is still experimental because there are no data from prospective randomized trials with large samples. In addition, OMBC, even the indolent behavior, is a widespread disease, where local treatments alone could not be sufficient. However, these preliminary results may identify subgroups of patients with more favorable outcomes and for whom the surgery could lead to long-term survival [13].

Table 1. Randomized trials that evaluate the efficacy of surgery in MBC.

Trial	Number of Patients	Site of Metastases	Biological Subtype	Site of Surgery	Outcome
Tata Memorial, NCT00193778	350	Bone and/or visceral	HR+/HER2− HR+/HER2+	- Modified radical mastectomy - Breast-conserving surgery - Palliative surgery upon progression	1. No differences in OS 2. Better locoregional PFS FOR surgery 3. Worse DPFS for surgery
MF0701, NCT00557986	274	Bone and/or lung and/or liver	HR+ 85.5% HER2+ 30.4% TN 7.3%	- Breast conserving surgery - Metastasectomy - Axillary lymph node dissection	1. Increase in median survival for surgery upfront 2. Superior survival for locoregional treatment in women with luminal tumors, age < 55 years, and solitary bone metastases
ECOG-ACRIN E 2108, NCT01242800	258	Bone and/or any organ system, including CNS	HR+/HER2− 60% HER2+ 26% TN 15%	- Breast-conserving therapy - Total mastectomy - Palliative surgery	1. No difference in OS and PFS 2. Possible detrimental effect of locoregional treatment in TN mBC 3. Increase of 2.5x risk of locoregional progression in patients who received systemic therapy without locoregional treatment
TBCRC 013, NCT00941759	127	Bone and/or any organ system, including CNS	HR+/HER2− HR+/HER2+ HR−/HER2+ HR−/HER2−	- Elective breast surgery - Palliative breast surgery	1. No improvement of PFS and OS for surgery in patients who have responded to first-line treatment

2.2. Radiotherapy

Patients with oligometastatic disease or with oligorecurrence in a single area could be treated with local therapy such as stereotactic body radiotherapy (SBRT), even associated with chemotherapy. Possible target lesions include brain, lung, liver, and lymph nodes.

Oligorecurrent metastases in the brain, lung, and liver can be definitively treated with SBRT. Instead, there are some controversies regarding lymph node oligometastases, thus further phase III trials are needed [42].

The use of stereotactic ablative radiotherapy (SABR) produces favorable outcomes, since it presents high accuracy to the target lesion, very conformal dose distributions, and delivers a highly ablative dose over a treatment duration of 1–5 treatments maximum.

Several works strengthen the use of SABR in OM disease, mostly randomized controlled trials (RCTs) [4].

Patients with a limited number of brain metastases and controlled extracranial disease may benefit from locoregional treatment combined with systemic therapy, which crosses the blood–brain barrier. Currently, stereotactic radiosurgery (SRS) is the recommended option for resected cavity and non-resected brain metastases [43] and achieves longer overall survival (OS) compared to whole-brain palliative irradiation [44,45].

Concerning lung OM disease, stereotactic techniques demonstrate a 2-year local control rate of 77.9% and a 2-year OS of 53.7%, according to a systematic review [46].

At the same time, a regional nodal recurrence after conservative breast treatment affects about 1% to 5.4% of patients with early-stage breast cancer [47–49]. A phase II study with SBRT or intensity-modulated radiation therapy for OMBC showed encouraging results [50]. Even though the principal site of metastases was the bone, several cases of lymph node metastases were treated with SBRT or intensity-modulated radiation therapy, without reporting severe toxicity. Furthermore, 90% of patients with oligorecurrence had an objective response to salvaging radiotherapy and the 3-year treated tumor control rate was 93% [51]. However, despite the lack of reports about SBRT for oligorecurrent lymph node metastases of breast cancer, this subgroup of patients seems to be well suited for SBRT, especially those who did not receive previous irradiation, because of the indolent behavior of the disease. Nonetheless, patients should be carefully monitored over time, because of the risk of late toxicities.

The research is moving forward, with an ongoing randomized phase II/III trial (NRG-BR002), which evaluates the role of these techniques in OMBC [42,52].

2.3. Systemic Treatments

Systemic treatment remains a milestone in the management of metastatic breast cancer.

Considering hormone receptor (HR) positive, HER2-negative metastatic breast cancers, certainly CDK4/6 inhibitors in combination with endocrine therapy have changed the paradigm of the treatment [53].

Concerns about the difference among the three CDK4/6 inhibitors involve the significant OS improvement, demonstrated from MONALEESA-3, MONALEESA-7, and MONARCH-2 trials, but not reported in PALOMA-1, PALOMA-3, and MONALEESA-2 trials [54–59].

As a result, a meta-analysis of all these randomized controlled trials evaluated the OS improvement among Palbociclib, Ribociclib and Abemaciclib, and focused on the efficacy of these compounds in some relevant subgroups of patients.

Of 5862 patients from MONALEESA-2, MONALEESA-3, and MONALEESA-7 trials, 2429 presented visceral (lung or liver) disease, 929 had bone-only disease, and 2504 had visceral and bone disease. Of 2845 patients, grouped by the number of metastases, 782 had only one metastatic site, 635 two, and 1428 three or more. The pooled results of the meta-analysis showed no heterogeneity for all these subgroups, with a statistically significant improvement in PFS with a similar hazard ratio [60].

Therefore, this meta-analysis demonstrates that CDK4/6 inhibitors plus endocrine therapy are beneficial in terms of PFS, regardless of the presence of visceral metastases, the number of metastatic sites, and the length of the treatment-free interval. Consequently, the pooled estimate for the overall population is also feasible for OMBC patients [60].

However, in luminal breast cancer, even after a first-line systemic treatment, OM disease could be persistent; therefore, due to the introduction and approval from FDA and EMA of Alpelisib, it is advisable to test the presence of PIK3CA mutation. Patients with PIK3CA mutation may benefit from Alpelisib plus Fulvestrant association, both with bone metastases and visceral metastases, as shown by the subgroup analysis of the SOLAR-1 study [61]. Instead, patients without the expression of PIK3CA mutation should receive a further line of hormonal treatment; this can be Everolimus plus Exemestane or Fulvestrant alone or, in selected patients, chemotherapy; confirmed data about the use of CDK4-6 inhibitors beyond progression are still unknown, and to date there are ongoing phase III studies comparing Alpelisib plus Fulvestrant versus Fulvestrant alone (CBYL719C2303 study-EPIK-B5).

In summary, a key role in the OMBC treatment is maintaining hormonal target therapy, reserving chemotherapy in cases of visceral crisis or widespread disease.

Unlike the luminal BC, often HER-2-like and triple-negative tumors have a different presentation since they have more aggressive behavior. Therefore, in these subtypes the strategy overlaps with a polymetastatic disease: in case of an HER-2 like OMBC, the use of anti-HER-2 molecules remains the first goal; instead, the current targets for triple-negative tumors are PD-L1 and BRCA mutations, and the use of Atezolizumab plus Nab-paclitaxel and Olaparib, respectively, showed better outcomes in terms of PFS and quality of life [62,63].

2.4. Combination of Radiotherapy and Systemic Treatment

Although CDK4/6 inhibitors are largely involved in the treatment of MBC, preliminary findings suggest a possible synergic effect of these compounds when combined with radiotherapy, especially in OM disease [64].

CDK4/6 inhibitors can act as a DNA double-strand break repair inhibitor, thus amplifying the anticancer effect of RT [65].

Therefore, the simultaneous administration of a radio-sensitizing drug could significantly improve symptoms and disease control. Despite the potential benefit of this combination, there is little literature on this topic, and clinicians could be frightened, since the radio-sensitizing effect may also increase the toxicity, involving healthy tissues as well [66,67]. The consequence might lead to, on one hand, improperly interrupting the systemic treatment or the radiotherapy.

Table 2 shows the preliminary results from small patient samples with the combination of CDK4/6 inhibitors with RT.

Hans et al. described five patients treated with Palbociclib and concurrent palliative RT without severe toxicity [68]: all patients experienced pain relief, but follow-up time and local control were not reported.

Meattini et al. described five patients treated with Ribociclib and concurrent palliative RT for bone metastases [69]: two patients developed grade 3–4 toxicity (one neutropenia and one vomit and diarrhea) and two needed temporary suspension of Ribociclib; radiotherapy was never suspended. At a 3-month assessment, three stable diseases and two partial responses were observed.

Chowdary et al. evaluated 16 patients treated with Palbociclib and RT for symptomatic metastases [64]. No side effect differences were found compared to the use of Palbociclib alone; all patients experienced prolonged pain control, and no local failures were described. However, only 31.3% of patients did not interrupt Palbociclib during the RT, while the other patients suspended the CDK4/6 inhibitor 14 days before or after RT, with a median interval of 5 days.

Ippolito et al. analyzed 16 patients treated with Palbociclib or Ribociclib concomitant to RT [70]. First, 68.7% of patients received palliative RT for bone metastases with a median dose of 30 Gy, while the remaining with OM disease were treated with higher doses (median 50 Gy). At 6.3 months follow-up, the only toxicity reported was neutropenia, apparently not worsened by radiotherapy, because it had already existed during the previous cycles of systemic treatment. Patients with bone metastases experienced all pain relief; the other subgroup developed complete responses (two patients with visceral and/or soft tissue), partial responses (two patients with bone disease), and stable disease (one patient with bone involvement) [71–76].

Two other retrospective analyses evaluated risks and benefits from the concomitant therapy with CDK4/6 inhibitors and RT. In one experience 16 patients under treatment with Palbociclib and radiotherapy were studied. At a follow-up of 14.7 months, none reported relevant acute or late toxicities: all reported that side effects were mild. All the patients achieved pain relief, and no local failures were developed [64]. The second study analyzed 18 patients treated with radiotherapy and concomitant CDK4/6 inhibitors for bone involvement. The hematologic toxicity was mild during the end of RT and the subsequent cycles of systemic treatment (grade 3–4 neutropenia) [72]; the other relevant side effect was grade 1 gastrointestinal toxicity. Three months after the end of RT, 88.9% of patients experienced pain relief, with no pain recurrence. With a median follow-up of 13.7 months, only one patient developed local recurrence. This study involves the largest cohort with concomitant CDK 4/6 inhibitors and RT published, but numbers are still limited.

These preliminary works suggest that the combination of CDK4/6 inhibitors and RT, particularly on bone metastases, is safe, with limited toxicities in terms of time and grade. The hematologic toxicity is comparable between the combination of these approaches and the medical treatment alone, while the gastrointestinal side effects could be more relevant; therefore, clinicians should be careful in case of RT of the abdominal or pelvic area.

Although the results of these trials are limited by the small number of the sample, the clinical and radiological outcomes are promising. Future studies with a larger population and a longer follow-up will validate these results [64,77].

Table 2. Trials that evaluate the efficacy of concomitant RT and CDK4/6-i in MBC.

Trial	Number of Patients	CDK4/6-I	Outcome
Hans et al.	5	Palbociclib	5 pain relief 1 stable disease
Meattini et al.	5	Ribociclib	3 stable disease 2 partial response
Chowdary et al.	16	Palbociclib	16 pain relief 0 local failures
Ippolito et al.	16	Palbociclib Ribociclib	16 pain relief 2 complete responses 2 partial responses 1 stable disease
Mudit et al.	16	Palbociclib	16 pain relief 0 local failures
Guerini et al.	18	Palbociclib Ribociclib Abemaciclib	16 pain relief 0 pain recurrence 17 local control 1 local recurrence

3. Conclusions

Even though metastatic breast cancer is considered incurable, OMBC presents a better prognosis [78].

Regardless of the lack of substantial data, this subset of patients could be treated with curative intent, mostly young women for whom a multidisciplinary aggressive approach appears suitable [3,78].

For these patients with a favorable nature for their disease, a multidisciplinary aggressive approach might improve survival [78].

Specifically, a combination of local and systemic treatment can achieve such long-term effects [13].

Local ablative options (radiotherapy/surgery) play a key role in this setting, as can be assumed from retrospective trials, but these encouraging results need confirmation by prospective randomized studies [78].

Moreover, preliminary data suggest an increase of disease-free survival after surgery on distant metastases; however, the selection of the appropriate candidates concerns the biology of the disease, and unfortunately, valuable comparative data are still missing. For this reason, surgery on breast cancer metastases remains an experimental approach.

Systemic therapy, e.g., the use of CDK4/6 inhibitors for HR+/HER2 negative BC, leads to an increase of PFS and OS in all the subgroups, with favorable toxicity.

Therefore, combined strategies increase the probability of producing results such as tumor-size reduction, long-lasting responses, and, eventually, cure [79].

All of these treatment strategies present a higher rate of success when the metastatic disease is detected early, so it is crucial to involve modern imaging equipment and liquid biopsies to model a personalized and multidisciplinary treatment [13].

4. Future Directions

The lack of strong data concerning the management of OMBC clearly emerges, due to the quality and heterogeneity of the systematic reviews and meta-analyses.

However, the increasing interest in the OM phenotype is emerging, and several prospective phase II/III randomized controlled trials involving new strategies for OMBC are ongoing (Table 3). A phase III study in the Netherlands (NCT01646034) is evaluating the role of high-dose chemotherapy with carboplatin, thiotepa, and cyclophosphamide in homologous recombination-deficient OMBC, since it seems that these tumors are particularly sensitive to alkylating agents which disrupt double-stranded DNA. Several trials are assessing the use of SABR and/or traditional surgery associated with systemic therapy in the first-line setting for newly diagnosed OMBC (e.g., CLEAR, NCT03750396; STEREO-SEIN, NCT02089100; NCT02364557). For instance, a pilot phase I study in Australia is evaluating the role of SABR followed by 6 months of anti-PD1 therapy with pembrolizumab, intending to show both safety and enhanced immune activation (BOSTON-II, NCT02303366).

The comparison of these trial results is weakened by the different definition of 'oligometastatic disease', which could include from two to five distant lesions. For further future studies, it would be reasonable to employ a universal definition of 'oligometastatic' within the breast cancer investigative community [3].

Table 3. Ongoing trials in oligometastatic BC.

Trial	Objective	Site of Metastases
NCT01646034	Role of high-dose polychemotherapy in HRD OMBC	1 to 3 distant metastatic lesions, with or without primary tumor, local recurrence, or locoregional lymph node metastases, including the ipsilateral axillary, parasternal, and periclavicular regions
CLEAR, NCT03750396	Local treatment (including surgical resection, stereotactic body radiotherapy, palliative radiotherapy, and radiofrequency ablation) in addition to endocrine treatment as 1st line for HR+/HER2- OMBC	≤2 lesions in single organ or site (lung, bone, liver, adrenal glands, distant LNs)
STEREO-SEIN, NCT02089100	Role of metastases SBRT with curative intent in de novo oligometastatic disease	≤5 metastatic lesions (measurable or not) No brain metastases
NCT02364557	Use of SABR and/or traditional surgery in addition to standard of care systemic therapy in the first-line setting for newly diagnosed OMBC	≤4 metastases in lung, bone, spine, abdominal-pelvic (lymph node/adrenal gland), liver, mediastinal/cervical lymph node
BOSTON-II, NCT02303366	Role of SABR followed by 6 months of anti-PD1 therapy with pembrolizumab, intending to show both safety and enhanced immune activation	1 to 5 metastases No evidence of visceral metastases in liver or brain

Author Contributions: Conceptualization, A.F.; methodology, A.P., G.F., F.M., I.P.; resources, A.F. and V.B.; writing—review and editing V.B., A.F.; supervision, R.M., F.C. and G.S. All authors have read and agreed to the published version of the manuscript.

Funding: This research received no external funding.

Institutional Review Board Statement: Not applicable.

Informed Consent Statement: Not applicable.

Data Availability Statement: Not applicable.

Conflicts of Interest: The authors declare no conflict of interest.

References

1. Henry, N.L.; Shah, P.D.; Haider, I.; Freer, P.E.; Jagsi, R.; Sabel, M.S. Cancer of the Breast. *Abeloff's Clin. Oncol.* **2020**, *12*, 1560–1603.
2. O'Shaughnessy, J. Extending Survival with Chemotherapy in Metastatic Breast Cancer. *Oncology* **2005**, *10*, 20–29. [CrossRef]
3. Makhlin, I.; Fox, K. Oligometastatic Breast Cancer: Is This a Curable Entity? A Contemporary Review of the Literature. *Curr. Oncol. Rep.* **2020**, *22*, 1–10. [CrossRef]

4. Al-Shafa, F.; Arifin, A.J.; Rodrigues, G.B.; Palma, D.A.; Louie, A.V. A Review of Ongoing Trials of Stereotactic Ablative Radiotherapy for Oligometastatic Cancers: Where Will the Evidence Lead? *Front. Oncol.* **2019**, *9*, 543. [CrossRef]
5. Palma, D.A.; Louie, A.V.; Rodrigues, G.B. New Strategies in Stereotactic Radiotherapy for Oligometastases. *Clin. Cancer Res.* **2015**, *21*, 5198–5204. [CrossRef]
6. Huang, F.; Wu, G.; Yang, K. Oligometastasis and oligo-recurrence. *Radiat. Oncol.* **2014**, *9*, 230. [CrossRef] [PubMed]
7. Pagani, O.; Senkus, E.; Wood, W.; Colleoni, M.; Cufer, T.; Kyriakides, S.; Costa, A.; Winer, E.P.; Cardoso, F.; Force, E.-M.T. International guidelines for management of metastatic breast cancer: Can metastatic breast cancer be cured? *J. Natl. Cancer Inst.* **2010**, *102*, 456–463. [CrossRef]
8. Cardoso, F.; Costa, A.; Senkus, E.; Aapro, M.; Andre, F.; Barrios, C.H.; Bergh, J.; Bhattacharyya, G.; Biganzoli, L.; Cardoso, M.J.; et al. 3rd ESO-ESMO International Consensus Guidelines for Advanced Breast Cancer (ABC 3). *Ann. Oncol.* **2017**, *28*, 16–33. [CrossRef] [PubMed]
9. Jain, S.K.; Dorn, P.L.; Chmura, S.J.; Weichselbaum, R.R.; Hasan, Y. Incidence and implications of oligometastatic breast cancer. *J. Clin. Oncol.* **2012**, *30*, e11512. [CrossRef]
10. Niibe, Y.; Hayakawa, K. Oligometastases and Oligo-recurrence: The New Era of Cancer Therapy. *Jpn. J. Clin. Oncol.* **2010**, *40*, 107–111. [CrossRef] [PubMed]
11. Correa, R.J.M.; Salama, J.K.; Milano, M.T.; Palma, D.A. Stereotactic body radiotherapy for oligometastasis opportunities for biology to guide clinical management. *Cancer J.* **2016**, *22*, 247–256. [CrossRef] [PubMed]
12. Reyes, D.K.; Pienta, K.J. The biology and treatment of oligometastatic cancer. *Oncotarget* **2015**, *6*, 8491–8524. [CrossRef] [PubMed]
13. Westphal, T.; Gampenrieder, S.P.; Rinnerthaler, G.; Greil, R. Cure in metastatic breast cancer. *Memo Mag. Eur. Med. Oncol.* **2018**, *11*, 172–179. [CrossRef]
14. Divisi, D.; Barone, M.; Zaccagna, G.; Gabriele, F.; Crisci, R. Surgical approach in the oligometastatic patient. *Ann. Transl. Med.* **2018**, *6*, 94. [CrossRef]
15. Criscitiello, C.; Giuliano, M.; Curigliano, G.; Laurentiis, M.D.; Arpino, G.; Carlomagno, N.; Placido, S.D.; Golshan, M.; Santangelo, M. Surgery of the primary tumor in de novo metastatic breast cancer: To do or not to do? *Eur. J. Surg. Oncol.* **2015**, *41*, 1288–1292. [CrossRef]
16. Harris, E.; Barry, M.; Kell, M.R. Meta-analysis to determine if surgical resection of the primary tumour in the setting of stage IV breast cancer impacts on survival. *Ann. Surg. Oncol.* **2013**, *20*, 2828–2834. [CrossRef]
17. Warschkow, R.; Güller, U.; Tarantino, I.; Cerny, T.; Schmied, B.M.; Thuerlimann, B.; Joerger, M. Improved Survival after Primary Tumor Surgery in Metastatic Breast Cancer: A Propensity-adjusted, Population-based SEER Trend Analysis. *Ann. Surg.* **2016**, *263*, 1188–1198. [CrossRef]
18. Badwe, R.; Hawaldar, R.; Nair, N.; Kaushik, R.; Parmar, V.; Siddique, S.; Budrukkar, A.; Mittra, I.; Gupta, S. Locoregional treatment versus no treatment of the primary tumour in metastatic breast cancer: An open-label randomised controlled trial. *Lancet Oncol.* **2015**, *16*, 1380–1388. [CrossRef]
19. Soran, A.; Ozmen, V.; Ozbas, S.; Karanlik, H.; Muslumanoglu, M.; Igci, A.; Canturk, Z.; Utkan, Z.; Ozaslan, C.; Evrensel, T. Randomized Trial Comparing Resection of Primary Tu-mor with No Surgery in Stage IV Breast Cancer at Presentation: Protocol MF07-01. *Ann. Surg. Oncol.* **2018**, *25*, 3141–3149. [CrossRef]
20. Khan, S.A.; Zhao, F.; Solin, L.J.; Goldstein, L.J.; Cella, D.; Basik, M.; Golshan, M.; Julian, T.B.; Pockaj, B.A.; Lee, C.A. A randomized phase III trial of systemic therapy plus early local therapy versus systemic therapy alone in women with de novo stage IV breast cancer: A trial of the ECOG-ACRIN Research Group (E2108). *J. Clin. Oncol.* **2020**, *38*, LBA2. [CrossRef]
21. King, T.A.; Lyman, J.; Gonen, M.; Reyes, S.; Hwang, R.S.; Liu, M.C.; Boughey, J.C.; Jacobs, L.K.; McGuire, K.P.; et al. A prospective analysis of surgery and survival in stage IV breast cancer (TBCRC 013). *J. Clin. Oncol.* **2016**, *34*, 1006. [CrossRef]
22. Raab, R.; Nussbaum, K.T.; Behrend, M.; Weimann, A. Liver metastases of breast cancer: Results of liver resection. *Anticancer Res.* **1998**, *18*, 2231–2233.
23. Pocard, M.; Pouillart, P.; Asselain, B.; Salmon, R.-J. Hepatic resection in metastatic breast cancer: Results and prognostic factors. *Eur. J. Surg. Oncol.* **2000**, *26*, 155–159. [CrossRef] [PubMed]
24. Yoshimoto, M.; Tada, T.; Saito, M.; Takahashi, K.; Makita, M.; Uchida, Y.; Kasumi, F. Surgical treatment of hepatic metastases from breast cancer. *Breast Cancer Res. Treat.* **2000**, *59*, 177–184. [CrossRef]
25. Pocard, M.; Pouillart, P.; Asselain, B.; Falcou, M.C.; Salmon, R.J. Hepatic resection for breast cancer metastases: Results and prognosis (65cases). *Ann. Chir.* **2001**, *126*, 413–420. [CrossRef]
26. Ercolani, G.; Zanello, M.; Serenari, M.; Cescon, M.; Cucchetti, A.; Ravaioli, M.; Gaudio, M.D.; D'Errico, A.; Brandi, G.; Pinna, A.D. Ten-year survival after liver resection for breast metastases: A single-center experience. *Dig. Surg.* **2018**, *4*, 372–380. [CrossRef] [PubMed]
27. Elias, D.; Maisonnette, F.; Druet-Cabanac, M.; Ouellet, J.F.; Guinebretiere, J.M.; Spielmann, M.; Delaloge, S. An attempt to clarify indications for hepatectomy for liver metastases from breast cancer. *Am. J. Surg.* **2003**, *185*, 158–164. [CrossRef]
28. Weinrich, M.; Weiß, C.; Schuld, J.; Rau, B.M. Liver Resections of Isolated Liver Metastasis in Breast Cancer: Results and Possible Prognostic Factors. *HPB Surg.* **2014**, *2014*, 893829. [CrossRef]
29. Ercolani, G.; Grazi, G.L.; Ravaioli, M.; Ramacciato, G.; Cescon, M.; Varotti, G.; Del Gaudio, M.; Vetrone, G.; Pinna, A.D. The role of liver resections for noncolorectal, nonneuroendocrine metastases: Experience with 142 observed cases. *Ann. Surg. Oncol.* **2005**, *12*, 459–466. [CrossRef]

30. Vlastos, G.; Smith, D.L.; Singletary, S.E.; Mirza, N.Q.; Tuttle, T.M.; Popat, R.J.; Curley, S.A.; Ellis, L.M.; Roh, M.S.; Vauthey, J.N. Long-term survival after an aggressive surgical approach in patients with breast cancer hepatic metastases. *Ann. Surg. Oncol.* **2004**, *11*, 869–874. [CrossRef] [PubMed]
31. Sakamoto, Y.; Yamamoto, J.; Yoshimoto, M.; Kasumi, F.; Kosuge, T.; Kokudo, N.; Makuuchi, M. Hepatic resection formetastatic breast cancer: Prognostic analysis of 34 patients. *World J. Surg.* **2005**, *29*, 524–547. [CrossRef] [PubMed]
32. Adam, R.; Aloia, T.; Krissat, J.; Bralet, M.P.; Paule, B.; Giacchetti, S.; Delvart, V.; Azoulay, D.; Bismuth, H.; Castaing, D. Is liver re-section justified for patients with hepatic metastases from breast cancer? *Ann. Surg.* **2006**, *244*, 897–907. [CrossRef] [PubMed]
33. Margonis, G.A.; Buettner, S.; Sasaki, K.; Kim, Y.; Ratti, F.; Russolillo, N.; Ferrero, A.; Berger, N.; Gamblin, T.C.; Poultsides, G.; et al. The role of liver directed surgery in patients with hepatic metastasis from primary breast cancer: A multi-institutional analysis. *HPB* **2016**, *18*, 700–705. [CrossRef]
34. Ye, T.; Yang, B.; Tong, H.; Zhang, Y.; Xia, J. Long-term outcomes of surgical resection for liver metastasis from breast cancer. *Hepatogastroenterology* **2015**, *62*, 688–692. [PubMed]
35. Kobryn, E.; Kobryn, K.; Wroblewski, T.; Kobryn, K.; Pietrzak, R.; Rykowski, P.; Ziarkiewicz-Wroblewska, B.; Lamparski, K.; Zieniewicz, K.; Patkowski, W. Is there a rationale for aggressive breast cancer liver metas-tases resections in Polish female patients? Analysis of overall survival following hepatic resection at a single centre in Poland. *Ann. Agric. Environ. Med.* **2016**, *23*, 683–687. [CrossRef] [PubMed]
36. Zegarac, M.; Nikolic, S.; Gavrilovic, D.; Jevric, M.; Kolarevic, D.; Nikolic-Tomasevic, Z.; Kocic, M.; Djurisic, I.; Inic, Z.; Ilic, V.; et al. Prognostic factors for longer disease free survival and overall survival after surgical resection of isolated liver metastasis from breast cancer. *J. BUON* **2013**, *18*, 859–865.
37. D'Angelica, M. Hepatic resection for metastatic breast cancer: An exercise in selection bias. *HPB* **2016**, *18*, 631–632. [CrossRef]
38. Hoffmann, K.; Franz, C.; Hinz, U.; Schirmacher, P.; Herfarth, C.; Eichbaum, M.; Büchler, M.W.; Schemmer, P. Liver Resection for Multimodal Treatment of Breast Cancer Metastases: Identification of Prognostic Factors. *Ann. Surg. Oncol.* **2010**, *17*, 1546–1554. [CrossRef]
39. Friedel, G.; Pastorino, U.; Ginsberg, R.J.; Goldstraw, P.; Johnston, M.; Pass, H.; Putnam, J.B.; Toomes, H. International Registry of Lung Metastases L. Results of lung metastasectomy from breast cancer: Prognostic criteria on the basis of 467 cases of the International Registry of Lung Metastases. *Eur. J. Cardiothorac. Surg.* **2002**, *22*, 335–344. [CrossRef]
40. Livartowski, A.; Chapelier, A.; Beuzeboc, P.; Dierick, A.; Asselain, B.; Dartevelle, P.; Pouillart, P. Surgical excision of pulmonary metastasis of cancer of the breast: Apropos of 40 patients. *Bull. Cancer* **1998**, *85*, 799–802.
41. Fan, J.; Chen, D.; Du, H.; Shen, C.; Che, G. Prognostic factors for resection of isolated pulmonary metastases in breast cancer patients: A systematic review and meta-analysis. *J. Thorac. Dis.* **2015**, *7*, 1441–1451. [PubMed]
42. Matsushita, H.; Jingu, K.; Umezawa, R.; Yamamoto, T.; Ishikawa, Y.; Takahashi, N.; Katagiri, Y.; Kadoya, N. Stereotactic Radiotherapy for Oligometastases in Lymph Nodes—A Review. *Technol. Cancer Res. Treat.* **2018**, *17*, 1–8. [CrossRef]
43. National Comprehensive Cancer Network. Central Nervous System Cancers (Version 2.2018). Available online: https://www.nccn.org/professionals/physician_gls/pdf/cns.pdf (accessed on 21 February 2019).
44. Gondi, V.; Hermann, B.P.; Mehta, M.P.; Tomé, W.A. Hippocampal dosimetry predicts neurocognitive function impairment after fractionated stereotactic radiotherapy for benign or low-grade adult brain tumors. *Int. J. Radiat. Oncol. Biol. Phys.* **2013**, *85*, 348–354. [CrossRef] [PubMed]
45. Li, J.; Bentzen, S.M.; Renschler, M.; Mehta, M.P. Regression after Whole-Brain Radiation Therapy for Brain Metastases Correlates with Survival and Improved Neurocognitive Function. *J. Clin. Oncol.* **2007**, *25*, 1260–1266. [CrossRef] [PubMed]
46. Ashworth, A.; Rodrigues, G.; Boldt, G.; Palma, D. Is there an oligometastatic state in non-small cell lung cancer? A systematic review of the literature. *Lung Cancer* **2013**, *82*, 197–203. [CrossRef] [PubMed]
47. Pejavar, S.; Wilson, L.D.; Haffty, B.G. Regional nodal recurrence in breast cancer patients treated with conservative surgery and radiation therapy (BCSþRT). *Int. J. Radiat. Oncol. Biol. Phys.* **2006**, *66*, 1320–1327. [CrossRef]
48. Whelan, T.J.; Olivotto, I.A.; Parulekar, W.R.; Ackerman, I.; Chua, B.H.; Nabid, A.; Katherine, A.; Vallis, M.B.; White, J.R.; Rousseau, P. Regional nodal irradiation in early-stage breast cancer. *N. Engl. J. Med.* **2015**, *373*, 307–316. [CrossRef] [PubMed]
49. Stranzl, H.; Peintinger, F.; Ofner, P.; Prettenhofer, U.; Mayer, R.; Hackl, A. Regional Nodal Recurrence in the Management of Breast Cancer Patients with One to Three Positive Axillary Lymph Nodes. *Strahlenther. Onkol.* **2004**, *180*, 623–628. [CrossRef]
50. Trovo, M.; Furlan, C.; Polesel, J.; Fiorica, F.; Arcangeli, S.; Giaj-Levra, N.; Alongi, F.; Conte, A.D.; Militello, L.; Muraro, E.; et al. Radical radiation therapy for oligometastatic breast cancer: Results of a prospective phase II trial. *Radiother. Oncol.* **2018**, *126*, 177–180. [CrossRef] [PubMed]
51. Miyata, M.; Ohguri, T.; Yahara, K.; Yamaguchi, S.; Imada, H.; Korogi, Y. Salvage radiotherapy for second oligo-recurrence in patients with breast cancer. *J. Radiat. Res.* **2017**, *59*, 58–66. [CrossRef]
52. NRG Oncology. Available online: https://www.nrgoncology.org/Clinical-Trials/NRG-BR002 (accessed on 11 February 2021).
53. Rugo, H.S.; Rumble, R.B.; Macrae, E.; Barton, D.L.; Connolly, H.K.; Dickler, M.N.; Fallowfield, L.; Fowble, B.; Ingle, J.N.; Jahanzeb, M.; et al. Endocrine Therapy for Hormone Receptor–Positive Metastatic Breast Cancer: American Society of Clinical Oncology Guideline. *J. Clin. Oncol.* **2016**, *34*, 3069–3103. [CrossRef]
54. Turner, N.C.; Slamon, D.J.; Ro, J.; Bondarenko, I.; Im, S.-A.; Masuda, N.; Colleoni, M.; DeMichele, A.; Loi, S.; Verma, S.; et al. Overall Survival with Palbociclib and Fulvestrant in Advanced Breast Cancer. *N. Engl. J. Med.* **2018**, *379*, 1926–1936. [CrossRef]

55. Hortobagyi, G.N.; Stemmer, S.M.; Burris, H.A.; Yap, Y.S.; Sonke, G.S.; Paluch-Shimon, S.; Campone, M.; Petrakova, K.; Blackwell, K.L.; Winer, E.P.; et al. Updated results from MONALEESA-2, a phase III trial of first-line ribociclib plus letrozole versus placebo plus letrozole in hormone receptor-positive, HER2-negative advanced breast cancer. *Ann. Oncol.* **2018**, *29*, 1541–1547. [CrossRef] [PubMed]
56. Im, S.-A.; Lu, Y.-S.; Bardia, A.; Harbeck, N.; Colleoni, M.; Franke, F.; Chow, L.; Sohn, J.; Lee, K.-S.; Campos-Gomez, S.; et al. Overall Survival with Ribociclib plus Endocrine Therapy in Breast Cancer. *N. Engl. J. Med.* **2019**, *381*, 307–316. [CrossRef] [PubMed]
57. Slamon, D.J.; Neven, P.; Chia, S.; Fasching, P.A.; De Laurentiis, M.; Im, S.-A.; Petrakova, K.; Bianchi, G.V.; Esteva, F.J.; Martín, M.; et al. Overall Survival with Ribociclib plus Fulvestrant in Advanced Breast Cancer. *N. Engl. J. Med.* **2020**, *382*, 514–524. [CrossRef]
58. Sledge, G.W.; Toi, M.; Neven, P.; Sohn, J.; Inoue, K.; Pivot, X.; Burdaeva, O.; Okera, M.; Masuda, N.; Kaufman, P.A.; et al. The E_ect of Abemaciclib plus Fulvestrant on Overall Survival in Hormone Receptor-Positive, ERBB2-Negative Breast Cancer That Progressed on Endocrine Therapy-MONARCH 2: A Randomized Clinical Trial. *JAMA Oncol.* **2019**, *6*, 116–124. [CrossRef]
59. Finn, R.S.; Boer, K.; Bondarenko, I.; Patel, R.; Pinter, T.; Schmidt, M.; Shparyk, Y.V.; Thummala, A.; Voitko, N.; Bananis, E.; et al. Overall survival results from the randomized phase 2 study of palbociclib in combination with letrozole versus letrozole alone for first-line treatment of ER+/HER2− advanced breast cancer (PALOMA-1, TRIO-18). *Breast Cancer Res. Treat.* **2020**, *183*, 419–428. [CrossRef]
60. Rossi, V.; Berchialla, P.; Giannarelli, D.; Nisticò, C.; Ferretti, G.; Gasparro, S.; Russillo, M.; Catania, G.; Vigna, L.; Mancusi, R.L.; et al. Should All Patients with HR-Positive HER2-Negative Metastatic Breast Cancer Receive CDK 4/6 Inhibitor as First-Line Based Therapy? A Network Meta-Analysis of Data from the PALOMA 2, MONALEESA 2, MONALEESA 7, MONARCH 3, FALCON, SWOG and FACT Trials. *Cancers* **2019**, *26*, 1661. [CrossRef]
61. André, F.; Ciruelos, E.; Rubovszky, G.; Campone, M.; Loibl, S.; Rugo, H.S.; Iwata, H.; Conte, P.; Mayer, I.A.; Kaufman, B.; et al. Alpelisib for PIK3CA-Mutated, Hormone Receptor–Positive Advanced Breast Cancer. *N. Engl. J. Med.* **2019**, *380*, 1929–1940. [CrossRef]
62. Schmid, P.; Adams, S.; Rugo, H.S.; Schneeweiss, A.; Barrios, C.H.; Iwata, H.; Diéras, V.; Hegg, R.; Im, S.A.; Shaw Wright, G.; et al. Atezolizumab and Nab-Paclitaxel in Advanced Triple-Negative Breast Cancer. *N. Engl. J. Med.* **2018**, *379*, 2108–2121. [CrossRef] [PubMed]
63. Robson, M.; Im, S.-A.; Senkus, E.; Xu, B.; Domchek, S.M.; Masuda, N.; Delaloge, S.; Li, W.; Tung, N.; Armstrong, A.; et al. Olaparib for Metastatic Breast Cancer in Patients with a Germline BRCA Mutation. *N. Engl. J. Med.* **2017**, *377*, 523–533. [CrossRef]
64. Chowdhary, M.; Sen, N.; Chowdhary, A.; Usha, L.; Cobleigh, M.A.; Wang, D.; Patel, K.R.; Barry, P.N.; Rao, R.D. Safety and Efficacy of Palbociclib and Radiation Therapy in Patients with Metastatic Breast Cancer: Initial Results of a Novel Combination. *Adv. Radiat. Oncol.* **2019**, *4*, 453–457. [CrossRef] [PubMed]
65. Huang, C.-Y.; Hsieh, F.-S.; Wang, C.-Y.; Chen, L.-J.; Chang, S.-S.; Tsai, M.-H.; Hung, M.-H.; Kuo, C.-W.; Shih, C.-T.; Chao, T.-I.; et al. Palbociclib enhances radiosensitivity of hepatocellular carcinoma and cholangiocarcinoma via inhibiting ataxia telangiectasia–mutated kinase–mediated DNA damage response. *Eur. J. Cancer* **2018**, *102*, 10–22. [CrossRef]
66. Kawamoto, T.; Shikama, N.; Sasai, K. Severe acute radiation-induced enterocolitis after combined palbociclib and palliative radiotherapy treatment. *Radiother. Oncol.* **2019**, *131*, 240–241. [CrossRef] [PubMed]
67. Messer, J.A.; Ekinci, E.; Patel, T.A.; Teh, B.S. Enhanced dermatologic toxicity following concurrent treatment with palbociclib and radiation therapy: A case report. *Rep. Pract. Oncol. Radiother.* **2019**, *24*, 276–280. [CrossRef] [PubMed]
68. Hans, S.; Cottu, P.; Kirova, Y.M. Preliminary results of the association of Palbociclib and radiotherapy in metastatic breast cancer patients. *Radiother. Oncol.* **2018**, *126*, 181. [CrossRef] [PubMed]
69. Meattini, I.; Desideri, I.; Scotti, V.; Simontacchi, G.; Livi, L. Ribociclib plus letrozole and concomitant palliative radiotherapy for metastatic breast cancer. *Breast* **2018**, *42*, 1–2. [CrossRef]
70. Ippolito, E.; Greco, C.; Silipigni, S.; Dell'Aquila, E.; Petrianni, G.M.; Tonini, G.; Fiore, M.; D'Angelillo, R.M.; Ramella, S. Concurrent radiotherapy with palbociclib or ribociclib for metastatic breast cancer patients: Preliminary assessment of toxicity. *Breast* **2019**, *46*, 70–74. [CrossRef]
71. Finn, R.S.; Martin, M.; Rugo, H.S.; Jones, S.; Im, S.-A.; Gelmon, K.; Harbeck, N.; Lipatov, O.N.; Walshe, J.M.; Moulder, S.; et al. Palbociclib and Letrozole in Advanced Breast Cancer. *N. Engl. J. Med.* **2016**, *375*, 1925–1936. [CrossRef] [PubMed]
72. Cristofanilli, M.; Turner, N.C.; Bondarenko, I.; Ro, J.; Im, S.-A.; Masuda, N.; Colleoni, M.; DeMichele, A.; Loi, S.; Verma, S.; et al. Fulvestrant plus palbociclib versus fulvestrant plus placebo for treatment of hormone-receptor-positive, HER2-negative metastatic breast cancer that progressed on previous endocrine therapy (PALOMA-3): Final analysis of the multicentre, double-blind, phase 3 randomised controlled trial. *Lancet Oncol.* **2016**, *17*, 425–439. [CrossRef]
73. O'Shaughnessy, J.; Petrakova, K.; Sonke, G.S.; Conte, P.; Arteaga, C.L.; Cameron, D.A.; Hart, L.L.; Villanueva, C.; Jakobsen, E.; Beck, J.T.; et al. Ribociclib plus letrozole versus letrozole alone in patients with de novo HR+, HER2− advanced breast cancer in the randomized MONALEESA-2 trial. *Breast Cancer Res. Treat.* **2018**, *168*, 127–134. [CrossRef]
74. Tripathy, D.; Im, S.-A.; Colleoni, M.; Franke, F.; Bardia, A.; Harbeck, N.; Hurvitz, S.A.; Chow, L.; Sohn, J.; Lee, K.S.; et al. Ribociclib plus endocrine therapy for premenopausal women with hormone-receptor-positive, advanced breast cancer (MONALEESA-7): A randomised phase 3 trial. *Lancet Oncol.* **2018**, *19*, 904–915. [CrossRef]

75. Sledge, G.W., Jr.; Toi, M.; Neven, P.; Sohn, J.; Inoue, K.; Pivot, X.; Burdaeva, O.; Okera, M.; Masuda, N.; Kaufman, P.A.; et al. MONARCH 2: Abemaciclib in Combination with Fulvestrant in Women with HR+/HER2− Advanced Breast Cancer Who Had Progressed while Receiving Endocrine Therapy. *J. Clin. Oncol.* **2017**, *35*, 2875–2884. [CrossRef]
76. Goetz, M.P.; Toi, M.; Campone, M.; Sohn, J.; Paluch-Shimon, S.; Huober, J.; Park, I.H.; Trédan, O.; Chen, S.-C.; Manso, L.; et al. MONARCH 3: Abemaciclib As Initial Therapy for Advanced Breast Cancer. *J. Clin. Oncol.* **2017**, *35*, 3638–3646. [CrossRef]
77. Guerini, A.E.; Pedretti, S.; Salah, E.; Simoncini, E.L.; Maddalo, M.; Pegurri, L.; Pedersini, R.; Vassalli, L.; Pasinetti, N.; Peretto, G.; et al. A single-center retrospective safety analysis of cyclin-dependent kinase 4/6 inhibitors concurrent with radiation therapy in metastatic breast cancer patients. *Sci. Rep.* **2020**, *10*, 1–8. [CrossRef] [PubMed]
78. Kwapisz, D. Oligometastatic breast cancer. *Breast Cancer* **2018**, *26*, 138–146. [CrossRef] [PubMed]
79. Kent, C.L.; McDuff, S.G.R.; Salama, J.K. Oligometastatic breast cancer: Where are we now and where are we headed?—A narrative review. *Ann. Palliat. Med.* **2021**, *10*, 5954–5968. [CrossRef]

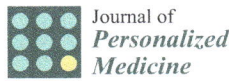

Review

Breast Cancer-Related Lymphedema: Recent Updates on Diagnosis, Severity and Available Treatments

Marco Pappalardo [1], Marta Starnoni [1,2,*], Gianluca Franceschini [3], Alessio Baccarani [1] and Giorgio De Santis [1]

1. Division of Plastic and Reconstructive Surgery, Department of Medical and Surgical Sciences, Modena Policlinico Hospital, University of Modena and Reggio Emilia, 41124 Modena, Italy; marco.pappalardo@unimore.it (M.P.); alessio.baccarani@unimore.it (A.B.); giorgio.desantis@unimore.it (G.D.S.)
2. Clinical and Experimental Medicine PhD Program, University of Modena and Reggio Emilia, 41124 Modena, Italy
3. Multidisciplinary Breast Center, Department of Woman and Child Health and Public Health, Fondazione Policlinico Universitario Agostino Gemelli IRCCS, Università Cattolica del Sacro Cuore, Largo A. Gemelli, 8-00168 Rome, Italy; gianlucafranceschini70@gmail.com
* Correspondence: martastarn@gmail.com

Abstract: Breast cancer-related lymphedema (BCRL) represents a global healthcare issue affecting the emotional and life quality of breast cancer survivors significantly. The clinical presentation is characterized by swelling of the affected upper limb, that may be accompanied by atrophic skin findings, pain and recurrent cellulitis. Cardinal principles of lymphedema management are the use of complex decongestive therapy and patient education. Recently, new microsurgery procedures have been reported with interesting results, bringing in a new opportunity to care postmastectomy lymphedema. However, many aspects of the disease are still debated in the medical community, including clinical examination, imaging techniques, patient selection and proper treatment. Here we will review these aspects and the current literature.

Keywords: breast cancer; lymphedema; lymphaticovenous anastomosis; vascularized lymph node transfer; lymphatic microsurgery; radiotherapy

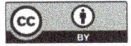

1. Introduction

Breast cancer-related lymphoedema (BCRL) remains a significant clinical issue for breast cancer survivors in that it causes severe physical and psychological discomfort. With the ever-increasing incidence of breast cancer, more patients are undergoing breast surgery that may include sentinel lymph node biopsy (SLNB) and/or axillary lymph node dissection (ALND) [1,2]. Chest wall radiotherapy is also commonly performed in patients with previous ALND, whereas axillary radiotherapy is sometimes indicated as an alternative to ALND in selected patients [3,4]. Both axillary surgery or radiotherapy can cause lymphedema with significant impairment of the normal lymphatic drainage producing an abnormal collection of protein-rich fluid within the upper limb. Despite improved early detection and evolving approaches to minimize surgical intervention increasing conservative surgery procedures with fewer ALND [5]; BCRL remains however a significant healthcare burden [6].

According to reports the incidence of BCRL varies and is approximately 20% at one year and increases to 40% at ten years after breast cancer treatment with a cumulative incidence of 28% [4,7]. Indeed, lymphedema is significantly more likely to occur following ALND than after SLNB alone [8,9]. Lymphedema can to develop within days postoperatively and can continue to present until 11 years after breast cancer treatment [10].

The impact of a lower quality-of-life on patients with lymphedema is unquestionable and there is a higher likelihood of poorer general health [11]. Besides, complications of lymphedema including repeated episodes of cellulitis and ulceration, may require antibiotic therapy and hospitalization.

Cardinal principles of lymphedema treatment are patient education and control of concomitant diseases that may worsen swelling. Upper limb swelling is primarily controlled through the use of complex decongestive therapy (CDT) such as manual lymphatic drainage, bandages, compression garments and individualized exercises to reduce limb swelling [12]. Historical surgical treatments for lymphedema such as Homans' operation and Charles' procedure are palliative and nowadays largely abandoned [13]. Instead, a more recent volume reduction approach is circumferential liposuction [14,15]. In recent years, microsurgical and supermicrosurgical techniques, such as lymphaticovenous anastomosis (LVA) [16,17] and vascularized lymph node transfer (VLNT) [18] have gained popularity as they can potentially reconstitute lymphatic flow and, ideally, reduce the use of compression garments.

The recent introduction of severity staging using lymphoscintigraphy [19,20], and indocyanine green (ICG) [16,21] has helped the patient selection and improved the reported outcomes as it allows preoperatively to evaluate the lymphatic obstruction and the lymphatic flow patterns. This review article will focus on the current issues and debates in BCRL including diagnosis, severity, patient selection criteria and type of treatment available.

2. Diagnosis of BCRL and Clinical Symptoms

In order to properly manage upper limb lymphedema, the physician should first have a detailed knowledge of the diagnosis and severity of the disease. Traditionally health-care professionals have clinically diagnosed BCRL with subjective interpretations of swelling [22]. Diagnosis of upper limb lymphedema depends on a combination of comprehensive history, physical examination with subjective/objective symptoms and physiologic measures [6]. The patient's medical history including risk evaluation, medical conditions and medications that may cause edema should be meticulously reviewed. The differential diagnosis of BCRL is wide and can include: infection, congestive heart failure, primary/recurrent malignancy, vascular anomalies, electrolyte imbalances, hypoproteinemia, renal or hepatic failure, and peripheral neuropathies [23]. The common subjective clinical symptoms of patients with lymphedema in the upper limb are swelling, numbness, heaviness, tightness, stiffness, decreased coordination and mobility, limb fatigue or weakness. However, symptom presentation is broad and not all patients experience these symptoms. Next, during the physical examination, evaluation of the swollen limb should provide information regarding size, presence of scars, comparison with the healthy limb, skin condition and sensation. Objective clinical signs can include skin changes such as reddening, hyperkeratosis, thickening/firmness of tissues. Pitting edema is commonly seen at the end of the latent phase, with a depression formed in the skin after a fingertip pressure as the lymph is pushed into the surroundings. Later, non-pitting edema is characterized by hypertrophied adipose tissue with fibrosis. Stemmer's test is commonly performed and it is considered positive when it is difficult or impossible to pinch the skin at the base of the toes or at proximal phalanx of the fingers due to severe fibrosis. Patients with BCRL are susceptible to recurrent episodes of cellulitis that may increase adipose tissue deposition [24].

Limb volumetric measurements are considered the mainstay of the diagnosis and to track the progression of the disease. Many non-invasive tools such as tape circumferential measurements, water displacement, perometry, bioimpedence spectroscopy and three-dimensional laser scanning are available to measure lymphedema (Table 1). However, there is not a universally accepted method.

Table 1. Comparison between Different Diagnostic Tools for the Diagnosis of Breast Cancer-related Lymphedema.

Diagnostic Tool	Lymphedema Features	Advantages	Disadvantages
Circumferential Measurements	• Circumferential difference	• Easy and economic • To monitor the progress of the disease	• Not provide a precise volume assessment
Water displacement	• water overflow	• Reliable • Validated	• Hygienic concerns • Not provide information about swelling localization • Contraindicated in patients with open wounds
Perometry	• Infrared scanning with calculation of multiple areas of the limb	• To measure bilateral lymphedema • To localize swelling • To detect 3% limb volume change	• Not available in all centers • Expensive
Bioimpedence Spectroscopy	• Impedance Ratio between the limbs. Lymphedema Index (L-Dex) ratio	• Safe, painless and rapid • Early detection of lymphedema • Repeatable	• Not appropriate for bilateral lymphedema • Expensive
Three-Dimensional Laser Scanner	• Real-time digital reconstruction of 3D upper limb	• Able to identify extremely small variations of arm volume	• High costs • Difficulty in arm reference points detection and acquisition • Time-consuming for software elaboration
Computed Tomography	• Skin thickening • Honeycombing • Fat lobules	• Objective method for limb volume	• Radiation exposure • Expensive
Lymphoscintigraphy	• Axillary/Elbow LNs • Lymphatic ducts • Dermal backflow	• Gold standard for the diagnosis • Provide assessment of the lymphatic obstruction severity (partial or total) • Allows assessment of deep lymph flows	• No standardized protocol • Occasional fuzzy images • No detailed information on subdermal lymphatics
ICG Lymphography	• Superficial Lymphatic ducts • Dermal backflow	• Detailed visualization of superficial lymphatic ducts • Visualization and mark of lymphatic ducts intra-operatively • No radiation exposure	• Can only visualize lymphatics about 1.5 cm into the subcutaneous tissue
Magnetic Resonance Lymphangiography	• Lymphatics • Fat deposition • Muscle compartments • Precise limb volume	• No radiation exposure • Good information on the lymphatics function	• No available in all centers • Technically demanding • Expensive

LNs: lymph nodes; CT: computed tomography; MR: magnetic resonance.

2.1. Tape Circumferential Measurements

Circumferential limb measurements at designated anatomic distances are the most common and easy method for quantification of lymphedema by measuring limb size or girth. Generally, a circumferential difference of greater than 2 cm or a volumetric differential of more than 200 mL is considered significant [25]. Sequential circumference measurements measured at standardized anatomical locations are widely used. The distance of each designated point is measured and total upper limb volume calculated based on the truncated cone formula [26].

Cheng et al. have described a sequence of measurements at 10 cm proximal and distal to the elbow [27,28]. These data are compared to the healthy limb, producing a quantitative limb measurement of lymphedema as well as a tool to check the progress during the follow-up.

Tape limb circumferential measurements are considered an easy and practical method for monitoring the progress of lymphedema. However, several critiques have been moved against this tool for not allowing a precise assessment of limb volume. Conversely, a study showed that circumferential and CT measurements are highly complementary in the assessment of volume in the lymphedematous limb [29].

2.2. Water Displacement

Water displacement offers perhaps the most precise tool for the assessment of the limb volume; however, this method is impractical in clinical setting and thus seldom used. In this procedure, the patients immerse the lymphedematous limb in a container full of water. The water overflow is transferred in another box, then it is weighed and measured. Disadvantage of this method include: (1) hygienic concerns, (2) it does not provide information about swelling location, (3) is contraindicated in patients with open wounds. It is thus rarely used in clinical practice.

2.3. Perometry

Perometry uses an infrared optoelectronic device that can measure the volume of the swollen limb and then compared to the healthy limb. The perometer works using infrared scanning to calculate the circumference of multiple areas of the limb [30] creating a 3-D image of the limb, with the limb volume calculated in ml. A great advantage of the perometer is its capacity: (1) to measure bilateral lymphedema, (2) to localize swelling, and (3) to detect a 3% limb volume change [31].

2.4. Bioimpedence Spectroscopy

Bioimpedence spectroscopy (BIS) calculates the rate of electrical current transmission through the tissues by comparing impedance and resistance in the extracellular fluid between the lymphedematous limb and the healthy limb using a low-level current (<30 kHz) [32]. Advantages of this method are: (1) it is safe, painless and rapid, (2) provides objective data even for the early detection of lymphedema and (3) it is repeatable. BIS uses the impedance ratio values between the lymphedema and the healthy limb, with the latter acting as a control, to calculate the Lymphedema Index (L-Dex) ratio. L-Dex outside the range (-10 to $+10$) reveals early signs of lymphedema. L-Dex value increases of +10 units from baseline also support the diagnosis of lymphedema. A disadvantage is that BIS is not useful for assessing bilateral limb lymphedema.

2.5. Three-Dimensional Laser Scanning

Recently, three-dimensional laser scanning has been used as a promising method for the measurement of upper limb volume [33,34]. This tool allows real-time reconstruction of 3D upper limb images. Three-dimensional laser scanners showed similar accuracy and reproducibility compared to water displacement for the measurement of arm volume [33,34]. Indeed the technique shows higher intra-rater reliability compared to water displacement. Furthermore, three-dimensional laser scanners are able to identify very small differences of limb volume, including increases or reductions of swelling as a consequence of CDT [35]. Conversely, the high costs of the devices, difficulties in the detection of upper limb reference points and time-consuming nature for the elaboration of data are the main issues of this tool. A recent study showed the reproducibility and reliability of three-dimensional laser scanner compared to tape circumferential measurements to assess arm volume in BCRL patients before and after CDT pointing out the easy learning curve of this method [36].

2.6. Lymphoscintigraphy

Lymphoscintigraphy is currently the 'gold standard' imaging technique for the diagnosis of extremity lymphedema when the clinical diagnosis is uncertain and, indeed, provides a clear image of the lymphatic drainage status of the upper limb [37,38]. Lymphoscintigraphy involves injection of a radiotracer in the hand and analysis of proximal lymph node uptake. It is, generally, performed as a qualitative analysis to evaluate the following features: (1) presence or absence of axillary/elbow lymph node uptake; (2) presence of linear, dilated or absent lymphatic ducts; (3) presence and location of dermal backflow. Some centers have reported also quantitative analysis based on decay-adjusted uptake and lymphatic transport index; however these are not commonly performed [39,40]. Recently, single photon emission computed tomography-computed tomography (SPECT-CT) lymphoscintigraphy has been used for the diagnosis of lymphedema providing 3-D live images of lymph flow [38,41,42]. A recent study reported significant association between the type of dermal backflow, the lymph flow pathways, and the visualization of lymph nodes around the clavicle [42].

2.7. Computed Tomography (CT)

This imaging study is able to differentiate between lymphedema, cellulitis, and generalized edema [43]. CT can detect lymphedema features including skin thickening, honeycombing or presence of fat lobules. It provides a standardized and reproducible method to measure the limb volume providing a 3-D representation of the lymphedematous limb [29].

2.8. Indocyanine Green (ICG) Lymphography

Nowadays, indocyanine green (ICG) lymphography is the most used imaging modality for the assessment of the severity and treatment in extremity lymphedema. This imaging technique involves the intradermal injection in the distal limb of the fluorescent dye ICG. Using a near-infrared camera, a laser light source is able to show the fluorescence in the dye when functioning lymphatics are present. Instead, non-functioning lymphatics will not be visualized. Several advantages have been described for ICG lymphography such as: (1) less invasiveness without radiation and (2) the capacity to clearly observe superficial lymphatic channels in real time bedside or even intraoperatively [44]. However, the main drawback of this imaging technique is its inability to visualize deep lymphatic at more than 1 cm in depth.

2.9. Magnetic Resonance Lymphangiography

Magnetic resonance (MR) lymphangiography is a safe imaging technique, with high spatial resolution with the possibility to provide visualization of the function of the lymphatics. Additional MR lymphangiography features include: (1) the amount of fat deposition, (2) the muscle compartments and (3) precise limb volume [45].

3. Severity of BCRL and Patient Selection

Since the severity of lymphedema starts from a soft pitting edema to an irreversible non-pitting edema with fatty and fibrotic deposition, it is imperative to understand the different lymphedema stages. A number of classifications and staging systems, based on clinical and imaging findings have been proposed in the medical literature. These classification systems are further explained in Table 2.

Table 2. Staging and Classification for the Severity of Breast Cancer-related Lymphedema.

Staging	Method	Staging Features	Characteristics
International Society of Lymphology (ISL)	• Physical findings	• 0: latent/sub-clinical • I: spontaneously reversible • II: spontaneously irreversible • III: lymphostatic elephantiasis	• Widely accepted
Campisi	• Physical findings	• I: initial/irregular edema, • II: persistent LE • III: persistent LE with lymphangitis • IV: fibrolymphedema • V: elephantiasis	• Rely primarily on physical findings
Arm Dermal Backflow	• ICG lymphography	• 0: No dermal backflow • 1: Splash pattern around the axilla • 2: Stardust limited between olecranon and axilla lymphangitis • 3: Stardust distal to olecranon • 4: Stardust involving the hand • 5: Diffuse and stardust pattern involving the entire limb	• Safe • Information regarding the lymphatic flow for LVA planning
MD Anderson	• ICG lymphography	• 0: No dermal backflow • 1: Many patent lymphatics and minimal dermal backflow • 2: Moderate number of patent lymphatics and segmental dermal backflow • 3: Few patent lymphatics with extensive dermal backflow • 4: Dermal backflow involving the hand • 5: ICG does not move proximally to injection site	• Safe • Information regarding the lymphatic flow for LVA planning
Cheng's Lymphedema grading	• Circumferential difference and lymphoscintigraphy	• 0: 0–9% • 1: 10–19% • 2: 20–29% • 3: 30–39% • 4: >40%	• Objective method
Taiwan Lymphoscintigraphy Staging	• Lymphoscintography	• L-0: Normal Lymphatic Drainage • P-1, P-2, P-3: Partial Obstruction • T-4, T-5, T-6: Total Obstruction	• Validated, Reliable

LE: Lymphedema; ICG: Indocyanine Green (ICG) Lymphography; LVA: Lymphovenous anastomosis.

3.1. International Society of Lymphology (ISL) Classification

The International Society of Lymphology (ISL) classification is the most widely used one and divides the severity of lymphedema into three stages [46]. Briefly, patients are classified as Stage 0 (latent or sub-clinical lymphedema) when lymphatic channels have been injured with impaired lymph transport, but swelling or edema is not measurable. Stage I (spontaneously reversible lymphedema) is considered with measurable swelling and pitting of the skin due to accumulation of lymph, which decreases with limb elevation or compression garments. Stage II (spontaneously irreversible lymphedema) occurs when significant adipose tissue deposition and protein-rich fluid accumulation prevent limb elevation alone or compression garments from being an effective method to reduce symptoms. In late Stage II, the limb may present increase of fat and fibrosis. Finally, Stage III (lymphostatic elephantiasis) is the most severe stage of lymphedema. It is characterized by severe swelling, excess deposition of fat and fibrosis and significant skin thickening in the form of acanthosis or hyperkeratosis.

Campisi et al. have published a similar classification with Stage I described as initial or irregular edema, Stage II defined as persistent lymphedema, Stage III as persistent lymphedema with lymphangitis, Stage IV as fibrolymphedema, and Stage V when elephantiasis is manifest [47].

3.2. NECST Classification

Mihara et al. have advocated a four-stage classification based on the pathological progression of post-mastectomy lymphedema. These stages are based on the histochemical changes of the lymphatic channels after axillary dissection. The changes in lymphatic channels were classified as normal, ectasis, contraction and sclerosis (NECST) [48].

3.3. Arm Dermal Backflow and MD Anderson Classifications

The Arm Dermal Backflow classification (ADB) [21,49], and the MD Anderson staging (MDA) [16] methods are widely used to define the severity of BCRL and both use ICG lymphangiography. The first was based on the examination of 20 patients, and the latter on 30 patients. Both staging systems include 6-stages of lymphedema severity, with stage 0 as normal linear lymphatics with no dermal backflow and stage 1–5 showing abnormal lymphatic patterns with various degrees of dermal backflow. Recently, Jørgensen et al., validated the two staging systems based on ICG lymphography, MDA Scale and ADB scale, in 237 unilateral BCRL [50]. They found near-perfect inter-rater and intra-rater agreement for both ICG lymphography staging and substantial agreement between the MDA and the ADB scales. Indeed, they found a slight correlation between the two ICG lymphography staging systems' results to conventional circumferential measurements. They concluded that the two ICG lymphography staging were reliable, safe tools with the MDA scale providing better disease stratification than the ADB scale.

3.4. Cheng's Lymphedema Grading and Taiwan Lymphoscintigraphy Staging

Cheng's Lymphedema Grading is a 5-grade classification that includes objective symptoms, limb volume measurements, and functional evaluation of lymphatic system using lymphoscintigraphy [51]. The five grades are divided based on the limb circumferential difference between the two limbs, the affected and non-affected as follows: grade 0 (<9%), grade I (10–19%), grade II (20–29%), grade III (30–39%) and grade IV (>40%).

Recently, the Taiwan Lymphoscintigraphy Staging has been validated and incorporated into the Cheng's Lymphedema Grading being it more objective and with the aim to offer a reliable and useful lymphedema staging system for diagnosis, severity and treatment of extremity lymphedema [19,20,37]. Patients selection for surgical treatment using the Cheng's Lymphedema Grading is as follow: Patients with Cheng's Grading 0 showing a range of circumferential difference between 0 and 10% and Taiwan Lymphoscintigraphy Stages L-0, P-1 or P-2 are suggested to be treated with compression garment treatment. Patients with Cheng's Grade I and early Grade II presenting respectively a circumferential difference range of 11–20% and 20–30% are commonly treated with LVA when presenting Taiwan Lymphoscintigraphy Stages P1–P3 and linear lymphatic ducts at ICG lymphography. Instead, when they show Taiwan Lymphoscintigraphy Stages P-3/T-4/T-5 with dermal backflow at ICG lymphography, they are suggested to be treated with VLN transfer. Patients with Cheng's Grade III and IV showing respectively a range of circumferential difference 30–40% and >40% with Lymphoscintigraphy Stages T4-T6, a single or double VLNT transfer is performed [52].

4. Treatments for BCRL

Current treatment options for BCRL include conservative and surgical treatments; however, determining the best treatment method for each patient remains challenging.

4.1. Conservative Treatments

CDT is widely accepted the universal first-line therapy for extremity lymphedema. It includes manual lymph drainage (MLD), skin care, specialized exercises, compression garments and self-education [6]. CDT is divided into Phase I Decongestion, and Phase II Maintenance and should be individualized to improve its effectiveness and contain costs.

Several advantages can be obtained by a CDT including: (1) reduction of lymphedema volume, pain and arm heaviness, (2) improvement of lymphatic drainage, (3) acceptable quality of life and (4) reduction of episodes of cellulitis [53,54]. Although conservative therapy alone may provide enough symptomatic relief, it depends essentially on patient compliance and their capacity to wear life-long compression garments.

4.1.1. Manual Lymphatic Drainage

Manual lymphatic drainage (MLD) is a massage method increasing the transport capacity of the lymph collectors and moving lymph fluid and protein absorption when the lymphatic ducts are still functioning. A meta-analysis showed that, compared with other CDT modalities, additional MLD is unlikely to produce a proper reduction in the lymphedematus limb circumference [55]. In the other hand, another systematic review found that when MLD was used in combination with compression garments, provide increased swelling reduction in BCRL patients compared to the compression bandages alone, especially for moderate lymphedema stages [56].

4.1.2. Compression Bandages and Compression Garments

Compression bandages are an important part of CDT maintaining the therapeutic effects of MLD. Compression bandages apply: (1) a resting pressure during the limb relaxed and (2) a working pressure when muscles contraction push the skin against resisting bandages. Low-stretch bandages produce the highest working pressure with multi-layered compression bandaging.

Compression garments are an essential part of CDT and with the aim to keep the volume reduction achieved with MLD and bandaging. Compression garments produce a two-way stretch in both longitudinal and transverse direction with the greatest pressure above the wrist and less pressure in the arm. The longitudinal pressure facilitates the joint movements. Generally, patients with BCRL wear a full arm sleeve and, frequently, a glove to prevent dermal backflow. There is no consensus regarding suitable compression values. Class 2 compression garments with 30–40 seamless are often recommended to be wear at least 12 h per day [19]. Of note, compression garments should be custom-made by a certified and experienced therapist in fitting garments for lymphedema patients.

4.1.3. Exercises and Life-Style

Exercises are an integral part of CDT with the aim (1) to promote lymph flow, (2) to mobilize the joints, and (3) to strengthen the muscles. It is widely known that participation in exercises during and after oncological treatment can improve the physical and psychosocial condition, ameliorating the quality-of-life [57]. Recent studies reported that gradual weight-lifting program does not worsen the risk of BCRL compared to patients without exercises [58,59].

4.2. Surgical Treatments

Many surgical procedures to treat BCRL have been propose as follow: (1) physiologic procedures (lymphaticovenous anastomosis, vascularized lymph node transfer) and (2) excisional procedures (reduction or liposuction) (Table 3).

Table 3. Available Treatments for Patients with Breast Cancer-Related Lymphedema.

Treatment	Indication	Advantages	Disadvantages
Complex Decongestive Therapy	• CLG 0-I	• Reduction lymphedema volume, pain and arm heaviness • Improvement lymphatic function • Acceptable quality of life • Reduction episodes of cellulitis	• It is a purely symptomatic treatment • Needs patient compliance • Life-long compression garments.
Lymphovenous anastomosis	• CLG I- early II	• Safe • Reduces of Circumference • Reduces callulitis	• Technically difficult • Needs supermicrosurgery instruments • Needs high resolution microscope • Needs ICG lymphography • Difficult to monitor the anastomoses patency
Vascularized Lymph Node Transfer	• CLG late II-III-IV	• Improvements in circumferential measurements, episodes of cellulitis, and quality of life	• Requires intraoperative techniques of greater complexity • Higher risk for postoperative re-exploration and the flap inset • Risk of donor-site lymphedema
Liposuction	• CLG III-IV	• Decrease limb size • Reduces episodes of cellulitis • Improve quality of life	• Risks of swelling recurrence • Life-long compression garments

CLG: Cheng's Lymphedema Grading.

4.2.1. Physiologic Procedures

In recent years, with the advent of microsurgical and supermicrosurgical techniques [60–64], lymphatic microsurgery procedures have gained popularity for the treatment of BCRL. Commonly practiced procedures include lymphovenous anastomosis (LVA) and vascularized lymph node (VLN) transfer. These surgeries try to deal with physiologic impairment resulted from cancer-related lymphedema and have the ability to provide venous shunting of lymphatic fluid bypassing areas of damaged lymphatics creating new lymphatic connections or by replacing the damaged lymph nodes and lymphatic channels [65].

Lymphovenous Anastomosis (LVA)

Lymphovenous anastomosis (LVA) is not a new procedure as it was initially described in 1969. It is a delicate supermicrosurgery technique, diverting lymph into the venous system bypassing proximal obstruction [66]. LVA has been shown to be especially beneficial in patients with early-stage upper limb lymphedema (Cheng's Grade I and early II) [16]. In a prospective study of 100 LVAs, symptomatic improvement was described in 96% of BCRL patients. Other advantages of LVA include decreased episodes of cellulitis. Recently, Cheng's group reported more effective lymph drainage in both proximal and distal sites using side-to-end LVA configuration compared with end-to-end LVA, without need of postoperative compression garment [17].

Previous studies have reported that LVA seems more effective in early-stage lymphedema due to the unavailability of functional lymphatic ducts in advanced stage lymphedema [16]. Therefore, advanced stage lymphedema was considered a relative contraindication for LVA [67]. However, recently Hong's group showed promising results using LVA for advanced stage lymphedema [68]. The authors pointed out the crucial role of preoperative magnetic resonance lymphangiography and ultrasound for the success of the procedure.

Prophylactic LVA have been also performed and has successfully prevented upper limb lymphedema in 23 patients who underwent oncologic resection for breast cancer treatment and ALND [69,70].

Disadvantages of these procedure include (1) its technical difficulty for the execution anastomosing lymphatic ducts with a diameter of 0.5–0.8 mm with subdermal venules of 0.6–1.0 mm in diameter. (2) the requirements of supermicrosurgery instruments, high resolution microscope, and ICG lymphography (3) difficulty to monitor the anastomoses patency. Reported complications of LVA include infection (3.9%), lymphorrea (4.1%) and necessity of reintervention (10%) [71].

Vascularized Lymph Node (VLN) Transfer

VLN transfer is the latest physiological procedure added to the treatment repertoire and it is commonly indicated in more advanced cases of lymphedema. Several donor sites have been described of VLN transfer including groin, submental, supraclavicular nodes, thoracic, and omental. In 2006 Becker et al. popularized for the first time the procedure with the publication of groin VLN transfer for postmastectomy lymphedema [72]. After that, Cheng and colleagues described anatomic and clinical application of both groin and submental VLN transfer transferred into the distal limb [28,73]. Three recipient sites have been described for upper limb lymphedema such as axilla, elbow and wrist. The decision of recipient site is taken based on the severity of the lymphedema, recipient vessel availability, and surgeon preference.

Recent studies have shown the benefit of VLN flap with significantly improvement of lymphedema limb without patent lymphatic ducts compared to CDT or LVA [74]. Indeed, microsurgical breast reconstruction do not improve the outcome of postmastectomy lymphedema [74,75]. A meta-analysis compared the outcome of VLN transfer and LVA in extremity lymphedema [71]. The result showed that although both procedures were both efficient in a short-term outcome, patients with VLN transfer presented significant better improvement in the long-term with good likelihood of discontinue to wear compression garments.

VLN transfer is suggested for Cheng's Grade II-IV who did not present patent lymphatic channels using ICG lymphography. Additional procedures such as flap debulking and liposuction following VLN transfer are suggested for Cheng's Grade III and IV. In a recent study, patients with different grades of bilateral limb lymphedema underwent LVA in the less severe limb and VLN transfer in the more severe limb. This individualized treatment achieved effective improvement in the reduction of each limb swelling and cellulitis, as well improvements in quality-of-life [76]. Although VLN transfer has shown favorable results, however it could carry the risk of donor site lymphedema [25,77,78]. Other complications include flap loss, lymphocele, infection, and wound healing complications.

4.2.2. Excisional Procedures

The first surgical method used to treat BCRL lymphedema was reported by Sistrunk in 1927 [79]. The excess skin and soft tissue were removed using a spindle-shaped incision in the medial region of the arm with removal of the deep fascia and creating a connection between superficial and deep lymphatics. Later, with Thompson a further step forward in the BCRL treatment was achieved using a lymphatic transposition method. A deepithelialized rectangular hinge skin flap was harvested from all length of the arm with the flap tip embedded near the neurovascular bundle with the aim to bridge the superficial and deep lymphatics [80].

Nowadays, excisional procedures, such radical reduction with preservation of perforators [81], and suction-assisted lipectomy [82] aim to eliminate the affected tissue in severe lymphedema stages. All excisional procedures produce the following advantages: (1) decrease limb size, (2) reduce episodes of cellulitis, and therefore improve the quality of life of the patients. Although these surgical procedures can be immediately effective to reduce the lymphedema volume, however they can carry some risks including wound complications, swelling recurrence, and the need for the patient to wear compression garments lifelong to prevent recurrence.

Liposuction

Fat accumulation is one of the pathologic findings of BCRL. Adipose tissue deposition is probably due because it is an endocrine organ in which complex structures of cytokine-activated cells, and chronic inflammation play a role [82]. However the pathophysiological mechanism of adipose tissue accumulation in lymphedema still remains controversial. Tashiro et al. reported adipose tissue alterations in extremity lymphedema using macroscopic and ultrasound findings [83]. They found in adipose tissue samples larger adipose lobules in lymphedema limb compared to non-lymphedema samples. Indeed, lymphedema samples presented hypertrophic changes of adipocytes and increased collagen fibres. Finally, adipose-derived stem cells and M2 macrophages were less in in lymphedema adipose tissue than in the healthy controls [83].

Liposuction is currently the most accepted excisional procedure. Brorson et al. showed that BCRL with nonpitting edema treated with liposuction presented 68% to 93% of fat, 32% of interstitial fluid, and 7% of lymph [84,85]. This excisional technique is able to remove fat producing significant arm reduction [84,86,87]. Indeed, a reduction in episodes of cellulitis was reported. A possible explanation of reduced cellulitis may be the increased skin blood flow after liposuction that could eliminate bacteria that entered through skin wounds [88]. However, the main drawback is the need to use life-long compression garments [84,89].

4.2.3. Combined Treatments

Due to lack of consensus among the experts regarding the most appropriate protocol for lymphedema treatment, each surgeon applies a surgical procedure based on his personal approach. A combined treatment have been proposed as an alternative to the single strategy [65,90]. Recently, Di Taranto et al., reported that patients with extremity lymphedema treated with combined VLN transfer, LVA and liposuction LVAs showed better improvement in terms of circumference reduction compared to patients treated only with VLN transfer and liposuction [91].

Later Baumeister et al. described a new method for the treatment of 28 BCRL patients in which autologous lymphatic grafting is initially performed to bypass the axilla reestablishing lymphatic flow and later on liposuction is performed as a second step [92] without the need for additional treatments.

5. Conclusions

BCRL is a debilitating and chronic and condition that can severely affect the patient's quality of life. An improvement in identification, prevention, and management of affected patients is imperative in reducing BCRL. A particular attention should be given to all stages of breast cancer treatment in order to reduce the incidence of BCRL. The use of new technologies for performing mastectomies and sentinel lymph node biopsy or axillary lymph node dissection could be useful [93–96]. Accurate physical examination and assessment of the lymphedema severity are essential to provide more predictable outcomes. A prompt management of the disease in a multidisciplinary team is the key to obtain good results [97–105]. Despite the fact lymphedema is still considered an incurable disease, in the last decade promising results with significant reduction of the limb swelling and improvement of psychosocial well-being have been shown.

Author Contributions: M.P.: Conceptualization, Writing. M.S.: Conceptualization, Writing. G.F.: Review, Supervision. A.B.: Review, Supervision. G.D.S.: Review, Supervision. All authors have read and agreed to the published version of the manuscript.

Funding: This research received no external funding.

Institutional Review Board Statement: Ethical review and approval were waived for this study, because this study is just a review of the literature.

Informed Consent Statement: Not applicable.

Data Availability Statement: Not applicable.

Conflicts of Interest: The authors declare no conflict of interest.

References

1. Starnoni, M.; Pinelli, M.; Franceschini, G.; De Santis, G. A Rare Case of Nipple-Areolar Complex Partial Necrosis following Micropigmentation: What to Learn? *Plast. Reconstr. Surg. Glob. Open* **2019**, *7*, e2494. [CrossRef]
2. Starnoni, M.; Baccarani, A.; Pinelli, M.; Pedone, A.; De Santis, G. Tattooing of the nipple-areola complex: What not to do. A case series. *Ann. Med. Surg.* **2020**, *55*, 305–307. [CrossRef]
3. Zhang, J.; Wang, C. Axillary radiotherapy: An alternative treatment option for adjuvant axillary management of breast cancer. *Sci. Rep.* **2016**, *6*, 26304. [CrossRef]
4. Rebegea, L.; Firescu, D.; Dumitru, M.; Anghel, R. The incidence and risk factors for occurrence of arm lymphedema after treatment of breast cancer. *Chirurgia* **2015**, *110*, 33–37.
5. Giuliano, A.E.; McCall, L.; Beitsch, P.; Whitworth, P.W.; Blumencranz, P.; Leitch, A.M.; Saha, S.; Hunt, K.K.; Morrow, M.; Ballman, K. Locoregional recurrence after sentinel lymph node dissection with or without axillary dissection in patients with sentinel lymph node metastases: The American College of Surgeons Oncology Group Z0011 randomized trial. *Ann. Surg.* **2010**, *252*, 426–432. [CrossRef]
6. Rockson, S.G. Lymphedema after Breast Cancer Treatment. *N. Engl. J. Med.* **2018**, *379*, 1937–1944. [CrossRef] [PubMed]
7. DiSipio, T.; Rye, S.; Newman, B.; Hayes, S. Incidence of unilateral arm lymphoedema after breast cancer: A systematic review and meta-analysis. *Lancet Oncol.* **2013**, *14*, 500–515. [CrossRef]
8. Wernicke, A.G.; Shamis, M.; Sidhu, K.K.; Turner, B.C.; Goltser, Y.; Khan, I.; Christos, P.J.; Komarnicky-Kocher, L.T. Complication rates in patients with negative axillary nodes 10 years after local breast radiotherapy after either sentinel lymph node dissection or axillary clearance. *Am. J. Clin. Oncol.* **2013**, *36*, 12–19. [CrossRef]
9. McLaughlin, S.A.; Wright, M.J.; Morris, K.T.; Giron, G.L.; Sampson, M.R.; Brockway, J.P.; Hurley, K.E.; Riedel, E.R.; Van Zee, K.J. Prevalence of lymphedema in women with breast cancer 5 years after sentinel lymph node biopsy or axillary dissection: Objective measurements. *J. Clin. Oncol.* **2008**, *26*, 5213–5219. [CrossRef]
10. Armer, J.M.; Stewart, B.R. Post-breast cancer lymphedema: Incidence increases from 12 to 30 to 60 months. *Lymphology* **2010**, *43*, 118–127.
11. Vassard, D.; Olsen, M.H.; Zinckernagel, L.; Vibe-Petersen, J.; Dalton, S.O.; Johansen, C. Psychological consequences of lymphoedema associated with breast cancer: A prospective cohort study. *Eur. J. Cancer* **2010**, *46*, 3211–3218. [CrossRef] [PubMed]
12. Badger, C.M.; Peacock, J.L.; Mortimer, P.S. A randomized, controlled, parallel-group clinical trial comparing multilayer bandaging followed by hosiery versus hosiery alone in the treatment of patients with lymphedema of the limb. *Cancer* **2000**, *88*, 2832–2837. [CrossRef]
13. Karri, V.; Yang, M.C.; Lee, I.J.; Chen, S.H.; Hong, J.P.; Xu, E.S.; Cruz-Vargas, J.; Chen, H.C. Optimizing outcome of charles procedure for chronic lower extremity lymphoedema. *Ann. Plast. Surg.* **2011**, *66*, 393–402. [CrossRef]
14. Boyages, J.; Kastanias, K.; Koelmeyer, L.A.; Winch, C.J.; Lam, T.C.; Sherman, K.A.; Munnoch, D.A.; Brorson, H.; Ngo, Q.D.; Heydon-White, A.; et al. Liposuction for Advanced Lymphedema: A Multidisciplinary Approach for Complete Reduction of Arm and Leg Swelling. *Ann. Surg. Oncol.* **2015**, *22* (Suppl. 3), S1263–S1270. [CrossRef] [PubMed]
15. Granoff, M.D.; Johnson, A.R.; Shillue, K.; Fleishman, A.; Tsai, L.; Carroll, B.; Donohoe, K.; Lee, B.T.; Singhal, D. A Single Institution Multi-Disciplinary Approach to Power-Assisted Liposuction for the Management of Lymphedema. *Ann. Surg.* **2020**. [CrossRef]
16. Chang, D.W.; Suami, H.; Skoracki, R. A prospective analysis of 100 consecutive lymphovenous bypass cases for treatment of extremity lymphedema. *Plast. Reconstr. Surg.* **2013**, *132*, 1305–1314. [CrossRef]
17. AlJindan, F.K.; Lin, C.Y.; Cheng, M.H. Comparison of Outcomes between Side-to-End and End-to-End Lymphovenous Anastomoses for Early-Grade Extremity Lymphedema. *Plast. Reconstr. Surg.* **2019**, *144*, 486–496. [CrossRef]
18. Pappalardo, M.; Patel, K.; Cheng, M.H. Vascularized lymph node transfer for treatment of extremity lymphedema: An overview of current controversies regarding donor sites, recipient sites and outcomes. *J. Surg. Oncol.* **2018**, *117*, 1420–1431. [CrossRef]
19. Cheng, M.H.; Pappalardo, M.; Lin, C.; Kuo, C.F.; Lin, C.Y.; Chung, K.C. Validity of the Novel Taiwan Lymphoscintigraphy Staging and Correlation of Cheng Lymphedema Grading for Unilateral Extremity Lymphedema. *Ann. Surg.* **2018**, *268*, 513–525. [CrossRef]
20. Pappalardo, M.; Lin, C.; Ho, O.A.; Kuo, C.F.; Lin, C.Y.; Cheng, M.H. Staging and clinical correlations of lymphoscintigraphy for unilateral gynecological cancer-related lymphedema. *J. Surg. Oncol.* **2020**, *121*, 422–434. [CrossRef]
21. Yamamoto, T.; Yamamoto, N.; Doi, K.; Oshima, A.; Yoshimatsu, H.; Todokoro, T.; Ogata, F.; Mihara, M.; Narushima, M.; Iida, T.; et al. Indocyanine green-enhanced lymphography for upper extremity lymphedema: A novel severity staging system using dermal backflow patterns. *Plast. Reconstr. Surg.* **2011**, *128*, 941–947. [CrossRef]
22. Czerniec, S.A.; Ward, L.C.; Refshauge, K.M.; Beith, J.; Lee, M.J.; York, S.; Kilbreath, S.L. Assessment of breast cancer-related arm lymphedema—Comparison of physical measurement methods and self-report. *Cancer Investig.* **2010**, *28*, 54–62. [CrossRef]
23. Tidhar, D.; Armer, J.M.; Bernas, M.; Stewart, B.R.; Feldamn, J.L.; Cormier, J.N. Clinical evaluation of lymphedema. In *Principles and Practice of Lymphedema Surgery*; Chang, D.W., Patel, K.M., Cheng, M.-H., Eds.; Elsevier: Beijing, China, 2015; pp. 51–59.

24. Lee, D.; Piller, N.; Hoffner, M.; Manjer, J.; Brorson, H. Liposuction of Postmastectomy Arm Lymphedema Decreases the Incidence of Erysipelas. *Lymphology* **2016**, *49*, 85–92. [PubMed]
25. Vignes, S.; Blanchard, M.; Yannoutsos, A.; Arrault, M. Complications of autologous lymph-node transplantation for limb lymphoedema. *Eur. J. Vasc. Endovasc. Surg.* **2013**, *45*, 516–520. [CrossRef]
26. Brorson, H.; Höijer, P. Standardised measurements used to order compression garments can be used to calculate arm volumes to evaluate lymphoedema treatment. *J. Plast. Surg. Hand Surg.* **2012**, *46*, 410–415. [CrossRef]
27. Lin, C.H.; Ali, R.; Chen, S.C.; Wallace, C.; Chang, Y.C.; Chen, H.C.; Cheng, M.H. Vascularized groin lymph node transfer using the wrist as a recipient site for management of postmastectomy upper extremity lymphedema. *Plast. Reconstr. Surg.* **2009**, *123*, 1265–1275. [CrossRef]
28. Cheng, M.H.; Chen, S.C.; Henry, S.L.; Tan, B.K.; Lin, M.C.; Huang, J.J. Vascularized groin lymph node flap transfer for postmastectomy upper limb lymphedema: Flap anatomy, recipient sites, and outcomes. *Plast. Reconstr. Surg.* **2013**, *131*, 1286–1298. [CrossRef] [PubMed]
29. Ho, O.A.; Chu, S.Y.; Huang, Y.L.; Chen, W.H.; Lin, C.Y.; Cheng, M.H. Effectiveness of Vascularized Lymph Node Transfer for Extremity Lymphedema Using Volumetric and Circumferential Differences. *Plast. Reconstr. Surg. Glob. Open* **2019**, *7*, e2003. [CrossRef]
30. Tierney, S.; Aslam, M.; Rennie, K.; Grace, P. Infrared optoelectronic volumetry, the ideal way to measure limb volume. *Eur. J. Vasc. Endovasc. Surg.* **1996**, *12*, 412–417. [CrossRef]
31. Stout Gergich, N.L.; Pfalzer, L.A.; McGarvey, C.; Springer, B.; Gerber, L.H.; Soballe, P. Preoperative assessment enables the early diagnosis and successful treatment of lymphedema. *Cancer* **2008**, *112*, 2809–2819. [CrossRef] [PubMed]
32. Ward, L.C. Bioelectrical impedance analysis: Proven utility in lymphedema risk assessment and therapeutic monitoring. *Lymphat. Res. Biol.* **2006**, *4*, 51–56. [CrossRef]
33. McKinnon, J.G.; Wong, V.; Temple, W.J.; Galbraith, C.; Ferry, P.; Clynch, G.S.; Clynch, C. Measurement of limb volume: Laser scanning versus volume displacement. *J. Surg. Oncol.* **2007**, *96*, 381–388. [CrossRef]
34. Cau, N.; Galli, M.; Cimolin, V.; Grossi, A.; Battarin, I.; Puleo, G.; Balzarini, A.; Caraceni, A. Quantitative comparison between the laser scanner three-dimensional method and the circumferential method for evaluation of arm volume in patients with lymphedema. *J. Vasc. Surg. Venous Lymphat. Disord.* **2018**, *6*, 96–103. [CrossRef]
35. Torres Lacomba, M.; Yuste Sánchez, M.J.; Zapico Goñi, A.; Prieto Merino, D.; Mayoral del Moral, O.; Cerezo Téllez, E.; Minayo Mogollón, E. Effectiveness of early physiotherapy to prevent lymphoedema after surgery for breast cancer: Randomised, single blinded, clinical trial. *BMJ* **2010**, *340*, b5396. [CrossRef]
36. De Sire, A.; Losco, L.; Cigna, E.; Lippi, L.; Gimigliano, F.; Gennari, A.; Cisari, C.; Chen, H.C.; Fusco, N.; Invernizzi, M. Three-dimensional laser scanning as a reliable and reproducible diagnostic tool in breast cancer related lymphedema rehabilitation: A proof-of-principle study. *Eur. Rev. Med. Pharmacol. Sci.* **2020**, *24*, 4476–4485. [CrossRef] [PubMed]
37. Pappalardo, M.; Cheng, M.H. Lymphoscintigraphy for the diagnosis of extremity lymphedema: Current controversies regarding protocol, interpretation, and clinical application. *J. Surg. Oncol.* **2020**, *121*, 37–47. [CrossRef] [PubMed]
38. Quartuccio, N.; Garau, L.M.; Arnone, A.; Pappalardo, M.; Rubello, D.; Arnone, G.; Manca, G. Comparison of 99m Tc-Labeled Colloid SPECT/CT and Planar Lymphoscintigraphy in Sentinel Lymph Node Detection in Patients with Melanoma: A Meta-Analysis. *J. Clin. Med.* **2020**, *9*, 1680. [CrossRef] [PubMed]
39. Yan, A.; Avraham, T.; Zampell, J.C.; Aschen, S.Z.; Mehrara, B.J. Mechanisms of lymphatic regeneration after tissue transfer. *PLoS ONE* **2011**, *6*, e17201. [CrossRef] [PubMed]
40. Modi, S.; Stanton, A.W.; Svensson, W.E.; Peters, A.M.; Mortimer, P.S.; Levick, J.R. Human lymphatic pumping measured in healthy and lymphoedematous arms by lymphatic congestion lymphoscintigraphy. *J. Physiol.* **2007**, *583*, 271–285. [CrossRef]
41. Quartuccio, N.; Siracusa, M.; Pappalardo, M.; Arnone, A.; Arnone, G. Sentinel Node Identification in Melanoma: Current Clinical Impact, New Emerging SPECT Radiotracers and Technological Advancements. An Update of the Last Decade. *Curr. Radiopharm.* **2020**, *13*, 32–41. [CrossRef] [PubMed]
42. Mikami, T.; Koyama, A.; Hashimoto, K.; Maegawa, J.; Yabuki, Y.; Kagimoto, S.; Kitayama, S.; Kaneta, T.; Yasumura, K.; Matsubara, S.; et al. Pathological changes in the lymphatic system of patients with secondary upper limb lymphoedema. *Sci. Rep.* **2019**, *9*, 8499. [CrossRef] [PubMed]
43. Shin, S.U.; Lee, W.; Park, E.A.; Shin, C.I.; Chung, J.W.; Park, J.H. Comparison of characteristic CT findings of lymphedema, cellulitis, and generalized edema in lower leg swelling. *Int. J. Cardiovasc. Imaging* **2013**, *29* (Suppl. 2), 135–143. [CrossRef] [PubMed]
44. Mihara, M.; Hara, H.; Araki, J.; Kikuchi, K.; Narushima, M.; Yamamoto, T.; Iida, T.; Yoshimatsu, H.; Murai, N.; Mitsui, K.; et al. Indocyanine green (ICG) lymphography is superior to lymphoscintigraphy for diagnostic imaging of early lymphedema of the upper limbs. *PLoS ONE* **2012**, *7*, e38182. [CrossRef] [PubMed]
45. Neligan, P.C.; Kung, T.A.; Maki, J.H. MR lymphangiography in the treatment of lymphedema. *J. Surg. Oncol.* **2017**, *115*, 18–22. [CrossRef]
46. Lymphology, I.S.o. The diagnosis and treatment of peripheral lymphedema: 2013 Consensus Document of the International Society of Lymphology. *Lymphology* **2013**, *46*, 1–11.
47. Campisi, C.; Davini, D.; Bellini, C.; Taddei, G.; Villa, G.; Fulcheri, E.; Zilli, A.; Da Rin, E.; Eretta, C.; Boccardo, F. Lymphatic microsurgery for the treatment of lymphedema. *Microsurgery* **2006**, *26*, 65–69. [CrossRef] [PubMed]

48. Mihara, M.; Hara, H.; Hayashi, Y.; Narushima, M.; Yamamoto, T.; Todokoro, T.; Iida, T.; Sawamoto, N.; Araki, J.; Kikuchi, K.; et al. Pathological steps of cancer-related lymphedema: Histological changes in the collecting lymphatic vessels after lymphadenectomy. *PLoS ONE* **2012**, *7*, e41126. [CrossRef] [PubMed]
49. Narushima, M.; Yamamoto, T.; Ogata, F.; Yoshimatsu, H.; Mihara, M.; Koshima, I. Indocyanine Green Lymphography Findings in Limb Lymphedema. *J. Reconstr. Microsurg.* **2016**, *32*, 72–79. [CrossRef]
50. Jørgensen, M.G.; Toyserkani, N.M.; Hansen, F.C.G.; Thomsen, J.B.; Sørensen, J.A. Prospective Validation of Indocyanine Green Lymphangiography Staging of Breast Cancer-Related Lymphedema. *Cancers* **2021**, *13*, 1540. [CrossRef]
51. Patel, K.M.; Lin, C.Y.; Cheng, M.H. A Prospective Evaluation of Lymphedema-Specific Quality-of-Life Outcomes Following Vascularized Lymph Node Transfer. *Ann. Surg. Oncol.* **2015**, *22*, 2424–2430. [CrossRef]
52. Pappalardo, M.; Cheng, M.-H. Lymphoscintigraphy Interpretation, Staging, and Lymphedema Grading. In *Principles and Practice of Lymphedema Surgery*, 2nd ed.; Cheng, M.-H., Chang, D.W., Patel, K.M., Eds.; Elsevier: San Leandro, CA, USA, 2021; pp. 39–51.
53. Mobarakeh, Z.S.; Mokhtari-Hesari, P.; Lotfi-Tokaldany, M.; Montazeri, A.; Heidari, M.; Zekri, F. Combined decongestive therapy and reduction of pain and heaviness in patients with breast cancer-related lymphedema. *Support Care Cancer* **2019**, *27*, 3805–3811. [CrossRef]
54. Ochalek, K.; Partsch, H.; Gradalski, T.; Szygula, Z. Do Compression Sleeves Reduce the Incidence of Arm Lymphedema and Improve Quality of Life? Two-Year Results from a Prospective Randomized Trial in Breast Cancer Survivors. *Lymphat. Res. Biol.* **2019**, *17*, 70–77. [CrossRef]
55. Huang, T.W.; Tseng, S.H.; Lin, C.C.; Bai, C.H.; Chen, C.S.; Hung, C.S.; Wu, C.H.; Tam, K.W. Effects of manual lymphatic drainage on breast cancer-related lymphedema: A systematic review and meta-analysis of randomized controlled trials. *World J. Surg. Oncol.* **2013**, *11*, 15. [CrossRef] [PubMed]
56. Ezzo, J.; Manheimer, E.; McNeely, M.L.; Howell, D.M.; Weiss, R.; Johansson, K.I.; Bao, T.; Bily, L.; Tuppo, C.M.; Williams, A.F.; et al. Manual lymphatic drainage for lymphedema following breast cancer treatment. *Cochrane Database Syst. Rev.* **2015**, CD003475. [CrossRef]
57. Hayes, S.C.; Reul-Hirche, H.; Turner, J. Exercise and secondary lymphedema: Safety, potential benefits, and research issues. *Med. Sci. Sports Exerc.* **2009**, *41*, 483–489. [CrossRef] [PubMed]
58. Ahmed, R.L.; Thomas, W.; Yee, D.; Schmitz, K.H. Randomized controlled trial of weight training and lymphedema in breast cancer survivors. *J. Clin. Oncol.* **2006**, *24*, 2765–2772. [CrossRef] [PubMed]
59. Panchik, D.; Masco, S.; Zinnikas, P.; Hillriegel, B.; Lauder, T.; Suttmann, E.; Chinchilli, V.; McBeth, M.; Hermann, W. Effect of Exercise on Breast Cancer-Related Lymphedema: What the Lymphatic Surgeon Needs to Know. *J. Reconstr. Microsurg.* **2019**, *35*, 37–45. [CrossRef] [PubMed]
60. Pappalardo, M.; Jeng, S.F.; Sadigh, P.L.; Shih, H.S. Versatility of the Free Anterolateral Thigh Flap in the Reconstruction of Large Defects of the Weight-Bearing Foot: A Single-Center Experience with 20 Consecutive Cases. *J. Reconstr. Microsurg.* **2016**, *32*, 562–570. [CrossRef]
61. Pappalardo, M.; Laurence, V.G.; Lin, Y.T. Chimeric Free Vascularized Metatarsophalangeal Joint with Toe Fillet Flap: A Technique for Reconstruction of the Posttraumatic Metacarpophalangeal Joint With Concomitant Soft Tissue Defect. *J. Hand Surg. Am.* **2018**, *43*, 193.e1–193.e6. [CrossRef]
62. Pappalardo, M.; Tsao, C.K.; Tsang, M.L.; Zheng, J.; Chang, Y.M.; Tsai, C.Y. Long-term outcome of patients with or without osseointegrated implants after resection of mandibular ameloblastoma and reconstruction with vascularized bone graft: Functional assessment and quality of life. *J. Plast. Reconstr. Aesthet. Surg.* **2018**, *71*, 1076–1085. [CrossRef]
63. Pappalardo, M.; Montesano, L.; Toia, F.; Russo, A.; Di Lorenzo, S.; Dieli, F.; Moschella, F.; Leto Barone, A.A.; Meraviglia, S.; Di Stefano, A.B. Immunomodulation in Vascularized Composite Allotransplantation: What Is the Role for Adipose-Derived Stem Cells? *Ann. Plast. Surg.* **2019**, *82*, 245–251. [CrossRef] [PubMed]
64. Di Stefano, A.B.; Pappalardo, M.; Moschella, F.; Cordova, A.; Toia, F. MicroRNAs in solid organ and vascularized composite allotransplantation: Potential biomarkers for diagnosis and therapeutic use. *Transplant Rev.* **2020**, *34*, 100566. [CrossRef]
65. Pappalardo, M.; Chang, D.W.; Masia, J.; Koshima, I.; Cheng, M.H. Summary of hands-on supermicrosurgery course and live surgeries at 8th world symposium for lymphedema surgery. *J. Surg. Oncol.* **2020**, *121*, 8–19. [CrossRef] [PubMed]
66. Yamamoto, T.; Yoshimatsu, H.; Narushima, M.; Yamamoto, N.; Koshima, I. Split intravascular stents for side-to-end lymphaticovenular anastomosis. *Ann. Plast. Surg.* **2013**, *71*, 538–540. [CrossRef] [PubMed]
67. Campisi, C.; Eretta, C.; Pertile, D.; Da Rin, E.; Macciò, A.; Campisi, M.; Accogli, S.; Bellini, C.; Bonioli, E.; Boccardo, F. Microsurgery for treatment of peripheral lymphedema: Long-term outcome and future perspectives. *Microsurgery* **2007**, *27*, 333–338. [CrossRef]
68. Cha, H.G.; Oh, T.M.; Cho, M.J.; Pak, C.S.J.; Suh, H.P.; Jeon, J.Y.; Hong, J.P. Changing the Paradigm: Lymphovenous Anastomosis in Advanced Stage Lower Extremity Lymphedema. *Plast. Reconstr. Surg.* **2021**, *147*, 199–207. [CrossRef] [PubMed]
69. Yamamoto, T.; Yamamoto, N.; Yamashita, M.; Furuya, M.; Hayashi, A.; Koshima, I. Efferent Lymphatic Vessel Anastomosis: Supermicrosurgical Efferent Lymphatic Vessel-to-Venous Anastomosis for the Prophylactic Treatment of Subclinical Lymphedema. *Ann. Plast. Surg.* **2016**, *76*, 424–427. [CrossRef]
70. Boccardo, F.M.; Casabona, F.; Friedman, D.; Puglisi, M.; De Cian, F.; Ansaldi, F.; Campisi, C. Surgical prevention of arm lymphedema after breast cancer treatment. *Ann. Surg. Oncol.* **2011**, *18*, 2500–2505. [CrossRef]
71. Basta, M.N.; Gao, L.L.; Wu, L.C. Operative treatment of peripheral lymphedema: A systematic meta-analysis of the efficacy and safety of lymphovenous microsurgery and tissue transplantation. *Plast. Reconstr. Surg.* **2014**, *133*, 905–913. [CrossRef]

72. Becker, C.; Assouad, J.; Riquet, M.; Hidden, G. Postmastectomy lymphedema: Long-term results following microsurgical lymph node transplantation. *Ann. Surg.* **2006**, *243*, 313–315. [CrossRef]
73. Ho, O.A.; Lin, C.Y.; Pappalardo, M.; Cheng, M.H. Comparisons of Submental and Groin Vascularized Lymph Node Flaps Transfer for Breast Cancer-Related Lymphedema. *Plast. Reconstr. Surg. Glob. Open* **2018**, *6*, e1923. [CrossRef] [PubMed]
74. Engel, H.; Lin, C.Y.; Huang, J.J.; Cheng, M.H. Outcomes of Lymphedema Microsurgery for Breast Cancer-related Lymphedema With or Without Microvascular Breast Reconstruction. *Ann. Surg.* **2018**, *268*, 1076–1083. [CrossRef] [PubMed]
75. Ho, O.A.; Lin, Y.L.; Pappalardo, M.; Cheng, M.H. Nipple-sparing mastectomy and breast reconstruction with a deep inferior epigastric perforator flap using thoracodorsal recipient vessels and a low lateral incision. *J. Surg. Oncol.* **2018**, *118*, 621–629. [CrossRef]
76. Cheng, M.H.; Tee, R.; Chen, C.; Lin, C.Y.; Pappalardo, M. Simultaneous Ipsilateral Vascularized Lymph Node Transplantation and Contralateral Lymphovenous Anastomosis in Bilateral Extremity Lymphedema with Different Severities. *Ann. Surg. Oncol.* **2020**. [CrossRef]
77. Viitanen, T.P.; Mäki, M.T.; Seppänen, M.P.; Suominen, E.A.; Saaristo, A.M. Donor-site lymphatic function after microvascular lymph node transfer. *Plast. Reconstr. Surg.* **2012**, *130*, 1246–1253. [CrossRef]
78. Pons, G.; Masia, J.; Loschi, P.; Nardulli, M.; Duch, J. A case of donor-site lymphoedema after lymph node-superficial circum flexiliac artery perforator flap transfer. *J. Plast. Reconstr. Aesth. Surg.* **2014**, *67*, 119–123. [CrossRef]
79. Sistrunk, W.E. Contribution to plastic surgery: Removal of scars by stages; an open operation for extensive laceration of the anal sphincter; the kondoleon operation for elephantiasis. *Ann. Surg.* **1927**, *85*, 185–193. [CrossRef] [PubMed]
80. Thompson, N. Buried dermal flap operation for chronic lymphedema of the extremities. Ten-year survey of results in 79 cases. *Plast. Reconstr. Surg.* **1970**, *45*, 541–548. [CrossRef]
81. Salgado, C.J.; Sassu, P.; Gharb, B.B.; Spanio di Spilimbergo, S.; Mardini, S.; Chen, H.C. Radical reduction of upper extremity lymphedema with preservation of perforators. *Ann. Plast. Surg.* **2009**, *63*, 302–306. [CrossRef]
82. Brorson, H. Liposuction in Lymphedema Treatment. *J. Reconstr. Microsurg.* **2016**, *32*, 56–65. [CrossRef]
83. Tashiro, K.; Feng, J.; Wu, S.H.; Mashiko, T.; Kanayama, K.; Narushima, M.; Uda, H.; Miyamoto, S.; Koshima, I.; Yoshimura, K. Pathological changes of adipose tissue in secondary lymphoedema. *Br. J. Dermatol.* **2017**, *177*, 158–167. [CrossRef]
84. Brorson, H.; Svensson, H. Liposuction combined with controlled compression therapy reduces arm lymphedema more effectively than controlled compression therapy alone. *Plast. Reconstr. Surg.* **1998**, *102*, 1058–1067. [CrossRef]
85. Brorson, H.; Ohlin, K.; Olsson, G.; Nilsson, M. Adipose tissue dominates chronic arm lymphedema following breast cancer: An analysis using volume rendered CT images. *Lymphat. Res. Biol.* **2006**, *4*, 199–210. [CrossRef] [PubMed]
86. Brorson, H.; Svensson, H.; Norrgren, K.; Thorsson, O. Liposuction reduces arm lymphedema without significantly altering the already impaired lymph transport. *Lymphology* **1998**, *31*, 156–172. [PubMed]
87. Brorson, H. Liposuction in arm lymphedema treatment. *Scand. J. Surg.* **2003**, *92*, 287–295. [CrossRef] [PubMed]
88. Brorson, H.; Svensson, H. Skin blood flow of the lymphedematous arm before and after liposuction. *Lymphology* **1997**, *30*, 165–172.
89. Brorson, H.; Svensson, H. Complete reduction of lymphoedema of the arm by liposuction after breast cancer. *Scand. J. Plast. Reconstr. Surg. Hand Surg.* **1997**, *31*, 137–143. [CrossRef]
90. Chang, D.W.; Masia, J.; Garza, R.; Skoracki, R.; Neligan, P.C. Lymphedema: Surgical and Medical Therapy. *Plast. Reconstr. Surg.* **2016**, *138*, 209S–218S. [CrossRef] [PubMed]
91. Di Taranto, G.; Bolletta, A.; Chen, S.H.; Losco, L.; Elia, R.; Cigna, E.; Rubino, C.; Ribuffo, D.; Chen, H.C. A prospective study on combined lymphedema surgery: Gastroepiploic vascularized lymph nodes transfer and lymphaticovenous anastomosis followed by suction lipectomy. *Microsurgery* **2021**, *41*, 34–43. [CrossRef]
92. Baumeister, R.G.H.; Wallmichrath, J.; Weiss, M.; Baumeister, S.H.C.; Frick, A. Microsurgical lymphatic vascular grafting and secondary liposuction: Results of combination treatment in secondary lymphedema. *Lymphology* **2020**, *53*, 38–47.
93. Baccarani, A.; Starnoni, M.; De Santis, G. Ultrasonic Cutting and Coagulating Device in Implant-based Breast Reconstruction. *Plast. Reconstr. Surg. Glob. Open* **2018**, *6*, e2020. [CrossRef]
94. Pinelli, M.; Starnoni, M.; De Santis, G. The Use of Cold Atmospheric Plasma Device in Flap Elevation. *Plast. Reconstr. Surg. Glob. Open* **2020**, *8*, e2815. [CrossRef] [PubMed]
95. Starnoni, M.; De Santis, G.; Pinelli, M. Fibula Free Flap Elevation without Tourniquet: Are Harmonic Scalpel Shears Useful? *Plast. Reconstr. Surg. Glob. Open* **2019**, *7*, e2409. [CrossRef] [PubMed]
96. Starnoni, M.; Pinelli, M.; De Santis, G. Setting of helium plasma device (J-Plasma) in flap elevation. *J. Vasc. Surg. Cases Innov. Tech.* **2020**, *6*, 446. [CrossRef] [PubMed]
97. Baccarani, A.; Aramini, B.; Casa, G.D.; Banchelli, F.; D'Amico, R.; Ruggiero, C.; Starnoni, M.; Pedone, A.; Stefani, A.; Morandi, U.; et al. Pectoralis Muscle Transposition in Association with the Ravitch Procedure in the Management of Severe Pectus Excavatum. *Plast. Reconstr. Surg. Glob. Open* **2019**, *7*, e2378. [CrossRef]
98. Benanti, E.; Starnoni, M.; Spaggiari, A.; Pinelli, M.; De Santis, G. Objective Selection Criteria between ALT and Radial Forearm Flap in Oral Soft Tissues Reconstruction. *Indian J. Plast. Surg.* **2019**, *52*, 166–170. [CrossRef]
99. Benanti, E.; De Santis, G.; Leti Acciaro, A.; Colzani, G.; Baccarani, A.; Starnoni, M. Soft tissue coverage of the upper limb: A flap reconstruction overview. *Ann. Med. Surg.* **2020**, *60*, 338–343. [CrossRef]
100. De Santis, G.; Mattioli, F.; Pinelli, M.; Martone, A.; Starnoni, M.; Fermi, M.; Presutti, L. Tip of the Tongue Reconstruction with Prelaminated Fasciomucosal Radial Forearm Free Flap. *Plast. Reconstr. Surg. Glob. Open* **2020**, *8*, e3226. [CrossRef]

101. Manfredini, B.; Morandi, U.; De Santis, G.; Catani, F.; Stefani, A.; Pinelli, M.; Baccarani, A.; Starnoni, M.; Artioli, F.; Aramini, B. Can surgery relieve pain and act as first-line treatment for a large metastasis of the sternum? *Int. J. Surg. Case Rep.* **2019**, *63*, 125–128. [CrossRef] [PubMed]
102. Starnoni, M.; Colzani, G.; De Santis, G.; Leti Acciaro, A. Management of Locked Volar Radio-ulnar Joint Dislocation. *Plast. Reconstr. Surg. Glob. Open* **2019**, *7*, e2480. [CrossRef]
103. Starnoni, M.; Colzani, G.; De Santis, G.; Acciaro, A.L. Median Nerve Injury Caused by Screw Malpositioning in Percutaneous Scaphoid Fracture Fixation. *Plast. Reconstr. Surg. Glob. Open* **2019**, *7*, e2292. [CrossRef] [PubMed]
104. Baccarani, A.; Pappalardo, M.; Starnoni, M.; De Santis, G. Plastic Surgeons in the Middle of the Coronavirus Disease 2019 Pandemic Storm in Italy. *Plast. Reconstr. Surg. Glob. Open* **2020**, *8*, e2889. [CrossRef] [PubMed]
105. Starnoni, M.; Baccarani, A.; Pappalardo, M.; De Santis, G. Management of Personal Protective Equipment in Plastic Surgery in the Era of Coronavirus Disease. *Plast. Reconstr. Surg. Glob. Open* **2020**, *8*, e2879. [CrossRef] [PubMed]

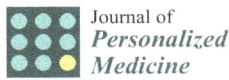

Article

Hormone Receptor Expression Variations in Normal Breast Tissue: Preliminary Results of a Prospective Observational Study

Giacomo Santandrea [1,2], Chiara Bellarosa [3], Dino Gibertoni [4], Maria C. Cucchi [5], Alejandro M. Sanchez [6,*], Gianluca Franceschini [6], Riccardo Masetti [6] and Maria P. Foschini [3,*]

1. Clinical and Experimental Medicine PhD Program, University of Modena and Reggio Emilia, 41121 Modena, Italy; giacomo.santandrea@ausl.re.it
2. Pathology Unit, Azienda USL-IRCCS di Reggio Emilia, 42122 Reggio Emilia, Italy
3. Unit of Anatomic Pathology at Bellaria Hospital, Department of Biomedical and Neuromotor Sciences, University of Bologna, 40126 Bologna, Italy; chiara.bellarosa@studio.unibo.it
4. Unit of Hygiene and Biostatistics, Department of Biomedical and Neuromotor Sciences, University of Bologna, 40126 Bologna, Italy; dino.gibertoni2@unibo.it
5. Breast Surgery Unit, Bellaria Hospital, AUSL Bologna, 40126 Bologna, Italy; mariacristina.cucchi@ausl.bo.it
6. Multidisciplinary Breast Center–Dipartimento Scienze della Salute della donna e del Bambino e di Sanità Pubblica, Fondazione Policlinico Universitario A. Gemelli IRCCS, 00168 Rome, Italy; gianluca.franceschini@policlinicogemelli.it (G.F.); riccardo.masetti@policlinicogemelli.it (R.M.)
* Correspondence: martin.sanchez@hotmail.it (A.M.S.); mariapia.foschini@unibo.it (M.P.F.); Tel.: +39-051-622-5523 (M.P.F.); Fax: +39-051-622-5759 (M.P.F.)

Abstract: Normal breast tissue undergoes great variations during a woman's life as a consequence of the different hormonal stimulation. The purpose of the present study was to examine the hormonal receptor expression variations according to age, menstrual cycle, menopausal state and body mass index. To this purpose, 49 tissue samples of normal breast tissue, obtained during surgery performed for benign and malignant conditions, were immunostained with Estrogen (ER), Progesterone (PR) and Androgen receptors (AR). In addition, Ki67 and Gross Cystic Disease Fluid Protein were studied. The data obtained revealed a great variability of hormone receptor expression. ER and AR generally increased in older and post-menopausal women, while young women presented a higher proliferative rate, evaluated with Ki67. PR increase was observed in women with BMI higher than 25. The different hormonal receptor expression could favor the development of breast cancer.

Keywords: breast cancer; normal breast; breast pathology; hormone receptor; hormone expression

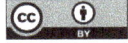

1. Introduction

Physiological variations in the expression of Estrogen receptor alpha (ER) and Progesterone receptor (PR) play an important role in breast in breast remodeling during physiological changes: from embryological development to puberty [1] as well as during menstrual cycle, pregnancy and even after menopause [2].

As it happens for physiological variations of breast glandular tissue, the expression of hormonal receptors is thought to be an underlying mechanism involved in breast cancer onset, with determinant variations induced by well-known risk factors, such as age [3,4] exogenous hormone use [5] or Body Mass Index (BMI) [6,7]. Indeed, breast cancer is now classified according to a combination of hormone receptor expression, Ki67 labelling index and HER2 [8,9].

Tot [10,11] proposed the theory of the "sick lobe", according to which breast cancer arises in a genetically predisposed breast epithelium. Tot based his theory on cytokeratin expression; nevertheless, hormone receptor expression variations occurring during life could predispose the breast epithelium to malignant transformation.

Furthermore, breast cancer presents differences in young pre-menopausal women and in older post-menopausal women [12], with ER negative cases being more frequently in the young.

Among hormonal receptors that are normally expressed in breast tissue, prior studies confirmed that the expression of ER and PR may be associated with subsequent breast cancer risk [5,13–18]. However, there is still scarce evidence regarding a larger panel of breast tissue receptors, including Androgen Receptor (AR), Gross Cystic Disease Fluid Protein 15 (GCDFP-15) and Ki67.

The aim of this study is to investigate the expression of ER, PR, AR, GCDFP-15 and Ki67 in breast normal tissue according to age, BMI, menstrual cycle and the onset of a breast neoplasm (benign vs. malignant).

2. Materials and Methods

2.1. Patients Selection

All patients who underwent surgery for benign or malignant breast lesions between June 2015 and January 2016 at the Breast Surgery Unit of Bellaria Hospital (Bologna, Italy), were asked to participate to the present study. Seventy-nine patients accepted.

Among them, 2 pre-menopausal patients who experienced post-chemotherapy menstrual cycle arrest and 28 patients who had only a little amount of normal glandular tissue, insufficient for the analyses, were excluded.

The 49 remaining patients constituted the study population and were grouped as follows:

- Group A: patients with regular menstrual cycle ($n = 22$), including 4 patients in contraceptive therapy, 1 in contraceptive therapy and breastfeeding;
- Group B: patients with absence of menstrual cycle and less than 60 years old ($n = 14$), including 3 patients who underwent hysterectomy;
- Group C: patients with absence of menstrual cycle aged 60 years or more ($n = 13$), including 1 patient in hormonal replacement therapy.

2.2. Tissue Selection Process

Histologic diagnoses and immunohistochemistry were obtained at the Section of Anatomic Pathology, Department of Biomedical and Neuromotor Sciences, University of Bologna, at Bellaria Hospital, Bologna, Italy. All tissues were fixed in 4% buffered formalin and paraffin embedded according to routine protocol. Serial 2µm sections were obtained from each block and stained with Haematoxylin and Eosin (H&E) for histologic evaluation.

Cases were retained for the present study when normal breast tissue was present around the lesion leading to surgery and the block containing the largest amount of normal breast tissue was selected for immunohistochemical studies. When possible, tissue obtained from the upper outer quadrant (UOQ) was chosen. Apocrine cysts, sclerosing adenosis and all the benign changes observed in aging breast were excluded from evaluation.

After histological evaluation on H&E, areas with at least 5 normal terminal ductular lobular units (TDLU) were selected for Tissue Micro-Arrays (TMA) construction. TMA were constructed following the technique described by Zimpfer et al. [19].

2.3. Tissue Immunohistochemical Evaluation

Immunohistochemical evaluation was made on TMA sections.

Evaluation and quantification of biomarkers was performed by counting the percentage of positive cells at 40x magnification. A minimum of 4 terminal-ductular-lobular units were evaluated for each marker. Immunohistochemical staining was performed on a Ventana Automatic Stainer (Ventana Medical Systems, Inc). The following pre-diluted antibodies were supplied by Ventana: Estrogen Receptor (ER) (clone SP1), Progesterone Receptor (clone 1E2), Androgen Receptor (clone SP107), Ki67 (clone 30-9) and Gross Cystic Disease Fluid Protein 15 (clone EP1582Y).

2.4. Statistical Analysis

For each patient who participated in the present study, the following data were collected: age, Body Mass Index (BMI), contraceptive therapy, post-menopausal hormonal replacement therapy, date of surgery, type of surgical procedure, and site and size of the lesion leading to surgery.

BMI was evaluated as a three-level categorical variable with cutoffs at 18.5 and 25 kg/m^2.

The variability of expression of ER, PGR, AR, GCDFP-15 and Ki-67 markers was very limited in the myoepithelial and stromal cells; therefore, it was evaluated only in the epithelial cells. Due to the limited population size and the skewed distribution of most markers (Figure S2), and although the hypothesis of normal distribution was not always rejected by the Shapiro–Wilk test (Table S1), median and interquartile range (IQR) were used as descriptive statistics. For each marker the percentage of patients with positive expression and the percentage of positive cells among positives were calculated. Comparisons of subgroups of patients according to the percentage of patients with positive expression were conducted using Fisher's exact test when the expected frequency of each cell was < 5, or using chi-square otherwise. The differences in the percentage of positive cells across subgroups defined by menstrual cycle and nature of lesions were evaluated by Mann–Whitney U test, and those across phenotypes and BMI subgroups by Kruskal–Wallis test. Post hoc analyses by Dunn's test with Holm adjustment for multiple comparisons were carried out after significant Kruskal–Wallis tests. Stata v.15.1 was used for all analyses, specifically the dunntest procedure [20] was used to perform the post hoc analyses. Statistical significance was set at $p = 0.05$.

3. Results

Descriptive statistics of the study population are reported in Table 1. The median age of patients was 50 years, with younger patients in group A and older patients in group C. Median BMI was lower in group A (22.81 kg/m^2) and higher in group C (27.92 kg/m^2). Most patients had a malignant diagnosis (75.0%), with a lower incidence in group A (61.9%). Only 5 patients, all in group A, were receiving contraceptive therapy and 1 patient (of group C) was under hormonal therapy.

Table 1. Characteristics of the study population.

	Study Population	Group A	Group B	Group C
Age; median (IQR)	50 (17)	42 (8)	54 (7)	66 (10)
BMI; median (IQR)	23.92 (4.7)	22.81 (2.9)	25.39 (3.9)	27.92 (5.5)
Malignant; n (%)	36 (75.0)	13 (61.9)	12 (85.7)	11 (84.6)

The observed expression of epithelial markers is reported in Table 2. AR and GCDFP-15 were expressed in the large majority of patients (84.2% and 72.2%, respectively), while Ki-67 (38.6%) and Estrogen receptor alpha (43.2%) showed lower prevalence.

Table 2. Epithelial expression of markers.

	Positive (%)	Median	Interquartile Range
ER	43.2	36	41.5
PGR	56.1	23	37
AR	84.2	30	26.5
GCDFP-15	72.2	55	70
Ki-67	38.6	3	6

GCDFP-15 and ER were the most evidenced markers (median rates of 55% and 36%, respectively). (Figure S1).

Most of the breast cancers here were ER positive, with 16 cases being Luminal A, 13 cases Luminal B cancers (two of which HER2 enriched) and 4 cases triple negative (TNBC) [8,9].

Hormone expression variations according to age:

There were significant differences among groups, specifically the proportion of positive cases for PR and AR was lower in group C. As for the distribution of expression among positive patients (Table 3), women in group A showed significantly lower values of GCDFP-15 with respect to group C (median: 30 vs. 90) and borderline lower values of ER with respect to group B (median: 8.5 vs. 48.5).

Table 3. Expression of hormone receptors according to age.

	Group A (%; Median)	Group B (%; Median)	Group C (%; Median)	p-Value	Post hoc Comparisons
ER	31.8%; 8.5	54.5%; 48.5	54.5%; 43	2.32; 0.314 *	5.9; 0.050; (none)
PR	85.0%; 27	55.6%; 16	8.3%; 2	<0.001	2.08; 0.354
AR	94.4%; 30	100.0%; 33.5	50.0%; 30	0.005	0.42; 0.809
GCDFP-15	57.9%; 30	85.7%; 65	90.0%; 90	0.157	9.42; 0.009 *;(A < C)
Ki-67	45.0%; 8	38.5%; 2	27.3%; 3	0.673	2.06; 0.357

* χ^2-test.

Hormone expression variations according to the menstrual cycle:

The proportions of positives for each marker evaluated in the 22 patients of group A were not significantly different for menstrual cycle phase; however, the expression of PR and Ki67 was remarkably higher in women in follicular phase (41.5 vs. 18 and 8.25 vs. 2.5, respectively) and not far from reaching statistical significance (Table 4).

Table 4. Expression of hormone receptors according to menstrual cycle.

	Follicular Phase	Luteinic Phase	p-Value	Test; p-Value
ER	40.0%; 16.5	33.3%; 8.5	0.570	0.71; 0.475
PR	88.9%; 41.5	88.9%; 18	1.000	1.68; 0.093
AR	100.0%; 34	85.7%; 35	0.467	−0.39; 0.698
GCDFP-15	75.0%; 20	44.4%; 35	0.335	−0.86; 0.389
Ki-67	25.0%; 8.25	44.4%; 2.5	0.620	1.88; 0.060

Hormone expression variations according to BMI:

ER positive cases increased with higher BMI, not significantly. PR positive cases were less frequent in the BMI ≥ 25 patients with respect to underweight and normal weight patients (33.3% vs. 75.0% and 73.7%; Fisher's exact test: p = 0.028, Table 5); on the contrary, underweight women showed a higher, but not significant, proportion of Ki-67 positives. The median values of expression did not differ according to BMI.

Table 5. Expression of hormone receptors according to BMI.

	BMI < 18.5	18.5 ≤ BMI < 25	BMI ≥ 25	p-Value	Test; p-Value
ER	20.0%; 3	40.9%; 36	52.9%; 48	0.423	1.64; 0.440
PR	75.0%; 16	73.7%; 32	33.3%; 19	0.028	0.43; 0.808
AR	100.0%; 16	85.7%; 34	75.0%; 30	0.568	1.51; 0.469
GCDFP-15	50.0%; 70	77.8%; 30	71.4%; 85	0.516	3.09; 0.214
Ki-67	80.0%; 5	38.1%; 3	27.8%; 3	0.104	0.74; 0.692

Hormone expression according to the type of lesion leading to surgery (benign versus malignant):

The proportion of Ki-67 positives was higher among patients who showed benign lesions than malignant lesions (66.7% vs. 25.8%, p = 0.032). The amount of hormone receptor expression did not change significantly for any marker (Table 6). Specifically, ER and PR expression was similar in breast tissue adjacent to benign and malignant lesions. Most patients included in the present study were affected by ER positive breast cancers.

Table 6. Expression of hormone receptors according to the nature of the treated lesion.

	Benign	Malignant	p-Value	Test; p-Value
ER	41.7%; 48	45.2%; 32	0.04; 0.836 *	1.11; 0.266
PR	63.6%; 16	51.7%; 27	0.723	0.21; 0.832
AR	90.9%; 22.5	80.8%; 30	0.646	−1.57; 0.117
GCDFP-15	54.6%; 25	79.2%; 70	2.24; 0.134 *	−1.28; 0.202
Ki-67	66.7%; 4	25.8%; 3	0.032	0.48; 0.630

* χ^2-test.

Examples of positivity obtained with ER, PR, AR and Ki67 are shown in Figure S1.

4. Discussion

The present study confirms the great variations in hormone receptor expression occurring in adult women. The data here shown reveal hormone receptors variations mainly according to age and BMI, while little changes were observed during the menstrual cycle. While ER, AR and GCDFP-15 were higher in post-menopausal patients, PR expression decreased as age increased, reaching very low values in patients older than 60 (Group C).

The ER increase in older women shown here is consistent to the data published by Lawson et al. [21] who observed higher ER levels in post-menopausal compared to pre-menopausal women.

The progressive increase in ER expression in older women lead to some considerations about the ER role in breast cancer development. Breast cancer is known to have a peak of incidence in the 6th decade of life. Moreover, hormonal receptor positive breast cancers, classified as Luminal A or Luminal B, according to the St. Gallen definition [8,9], are the most frequent cancer types encountered in elderly women [22].

The association between hormonal expression and cancer has been studied extensively. Khan et al. [14] observed a significant ER expression increase in normal breast tissue of patients who underwent surgery for breast cancer. Steroid hormone receptors play an important role in regulating cell cycle and cell proliferation [23]. In Luminal A and B breast cancer, ER binds to the CCND1 promoter favoring cell proliferative activity. The ER higher expression here observed in post-menopausal women can lead to ER-driven transcription of CCND1, that is a crucial factor in neoplastic transformation [23].

ER expression in our study showed a peak in group C (patients older than 60 y/o) while PR gradually reduces after the 6th decade of life, supporting the concept that estrogen plays a role in developing Luminal A and Luminal B cancers (typically ER+ and PR +/−). Moreover, in the present study, ER mean values observed in normal breast epithelial cells surrounding cancers were slightly higher than those found in normal breast tissue surrounding benign breast lesions.

Similar considerations can be done for AR. AR is expressed in the majority of breast cancers [24–26]. Cancers being ER/PR/HER2 negative but AR positive showed better outcome compared to those AR negative [24,25]. AR expression in our study was higher in older patients and significantly lower in younger patients. AR positive breast cancers, are also of apocrine histotype [27]. This finding is consistent with the present data that AR expression is paralleled by GCDFP-15 expression. GCDFP-15 is strongly expressed in Apocrine carcinomas which are well known to be AR positive [27,28]. This suggests that AR could promote the development of Apocrine carcinomas in post-menopausal women [24,25].

Ki67 showed higher expression in younger patients. Ki67, an antigen expressed in cells G1, S, G2 and M phases, is widely used in daily practice as proliferation marker. Higher levels in Ki67 in normal breast tissue from younger patients may be justified by a higher regenerating tissue levels under the influence of the periodic hormonal variation of the menstrual cycle.

Several studies demonstrated that a BMI greater than 25 kg/m^2 represents a risk factor for the development of breast cancer [29]. The risk of breast cancer raises significantly in obese women (BMI > 35 kg/m^2) compared to those having a BMI within normal ranges [6]. Estrogen circulating levels are significantly higher in overweight and obese patients which usually develop ER+ cancers; this, together with the evidence that expression of ER and PR levels is significantly higher in obese patients' breast cancers, led to the conclusion that estrogens could play a role in breast cancerogenesis [6,29,30]. In the present series, ER expression showed an increasing trend according to BMI even if it did not reach statistical significance. It should be underlined that, in our series women with BMI < 18.5 were predominantly in the group A (mean age < 42 y/o) while women in overweight group belonged from groups B (mean age 54 y/o) and C (mean age 66 y/o). Therefore, the increased ER expression could be related to the older age and not only to increasing BMI.

The limited number of young obese or overweight patients, in the pre-menopausal period, does not allow definitive conclusions to be drawn.

In the present study, hormonal expression variation according to menstrual cycle phase was not so evident as expected. The present data demonstrated a tendency for reduced hormonal expression from follicular to luteal phase. Data here shown, even if not reaching statistical significance, are in keeping with those of Battersby et al. [31] who observed a marked reduction in ER expression during the menstrual cycle, while PR did not show a significant variation. The same result was achieved by Khan et al. [32].

Among the limitations of the current study, its limited sample size prevented us from obtaining results with robust statistical significance; therefore, our findings should be carefully interpreted.

5. Conclusions

Our study highlighted a high variability in the expression of hormonal receptors in healthy breast epithelial cells. The combination of different expressions of ER, PR, AR, GCDP-15 and Ki67 could be a risk factor in the development of breast cancer. Even the molecular subtypes of breast cancer could be influenced by the normal expression of hormones at a certain age: for example, triple negative cancer are more frequent at younger age when we demonstrated that ER expression is at its lowest value. On the contrary, post-menopausal women's breasts, characterized by higher expression of ER, PR and AR in the epithelial component, tend to develop ER+/PR+/AR+ cancers.

Supplementary Materials: The following are available online at https://www.mdpi.com/article/10.3390/jpm11050387/s1, Table S1: Results of the Shapiro-Wilk test of normality conducted on the markers used in the study, Figure S1: Examples of positivities obtained with ER, PR, AR and Ki67, Figure S2: Histograms of markers used in the study.

Author Contributions: G.S., M.P.F.—Designed study, analysis and interpretation of data, drafted paper and revised it critically, approved the submitted version; C.B., D.G., M.C.C., A.M.S.—Designed study, analysed and interpretation of data, drafted paper; G.F., R.M.—Designed study, drafted paper and revised it critically, approved the submitted version. All authors have read and agreed to the published version of the manuscript.

Funding: This research received no external funding

Institutional Review Board Statement: The study was approved by the local ethics committee (number of study: Protocol Number: 15005/CE AUSL Bologna, Bologna, Italy). The study protocol conformed to the ethical guidelines of the World Medical Association Declaration of Helsinki and Ethical Principles for Medical Research Involving Human Subjects.

Informed Consent Statement: Informed consent was obtained from all subjects involved in the study.

Data Availability Statement: The data presented in this study are available on request from the corresponding author.

Conflicts of Interest: Disclosure of financial interests and potential conflicts of interest. MPF received grants from Roche, Devicor Mammotome as support for course organization and participation, and from MSD and Biocartis as speaker fee. All the remaining authors submitting this manuscript confirm and attest that they have no conflict of interest. There are no source of support in any form nor funding for this work. There are no financial relation-ships for this work.

References

1. Lteif, A.; Javed, A. Development of the Human Breast. *Semin. Plast. Surg.* **2013**, *27*, 005–012. [CrossRef]
2. Longacre, T.A.; Bartow, S.A. A Correlative Morphologic Study of Human Breast and Endometrium in the Menstrual Cycle. *Am. J. Surg. Pathol.* **1986**, *10*, 382–393. [CrossRef]
3. American Cancer Society. *Breast Cancer Facts & Figure 2015–Figure 2016*; American Cancer Society: Atlanta, GA, USA, 2015.
4. Howlader, N.A.; Krapcho, M.; Miller, D. SEER Cancer Statistics Review, 1975–2014; National Cancer Institute: Bethesda, MD, USA. Available online: https://seer.cancer.gov/csr/1975_2014/ (accessed on 2 February 2021).
5. Daly, A.; Rolph, R.; Cutress, R.; Copson, E.R. A Review of Modifiable Risk Factors in Young Women for the Prevention of Breast Cancer. *Breast Cancer Targets Ther.* **2021**, *13*, 241–257. [CrossRef]
6. Cheraghi, Z.; Poorolajal, J.; Hashem, T.; Esmailnasab, N.; Irani, A.D. Effect of Body Mass Index on Breast Cancer during Premenopausal and Postmenopausal Periods: A Meta-Analysis. *PLoS ONE* **2012**, *7*, e51446. [CrossRef]
7. Munsell, M.F.; Sprague, B.L.; Berry, D.A.; Chisholm, G.; Trentham-Dietz, A. Body Mass Index and Breast Cancer Risk According to Postmenopausal Estrogen-Progestin Use and Hormone Receptor Status. *Epidemiol. Rev.* **2014**, *36*, 114–136. [CrossRef] [PubMed]
8. Goldhirsch, A.; Winer, E.P.; Coates, A.S.; Gelber, R.D.; Piccart-Gebhart, M.; Thürlimann, B.; Senn, H.-J.; Albain, K.S.; André, F.; Bergh, J.; et al. Personalizing the treatment of women with early breast cancer: Highlights of the St Gallen International Expert Consensus on the Primary Therapy of Early Breast Cancer 2013. *Ann. Oncol.* **2013**, *24*, 2206–2223. [CrossRef]
9. Maisonneuve, P.; Disalvatore, D.; Rotmensz, N.; Curigliano, G.; Colleoni, M.; Dellapasqua, S.; Pruneri, G.; Mastropasqua, M.G.; Luini, A.; Bassi, F.; et al. Proposed new clinicopathological surrogate definitions of luminal A and luminal B (HER2-negative) intrinsic breast cancer subtypes. *Breast Cancer Res.* **2014**, *16*, R65. [CrossRef]
10. Tot, T. DCIS, cytokeratins, and the theory of the sick lobe. *Virchows Arch.* **2005**, *447*, 1–8. [CrossRef] [PubMed]
11. Tot, T. The Theory of the Sick Breast Lobe and the Possible Consequences. *Int. J. Surg. Pathol.* **2007**, *15*, 369–375. [CrossRef] [PubMed]
12. Eiriz, I.; Batista, M.V.; Tomás, T.C.; Neves, M.; Guerra-Pereira, N.; Braga, S. Breast cancer in very young women—a multicenter 10-year experience. *ESMO Open* **2021**, *6*, 100029. [CrossRef]
13. Santisteban, M.; Reynolds, C.; Fritcher, E.G.B.; Frost, M.H.; Vierkant, R.A.; Anderson, S.S.; Degnim, A.C.; Visscher, D.W.; Pankratz, V.S.; Hartmann, L.C. Ki67: A time-varying biomarker of risk of breast cancer in atypical hyperplasia. *Breast Cancer Res. Treat.* **2010**, *121*, 431–437. [CrossRef]
14. Khan, S.; Rogers, M.; Obando, J.; Tamsen, A. Estrogen receptor expression of benign breast epithelium and its association with breast cancer. *Cancer Res.* **1994**, *54*, 993–997.
15. Lydon, J.P.; Ge, G.; Kittrell, F.S.; Medina, D.; O'Malley, B.W. Murine mammary gland carcinogenesis is critically dependent on progesterone receptor function. *Cancer Res.* **1999**, *59*.
16. Huh, S.J.; Oh, H.; Peterson, M.A.; Almendro, V.; Hu, R.; Bowden, M.; Lis, R.L.; Cotter, M.B.; Loda, M.; Barry, W.T.; et al. The Proliferative Activity of Mammary Epithelial Cells in Normal Tissue Predicts Breast Cancer Risk in Premenopausal Women. *Cancer Res.* **2016**, *76*, 1926–1934. [CrossRef]
17. Oh, H.; Eliassen, A.H.; Wang, M.; Smith-Warner, S.; Beck, A.H.; Schnitt, S.J.; Collins, L.C.; Connolly, J.L.; Montaser-Kouhsari, L.; Polyak, K.; et al. Expression of estrogen receptor, progesterone receptor, and Ki67 in normal breast tissue in relation to subsequent risk of breast cancer. *NPJ Breast Cancer* **2016**, *2*, 16032. [CrossRef]
18. Tamimi, R.M.; Colditz, G.A.; Wang, Y.; Collins, L.C.; Hu, R.; Rosner, B.; Irie, H.Y.; Connolly, J.L.; Schnitt, S.J. Expression of IGF1R in normal breast tissue and subsequent risk of breast cancer. *Breast Cancer Res. Treat.* **2011**, *128*, 243–250. [CrossRef] [PubMed]
19. Zimpfer, A.; Schönberg, S.; Lugli, A.; Agostinelli, C.; Pileri, S.; Went, P.; Dirnhofer, S. Construction and validation of a bone marrow tissue microarray. *J. Clin. Pathol.* **2007**, *60*, 57–61. [CrossRef]
20. Dinno, A. Dunntest: Dunn's Test of Multiple Comparisons Using Rank Sums. Stata Software Package. 2014. Available online: http://www.alexisdinno.com/stata/dunntest.html (accessed on 22 July 2019).
21. Lawson, J.S.; Field, A.S.; Tran, D.D.; Houssami, N. Hormone replacement therapy use dramatically increases breast oestrogen receptor expression in obese postmenopausal women. *Breast Cancer Res.* **2001**, *3*, 342–345. [CrossRef]
22. Acheampong, T.; Kehm, R.D.; Terry, M.B.; Argov, E.L.; Tehranifar, P. Incidence Trends of Breast Cancer Molecular Subtypes by Age and Race/Ethnicity in the US From 2010 to 2016. *JAMA Netw. Open* **2020**, *3*, e2013226. [CrossRef] [PubMed]
23. Saha, S.; Dey, S.; Nath, S. Steroid Hormone Receptors: Links With Cell Cycle Machinery and Breast Cancer Progression. *Front. Oncol.* **2021**, *11*. [CrossRef]
24. Vera-Badillo, F.E.; Templeton, A.J.; De Gouveia, P.; Diaz-Padilla, I.; Bedard, P.L.; Al-Mubarak, M.; Seruga, B.; Tannock, I.F.; Ocana, A.; Amir, E. Androgen Receptor Expression and Outcomes in Early Breast Cancer: A Systematic Review and Meta-Analysis. *J. Natl. Cancer Inst.* **2014**, *106*, djt319. [CrossRef] [PubMed]
25. McNamara, K.; Yoda, T.; Takagi, K.; Miki, Y.; Suzuki, T.; Sasano, H. Androgen receptor in triple negative breast cancer. *J. Steroid Biochem. Mol. Biol.* **2013**, *133*, 66–76. [CrossRef] [PubMed]

26. Vidula, N.; Yau, C.; Wolf, D.; Rugo, H.S. Androgen receptor gene expression in primary breast cancer. *NPJ Breast Cancer* **2019**, *5*, 1–7. [CrossRef]
27. Cremonini, A.; Saragoni, L.; Morandi, L.; Corradini, A.G.; Ravaioli, C.; Di Oto, E.; Limarzi, F.; Sanchez, A.M.; Cucchi, M.C.; Masetti, R.; et al. Chromosome X aneusomy and androgen receptor gene copy number aberrations in apocrine carcinoma of the breast. *Virchows Archiv* **2021**, 1–10. [CrossRef]
28. Sun, X.; Zuo, K.; Yao, Q.; Zhou, S.; Shui, R.; Xu, X.; Bi, R.; Yu, B.; Cheng, Y.; Tu, X.; et al. Invasive apocrine carcinoma of the breast: Clinicopathologic features and comprehensive genomic profiling of 18 pure triple-negative apocrine carcinomas. *Mod. Pathol.* **2020**, *33*, 2473–2482. [CrossRef] [PubMed]
29. Tamaki, K.; Tamaki, N.; Terukina, S.; Kamada, Y.; Uehara, K.; Arakaki, M.; Miyashita, M.; Ishida, T.; McNamara, K.M.; Ohuchi, N.; et al. The Correlation between Body Mass Index and Breast Cancer Risk or Estrogen Receptor Status in Okinawan Women. *Tohoku J. Exp. Med.* **2014**, *234*, 169–174. [CrossRef]
30. Neuhouser, M.L.; Aragaki, A.K.; Prentice, R.L.; Manson, J.E.; Chlebowski, R.; Carty, C.L.; Ochs-Balcom, H.M.; Thomson, C.A.; Caan, B.J.; Tinker, L.F.; et al. Overweight, Obesity, and Postmenopausal Invasive Breast Cancer Risk: A Secondary Analysis of the Women's Health Initiative Randomized Clinical Trials. *JAMA Oncol.* **2015**, *1*, 611–621. [CrossRef]
31. Battersby, S.; Robertson, B.J.; Anderson, T.J.; King, R.J.; McPherson, K. Influence of menstrual cycle, parity and oral contraceptive use on steroid hormone receptors in normal breast. *Br. J. Cancer* **1992**, *65*, 601–607. [CrossRef]
32. Khan, S.A.; Rogers, M.A.M.; Khurana, K.K.; Meguid, M.M.; Numann, P.J. Estrogen Receptor Expression in Benign Breast Epithelium and Breast Cancer Risk. *J. Natl. Cancer Inst.* **1998**, *90*, 37–42. [CrossRef]

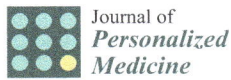
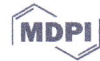

Review

Neoadjuvant Chemotherapy in Breast Cancer: An Advanced Personalized Multidisciplinary Prehabilitation Model (APMP-M) to Optimize Outcomes

Alba Di Leone [1,*], Daniela Terribile [1], Stefano Magno [1], Alejandro Martin Sanchez [1], Lorenzo Scardina [1], Elena Jane Mason [1], Sabatino D'Archi [1], Claudia Maggiore [2], Cristina Rossi [2], Annalisa Di Micco [2], Stefania Carnevale [3], Ida Paris [4], Fabio Marazzi [5], Valeria Masiello [5], Armando Orlandi [6], Antonella Palazzo [6], Alessandra Fabi [7], Riccardo Masetti [1] and Gianluca Franceschini [1]

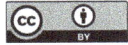

1. Multidisciplinary Breast Centre, Dipartimento Scienze della Salute della Donna e del Bambino e di Sanità Pubblica, Fondazione Policlinico Universitario A. Gemelli IRCCS, 00168 Rome, Italy; daniterribile@gmail.com (D.T.); stefano.magno@policlinicogemelli.it (S.M.); martin.sanchez@hotmail.it (A.M.S.); lorenzoscardina@libero.it (L.S.); elenajanemason@gmail.com (E.J.M.); sabatinodarchi@gmail.com (S.D.); riccardo.masetti@policlinicogemelli.it (R.M.); gianlucafranceschini70@gmail.com (G.F.)
2. Centre of Integrative Oncology—Multidisciplinary Breast Centre—Dipartimento Scienze della Salute della Donna e del Bambino e di Sanità Pubblica, Fondazione Policlinico Universitario A. Gemelli I RCCS, 00168 Rome, Italy; claud.maggiore@gmail.com (C.M.); cristina.rossi13@yahoo.it (C.R.); annalisadimicco@nutrimentidimindfulness.it (A.D.M.)
3. UOS Psicologia Clinica, Fondazione Policlinico Universitario A. Gemelli IRCCS, 00168 Rome, Italy; dott.stefaniacarnevale@gmail.com
4. Department of Woman and Child Health and Public Health, Woman Health Area, Fondazione Policlinico Universitario A. Gemelli I RCCS, 00168 Rome, Italy; ida.paris@policlinicogemelli.it
5. UOC di Radioterapia Oncologica, Dipartimento di Diagnostica per Immagini, Radioterapia Oncologica ed Ematologia, Fondazione Policlinico Universitario A. Gemelli I RCCS, 00168 Rome, Italy; fabio.marazzi@policlinicogemelli.it (F.M.); valeria.masiello@policlinicogemelli.it (V.M.)
6. Comprehensive Cancer Center, Multidisciplinary Breast Unit, Fondazione Policlinico Universitario Agostino Gemelli IRCCS, Largo Agostino Gemelli, 8, 00168 Rome, Italy; armando.orlandi@policlinicogemelli.it (A.O.); antonella.palazzo@policlinicogemelli.it (A.P.)
7. Medicina di Precisione in Senologia, Dipartimento Scienze della Salute della Donna e del Bambino e di Sanità Pubblica, Fondazione Policlinico Universitario A. Gemelli IRCCS, 00168 Rome, Italy; alessandra.fabi@policlinicogemelli.it
* Correspondence: alba.dileone@policlinicogemelli.it; Tel.: +39-3474980503; Fax: +39-0630156317

Abstract: Neoadjuvant chemotherapy is increasingly being employed in the management of breast cancer patients. Efforts and resources have been devoted over the years to the search for an optimal strategy that can improve outcomes in the neoadjuvant setting. Today, a multidisciplinary approach with the application of evidence-based medicine is considered the gold standard for the improvement of oncological results and patient satisfaction. However, several clinical complications and psychological issues due to various factors can arise during neoadjuvant therapy and undermine outcomes. To ensure that health care needs are adequately addressed, clinicians must consider that women with breast cancer have a high risk of developing "unmet needs" during treatment, and often require a clinical intervention or additional care resources to limit possible complications and psychological issues that can occur during neoadjuvant treatment. This work describes a multidisciplinary model developed at "Fondazione Policlinico Universitario Agostino Gemelli" (FPG) in Rome in an effort to optimize treatment, ease the application of evidence-based medicine, and improve patient quality of life in the neoadjuvant setting. In developing our model, our main goal was to adequately meet patient needs while preventing high levels of distress.

Keywords: breast cancer; neoadjuvant chemotherapy; multidisciplinary treatment; evidence-based medicine; personalized treatment; oncological outcomes; patient quality of life

1. Introduction

Breast cancer patients that exhibit high tumor-to-breast volume ratio, lymph node-positive disease, and aggressive biological features (high grade, hormone receptor-negative, HER2-positive, triple negative characterization) are more often candidates for neoadjuvant chemotherapy (NAC). Although large clinical trials have shown no differences in terms of overall and disease-free survival between adjuvant and neoadjuvant systemic therapy, NAC may provide important advantages [1,2]: tumor chemosensitivity can be assessed in vivo by monitoring the response to therapy, potentially allowing for the switching of therapies in case of non-responsiveness; downstaging of tumors often allows clinicians to favor breast-conserving surgery (BCS) over mastectomy and contain excision volumes, thus improving cosmetic results; downstaging of the axilla can allow for the avoidance of lymph node dissection in selected patients, reducing surgical morbidity [3] (Figure 1). Therapeutic regimens include anthracyclines (epirubicin, 100 mg/m^2), cyclophosphamide (500 mg/m^2; triweekly for 4 cycles) and taxanes (docetaxel, 70 mg/m^2; triweekly for 4 cycles); or carboplatin (100 mg/m^2; weekly for 12 cycles); taxanes are combined with targeted trastuzumab therapy in case of HER2-positivity.

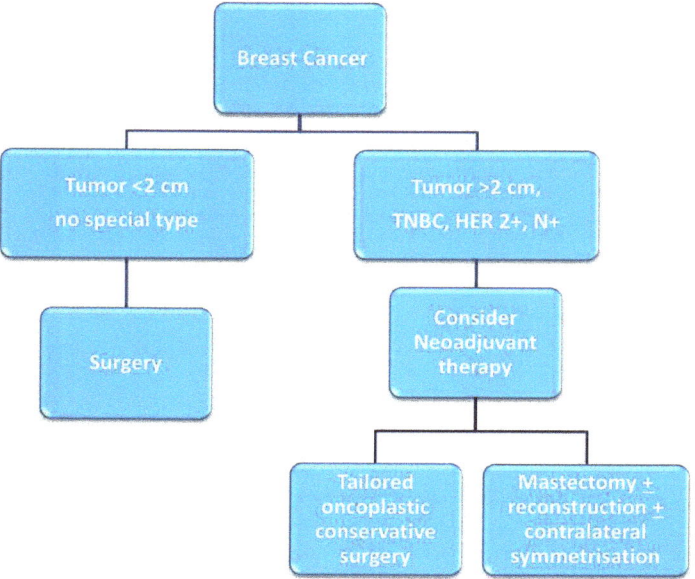

Figure 1. Decision-making process for neoadjuvant chemotherapy [4].

Specific evidence-based guidelines have been released to ensure that each patient treated in the neoadjuvant setting may receive the most effective, evidence-based chemotherapy regimen, in a personalized, multidisciplinary setting (Figure 2).

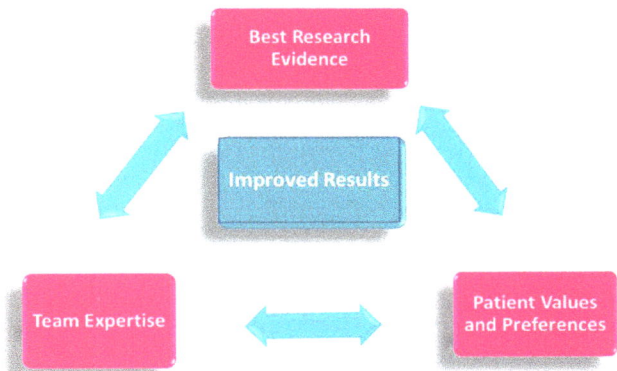

Figure 2. Evidence-based medicine in neoadjuvant chemotherapy.

Less attention has been devoted to addressing the specific "unmet needs" that patients may experience during treatment [5]. The benefits of a multimodal prehabilitation model are still emerging in recent studies, particularly during the preoperative period. During this window of opportunity, patients may be more receptive to health behavior changes in a structured support network [6].

In this paper, we present the details of an advanced, personalized, multidisciplinary prehabilitation protocol, which we have adopted in our Multidisciplinary Breast Center at Fondazione Policlinico Universitario Agostino Gemelli (FPG) in Rome since 1 May 2018 for patients scheduled to receive NAC.

This protocol allows patients to access not only the most appropriate, evidence-based chemotherapy regimen, but also specific interventions aimed at protecting their quality of life via the inclusion of lifestyle and nutrition counselling, along with psychological distress- and integrative oncology (IO)-complementary interventions [7].

2. Materials and Methods

Our breast unit treats approximately 1000 new breast cancer cases every year. Between 1 May 2018 and 31 December 2020, 250 patients were referred to our center for neoadjuvant treatment. The mean patient age was 53 (range 25–74), and 130 patients were premenopausal.

Our broad-based interdisciplinary team includes ten breast surgeons, two medical oncologists, two breast pathologists, five breast radiologists, three breast radiologic technicians, three psycho-oncologists, two nutritionists, two integrative oncology physicians, six certified breast care nurses, and one data manager, all exclusively devoted to the management of patients with breast disease. Other team members that devote at least 50% of their activity to breast pathology include three plastic surgeons, three additional medical oncologists, two radiation oncologists, two oncogeriatricians, two gynecologists, one geneticist, one cardiologist, and two palliative care specialists. All specialists regularly attend weekly multidisciplinary meetings (MDMs), in which all new cases of breast cancer are discussed [8]. In this setting, patients are also evaluated for enrollment in clinical trials [9].

During MDMs, the case of every patient is discussed in detail, and an individualized treatment plan is programmed in adherence to the latest practice guidelines. Out of 250 patients, 98 were scheduled for an appointment with the geneticist, 14 were referred for fertility counseling, and an appointment with a geriatrician was arranged for 34 elderly patients.

3. Breast Unit and Outpatient Neoadjuvant Care Prehabilitation Clinic

All patients receiving an indication to NAC are referred to the "outpatient neoadjuvant care prehabilitation clinic", where they are jointly taken care of by a "neoadjuvant oncologic treatment team" and a "neoadjuvant supportive care team". The first team explains the care plan designed by the multidisciplinary panel, and brings into focus the important aspects of their respective areas of expertise. At the end of the interview, the patients are directed to a follow-up examination by the supportive care team for a complete psychological, nutritional, and lifestyle assessment that will serve as a baseline for the upcoming treatment. As a result, the treatment is tailored to every patient in a multidisciplinary, holistic fashion [10]. When possible, every appointment is scheduled on the same day, to limit patient discomfort in returning to the hospital several times in the same week.

4. The Neoadjuvant Oncologic Treatment Team

In this setting, patients are welcomed by a team of experts consisting of a breast surgeon together with the patient's referring oncologist and breast nurse (Figure 3) [11].

This treatment team is in charge of reviewing the diagnostic workup, discussing the therapeutic plan, and explaining, scheduling, and monitoring additional interventions that may be relevant according to the age and specific medical features of each individual patient.

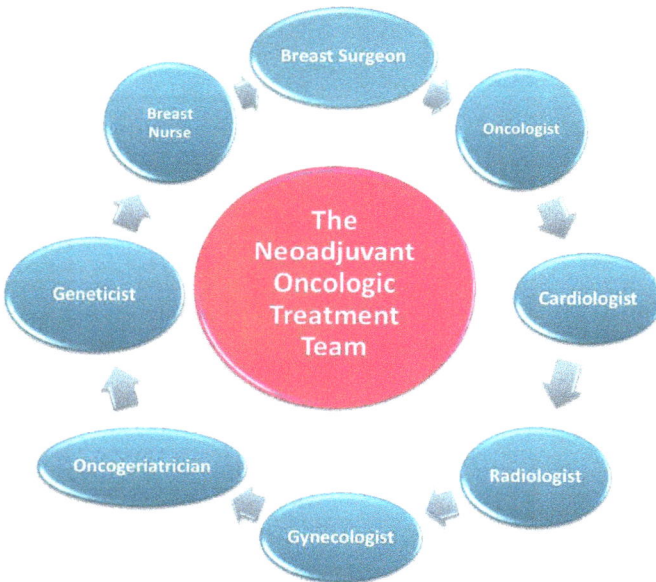

Figure 3. The neoadjuvant oncologic treatment team.

As a first step, the oncologic team reviews the diagnostic workup and schedules any additional appointments that may be required to complete it.

Every patient undergoing NAC in our breast center must have completed a full diagnostic panel that includes [12]:
- Clinical breast examination, mammography, breast ultrasound, and breast MRI;
- Ultrasound- or stereotactic-guided tissue sampling of breast lesions and suspicious lymph nodes. Markers are positioned in the breast tissue and pathologic lymph nodes

in order to ensure a correct pre-surgical localization in case of pathologic complete response or regression to a non-palpable lesion;
- Complete histopathological and prognostic characterization (ER, PgR, AR, Ki67, HER2 status);
- Photographical documentation of pre-NAC patient breasts. After clinical and ultrasound evaluation, the surgeon draws the tumor's projection and measurements on the skin surface and takes two photographs in frontal and lateral projection (Figure 4). Pictures are re-evaluated after NAC and assist in surgical planning [13];
- Systemic staging is completed by performing either a whole-body CT scan and bone scintigraphy, or a PET/CT scan.

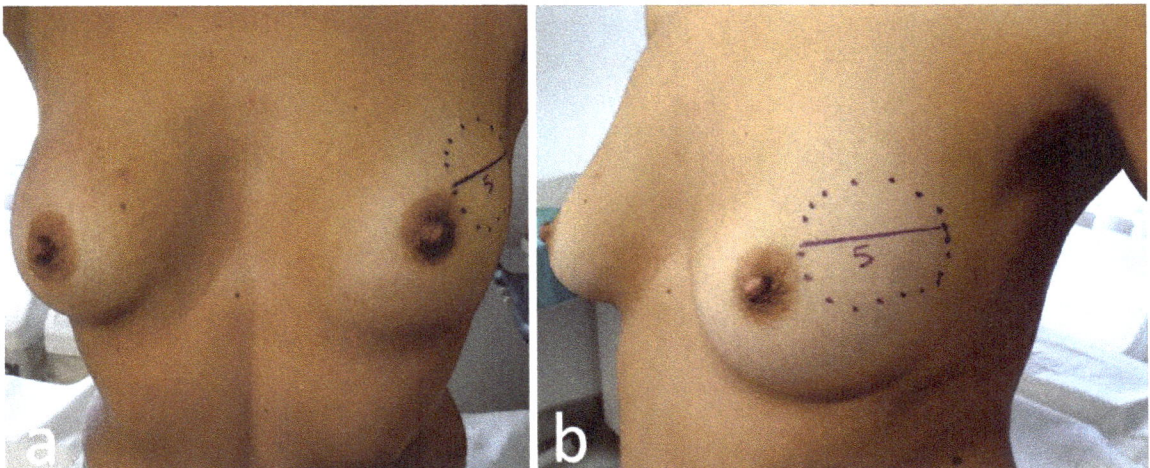

Figure 4. Frontal (**a**) and lateral (**b**) view of pre-neoadjuvant chemotherapy (NAC) breast with tumor projection and measurement (cm).

The team then reviews with the patient the global therapeutic plan [14]. The oncologist discusses with the patient the details of the chemotherapeutic regimen (previously defined at the MDM) and a date for the first session of NAC is set. An appointment for central venous catheter placement is also provided.

Based on age, general conditions, family history, and pathologic features of the tumor, the following additional interventions are discussed and eventually scheduled.

4.1. Cardiovascular Assessment

As conventional chemotherapy and targeted therapies are associated with an increased risk of cardiac damage [15], each patient scheduled for NAC undergoes preliminary cardiovascular assessment.

The development of cardiotoxicity, even if asymptomatic, not only adversely affects patient cardiac prognosis, but may significantly limit the proper completion of therapeutic protocols, especially if additional anticancer treatments become necessary after recovery/relapse of the disease [16]. Cardiovascular disease is now the second leading cause of long-term morbidity and mortality among cancer survivors, and the leading cause of death among female breast cancer survivors [17].

Our protocol ensures that a cardio-oncologist evaluates the patient via electrocardiogram and echocardiography before beginning treatment, and then periodically in relation to personal risk and ongoing pharmacological treatment. An adequate preliminary stratification of cardiotoxicity risk and the early identification and treatment of subclinical cardiac damage may help to avoid withdrawal of chemotherapy and prevent irreversible cardiovascular dysfunction.

4.2. Genetic Counselling

Because of recent media and popular culture coverage, general knowledge about breast cancer genetics has increased in recent years [18]. Genetic test results have also become increasingly relevant in selecting the most effective systemic therapy, thanks to the advent of PARP inhibitors for treatment of BRCA1/2-associated breast cancers. Genetic assessment has become equally relevant for the optimization of radiation therapy, with emerging concerns about radiation safety for the carriers of certain pathogenic mutations (e.g., TP53) [19].

In our model, indications to genetic testing are discussed for every patient during the MDM, taking into account patient age, family history, and the clinical features of the disease. If, according to current Italian and American guidelines [20,21], genetic testing is considered appropriate, an interview with the clinical geneticist is immediately scheduled [22]. The advantage of this approach is that patients who then undergo NAC have approximately six months to complete a full, well-rounded genetic evaluation before the scheduling of surgery. This allows us to tailor surgical choices based on the test results, avoiding the unnecessary double surgery that could derive from a positive test result obtained after breast-conserving surgery [23].

4.3. Multiparametric Geriatric Assessment in Elderly Patients

Elderly patients represent a very heterogeneous community in terms of life expectancy, comorbidities, and cognitive and social function, therefore it is crucial not to deny treatment based on age alone. In this framework, a multiparametric geriatric assessment is always appropriate, and is a convenient supplement in the evaluation of every elderly patient treated for breast cancer, as it can move the needle on proposed treatment.

A recent study by Okonji et al. reported that nearly 50% of fit elderly women with high-risk disease are undertreated [24]. The neoadjuvant use of chemotherapy is further neglected, with studies reporting higher toxicity rates and lower incidence of complete pathological response in patients aged over 65 [25]. However, although elderly patients are generally underrepresented in clinical trials, those with non-triple negative breast cancer show a prognosis comparable to younger patients in terms of overall survival [26]. An individualized care model must therefore be applied to select the elderly sub-population that could benefit from neoadjuvant chemotherapy, and monitor it closely during treatment to prevent toxicity in these fragile patients [27].

In our protocol, patients aged 70 years or older, whether or not they exhibit relevant comorbidities, are scheduled for a pre-treatment comprehensive geriatric assessment. The assessment is performed by a dedicated geriatrician with experience in breast oncology, who actively participates in our multidisciplinary team. Comorbidities, cognitive and psychological disorders, physical performance, risk factors, nutritional status, and general autonomy are comprehensively evaluated, and NAC is scheduled only in the event of oncogeriatric clearance. A second assessment is also scheduled at the end of chemotherapy.

4.4. Gynecologic and Fertility Counselling in Younger Patients

Chemotherapy and/or ovarian suppression can cause early (permanent or temporary) menopausal symptoms and reduce fertility. Many women are concerned about these issues, and it is important to provide them with proper counseling and treatment [28]. As regards menopausal symptoms, a large number of patients find these difficult to cope with, with a significant negative impact on their quality of life. Our gynecologists manage these symptoms using both traditional medicine and integrative care.

Fertility care should follow a multidisciplinary team-based approach, with strict interaction between medical oncologists, surgeons, and fertility specialists [29,30]. In our multidisciplinary prehabilitation care model, the main goal is to preserve the opportunity for family planning, offering oncofertility services in a timely manner without delaying chemotherapy.

The breast nurse follows the patient on this pathway and during the subsequent procedures for ovarian function and/or fertility preservation.

5. The Neoadjuvant Supportive Care Team

After completing the assessment with the "oncological treatment team", every patient is directed to a meeting with the "neoadjuvant supportive care team", which includes a nutritionist, a psycho-oncologist, and an integrative oncology expert (Figure 5) [31].

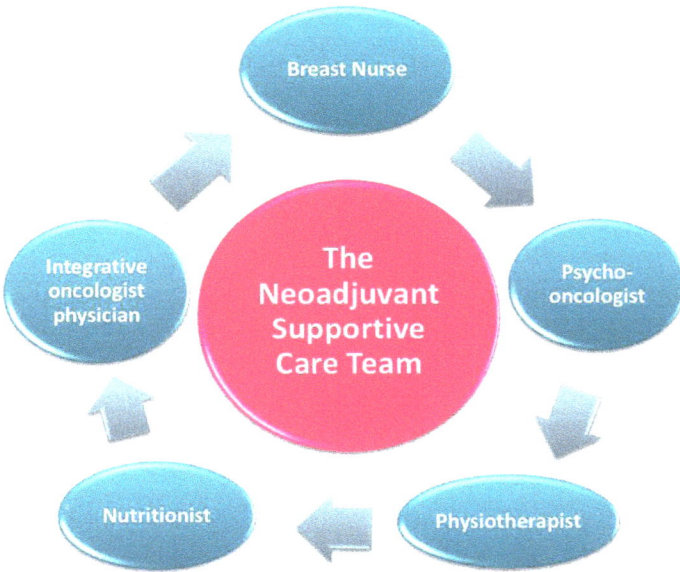

Figure 5. The neoadjuvant supportive care team.

A lifestyle interview is conducted, and anthropometric parameters and body composition analysis are measured via segmental multi frequency–bioelectrical impedance analysis (SMF-BIA).

Nutritional and physical activity screenings are performed in our unit just before the beginning and at the conclusion of oncologic treatments, and the impact of each type of intervention, from surgery to chemotherapy, on BMI, body composition, and metabolism is monitored during therapy. In this regard, patients are asked to keep a diary and send it regularly via email, and periodic video interviews are scheduled [32–34].

5.1. Lifestyle and Nutrition Counseling

Physical activity (PA), nutrition, body weight, and metabolism all play a key role in almost every aspect of cancer onset, progression, and management [35] (WCRF -World Cancer Research Fund 2018). However, nutritional screening is seldom performed even in high-quality breast units, and data on its value are still scarce [36–38].

Specific recommendations about diet and physical activity based on the most recent scientific evidence [35] are given to all patients, with the aim of relieving chemotherapy toxicity and improving quality of life and oncological outcomes [39,40]. Moreover, during and after treatments, patients are supported by a personalized nutritional approach and motivated to practice PA in order to decrease their disease recurrence risk [39,41]. PA during cancer treatments represents a powerful asset to improve therapy-induced conditions such as anxiety, depression, sleep disorders, lymphedema, cancer- and therapy-related fatigue, bone health, and overall quality of life [42–46].

5.2. Psychological Counselling

Chemotherapy generates a distress that, over time, can severely affect patient quality of life [47,48]. A recent study showed that post-NAC patients have a significantly higher level of distress compared to patients receiving chemotherapy after surgery [49]. Understanding the needs of patients undergoing NAC enables us to address the communication process more appropriately, provide psychological support, and build clinical and rehabilitation interventions in a more personalized way [47]. In line with NCCN guidelines, the diagnostic and therapeutic pathways of patients scheduled for NAC include a pre–post treatment psychological evaluation. Specific, psycho-oncological support should be given to patients undergoing chemotherapy. At the beginning of NAC, patients undergo a clinical psychological interview aimed at assessing their risk of oncological distress, and identifying both the dysfunctional psychological factors and the protective psychosocial factors that could affect treatment. The goal is to improve adaptation to the oncological disease and promote adherence to therapeutic treatments. In addition to the interview, a psychometric assessment is carried out through screening and the employment of clinical tools such as the Distress Thermometer (DT) [50], the Hospital Anxiety Depression Scale (HADS) [51] and the General Self-Efficacy Scale (GSES) [52].

In our breast center, we aim to validate a semi-structural interview, which leads to a holistic and trans-disciplinary measurement of the psychological state of the patients. The assessment allows us to identify patients who may benefit from a psychological support intervention, individual psychotherapy, or group therapy [53] (Figure 6).

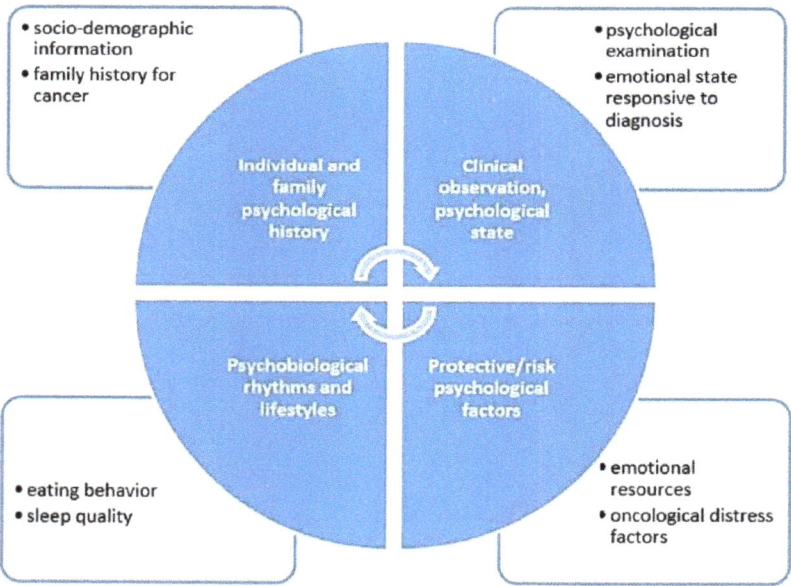

Figure 6. Psychological interview.

Emotional Eating Prevention during NAC

The impact of psychosocial factors such as worry, perceived risk, and perceived treatment efficacy on diet has been understudied in breast cancer patients [54]. The relationship between distress, weight change, and nutrition has been the subject of a fairly recent psycho-oncological study trend, with major studies conducted on patients at the end of their therapies. Our model proposes an integrative approach to identify emotional eating, a dietary pattern wherein people use food to help them deal with stressful situations and in response to negative emotions. Overweight individuals have been found to exhibit less effective coping skills in response to negative emotions, which leads them to emotionally eat more frequently [55]. Psychological disciplines can help to identify healthy and harmful habits, and promote changes in attitudes and healthy behaviors.

Psychological intervention based on the activation of self-efficacy in dietary behavior could favor the ability to adapt to oncological therapies through active participation in treatment, redefinition of problems, and the evaluation of alternative solutions. At the same time, the intervention acts in support of lifestyle changes and involves the activation of specific psychoeducational groups for patients who need to change their dietary behavior.

5.3. Integrative Oncology during Neoadjuvant Therapy

Our patients receive information about evidence-based complementary therapies available, in order to optimize the management of symptoms related either to the disease itself or to treatment toxicity: most frequently gastro-intestinal disorders, hot flashes, fatigue, insomnia, mucositis, peripheral neuropathy, anxiety, and mood disorders.

In accordance with the SIO (Society of Integrative Oncology) clinical guidelines for breast cancer patients [56] recently endorsed by the American Society of Clinical Oncology (ASCO) [7], personalized integrative care plans at the FPG Center for Integrative Oncology include mind–body interventions such as acupuncture, mindfulness-based protocols, qi gong, massage therapy, and other group programs like music therapy, art therapy, and therapeutic writing workshops.

5.3.1. Acupuncture

Acupuncture, well known as a branch of traditional Chinese medicine, represents a reliable, cost-effective, and safe procedure for symptom management, if performed properly and by a specialized practitioner. The NCCN recommends acupuncture for pain, fatigue, nausea/vomiting, and hot flashes [57]. For some of these symptoms, such as nausea/vomiting, acupuncture can be used as a valid option for patients who wish to avoid pharmacological treatment. For other conditions, including fatigue, hot flashes, and chemotherapy-induced peripheral neuropathy (CIPN), acupuncture should be considered when conventional treatments are ineffective, not available, or burdened by remarkable side effects.

In many patients experiencing hot flashes due to chemotherapy-induced ovarian failure and/or estrogen-blocking treatments, a course of 6–12 acupuncture treatments is associated with therapeutic effects that persist for six months or longer and do not appear to require prolonged treatment [58,59].

Chemotherapy-induced peripheral neuropathy is a challenging pain symptom to manage, and has been a hot topic for acupuncturists for a long time. A recent Cochrane review concluded that there was insufficient evidence to support or reject the use of acupuncture for neuropathic pain [60]. To date, some randomized phase II studies on the effects of acupuncture are very promising [61–63]. Recently published ESMO (European Society of Medical Oncology) guidelines on therapy-induced neurotoxicity [64] state that "Acupuncture might be considered in selected patients to treat CIPN symptoms "(grade II, C). Currently, our Center for Integrative Oncology is taking part in a multicenter clinical trial on acupuncture for chemotherapy-induced peripheral neuropathy (CIPN) in breast cancer.

5.3.2. Mindfulness

Mindfulness is defined as present-moment nonjudgmental awareness, and its practice can take the form of formal meditation, or more informal practices, such as simply remembering to be present as one undertakes day-to-day tasks. Mindfulness-based stress reduction (MBSR) has been shown to reduce distress and improve psychological well-being in patients with cancer [65–67]. Preliminary evidence suggests that MBSR may produce effects comparable to pharmacologic treatment for primary insomnia [68] and positively impact sleep quality and quantity in patients with cancer [69–71]. Randomized trials of mindfulness-based stress reduction report decreased fatigue, depression, anxiety, and fear of recurrence [72,73].

In addition, improvements have been noted in sleep [72,74], quality of life, and psychosocial adjustments [70], as well as in the long-term adverse effects associated with treatment [65].

6. Conclusions

Specific clinical complications and psychological issues due to the disease and therapies can occur during the course of neoadjuvant therapy, undermining outcomes.

We have therefore developed a multidisciplinary model to ease the application of evidence-based oncologic protocols, ensure patient-centered optimal treatment, prevent distress, and improve patient quality of life. Our model of intervention can encourage clinicians to personalize supportive care medicine and direct it towards precision medicine. The development of an appropriate clinical pathway, with multidisciplinary competence and the performance of standardized tasks, is essential in order to obtain a successful treatment and make the patient co-responsible for optimized results within the neoadjuvant setting. However, multidisciplinary prehabilitation trials in breast cancer patients undertaking NAC are necessary to confirm the efficacy of this model.

Author Contributions: Conceptualization, A.D.L., S.M. and D.T.; methodology, A.M.S. and A.P.; software, A.D.M. and S.C.; validation, F.M., V.M. and A.O.; formal analysis, C.R.; investigation, C.M.; resources, L.S.; data curation, E.J.M.; writing—original draft preparation, A.D.L.; writing—review and editing, G.F. and I.P.; visualization, A.F.; supervision, R.M.; project administration, S.D. All authors have read and agreed to the published version of the manuscript.

Funding: This research received no external funding.

Institutional Review Board Statement: The study was conducted according to the guidelines of the Declaration of Helsinki, and approved by the Institutional Review Board (or Ethics Committee) of Fondazione Universitaria Policlinico Agostino Gemelli IRCCS.

Informed Consent Statement: Not applicable.

Acknowledgments: In this section, you can acknowledge any support given which is not covered by the author contribution or funding sections. This may include administrative and technical support, or donations in kind (e.g., materials used for experiments).

Conflicts of Interest: The authors declare no conflict of interest.

References

1. Early Breast Cancer Trialists' Collaborative Group (EBCTCG). Long-Term outcomes for neoadjuvant versus adjuvant chemotherapy in early breast cancer: Meta-Analysis of individual patient data from ten randomised trials. *Lancet Oncol.* **2018**, *19*, 27–39. [CrossRef]
2. O'Halloran, N.; Lowery, A.; Curran, C.; McLaughlin, R.; Malone, C.; Sweeney, K.; Keane, M.; Kerin, M. A Review of the impact of neoadjuvant chemotherapy on breast surgery practice and outcomes. *Clin. Breast Cancer* **2019**, *19*, 377–382. [CrossRef]
3. Franceschini, G.; Di Leone, A.; Natale, M.; Sanchez, A.M.; Masetti, R. Conservative surgery after neoadjuvant chemotherapy in patients with operable breast cancer. *Ann. Ital. Chir.* **2018**, *89*, 290.
4. Franceschini, G.; Visconti, G.; Masetti, R. Oncoplastic breast surgery with oxidized regenerated cellulose: Appraisals based on five-year experience. *Breast J.* **2014**, *20*, 447–448. [CrossRef]

5. Lo-Fo-Wong, D.N.; de Haes, H.C.; Aaronson, N.K.; van Abbema, D.L.; den Boer, M.D.; van Hezewijk, M.; Immink, M.; Kaptein, A.A.; Menke-Pluijmers, M.B.; Reyners, A.K.; et al. Risk factors of unmet needs among women with breast cancer in the post-treatment phase. *Psychooncology* **2020**, *29*, 539–549. [CrossRef]
6. Brahmbhatt, P.; Sabiston, M.C.; Lopez, C.; Chang, E.; Goodman, J.; Jones, J.; McCready, D.; Randall, I.; Rotstein, S.; Santa Mina, D. Feasibility of prehabilitation prior to breast cancer surgery: A mixed-methods study. *Front. Oncol.* **2020**, *10*. [CrossRef]
7. Lyman, G.H.; Greenlee, H.; Bohlke, K.; Bao, T.; DeMichele, A.M.; Deng, G.E.; Fouladbakhsh, J.M.; Gil, B.; Hershman, D.L.; Mansfield, S.; et al. Integrative therapies during and after breast cancer treatment: ASCO endorsement of the SIO clinical practice guideline. *J. Clin. Oncol.* **2018**, *36*, 2647–2655. [CrossRef]
8. Franceschini, G.; di Leone, A.; Masetti, R. The breast unit update on advantages and the open issues. *Ann. Ital. Chir.* **2014**, *85*, 407–412. [PubMed]
9. Nardone, L.; Valentini, V.; Marino, L.; De Santis, M.C.; Terribile, D.; Franceschini, G.; Balducci, M.; Mantini, G.; Mattiucci, G.; Mulè, A.; et al. A feasibility study of neo-adjuvant low-dose fractionated radiotherapy with two different concurrent anthracycline-docetaxel schedules in stage IIA/B-IIIA breast cancer. *Tumori* **2012**, *98*, 79–85. [CrossRef]
10. Grimmett, C.; Bradbury, K.; Dalton, S.O.; Fecher-Jones, I.; Hoedjes, M.; Varkonyi-Sepp, J.; Short, C.E. The role of behavioral science in personalized multimodal prehabilitation in cancer. *Front. Psychol.* **2021**, *12*. [CrossRef]
11. Shao, J.; Rodrigues, M.; Corter, A.L.; Baxter, N.N. Multidisciplinary care of breast cancer patients: A scoping review of multidisciplinary styles, processes, and outcomes. *Curr. Oncol.* **2019**, *26*, e385–e397. [CrossRef]
12. Franceschini, G.; Terribile, D.; Fabbri, C.; Magno, S.; D'Alba, P.; Chiesa, F.; Di Leone, A.; Masetti, R. Management of locally advanced breast cancer: Mini-Review. *Minerva Chir.* **2007**, *62*, 249–255.
13. Salgarello, M.; Visconti, G.; Barone-Adesi, L.; Franceschini, G.; Masetti, R. Contralateral breast symmetrisation in immediate prosthetic breast reconstruction after unilateral nipple-sparing mastectomy: The tailored reduction/augmentation mammaplasty. *Arch. Plast. Surg.* **2015**, *42*, 302–308. [CrossRef]
14. Franceschini, G.; Sanchez, A.M.; Di Leone, A.; Magno, S.; Moschella, F.; Accetta, C.; Natale, M.; Di Giorgio, D.; Scaldaferri, A.; D'Archi, S.; et al. Update on the surgical management of breast cancer. *Ann. Ital. Chir.* **2015**, *86*, 89–99.
15. Shan, K.; Lincoff, A.M.; Young, J.B. Anthracycline-Induced cardiotoxicity. *Ann. Intern. Med.* **1996**, *125*, 47–58. [CrossRef]
16. Felker, G.M.; Thompson, R.E.; Hare, J.M.; Hruban, R.H.; Clemetson, D.E.; Howard, D.L.; Baughman, K.L.; Kasper, E.K. Underlying causes and long-term survival in patients with initially unexplained cardiomyopathy. *N. Engl. J. Med.* **2000**, *342*, 1077–1084. [CrossRef]
17. Patnaik, J.L.; Byers, T.; DiGuiseppi, C.; Dabelea, D.; Denberg, T.D. Cardiovascular disease competes with breast cancer as the leading cause of death for older females diagnosed with breast cancer: A retrospective cohort study. *Breast Cancer Res.* **2011**, *13*, R64. [CrossRef] [PubMed]
18. Tischler, J.; Crew, K.D.; Chung, W.K. Cases in precision medicine: The role of tumor and germline genetic testing in breast cancer management. *Ann. Intern. Med.* **2019**, *171*, 925–930. [CrossRef] [PubMed]
19. Katz, S.J.; Ward, K.C.; Hamilton, A.S.; McLeod, M.C.; Wallner, L.P.; Morrow, M.; Jagsi, R.; Hawley, S.T.; Kurian, A.W. Gaps in receipt of clinically indicated genetic counseling after diagnosis of breast cancer. *J. Clin. Oncol.* **2018**, *36*, 1218–1224. [CrossRef]
20. Associazione Italiana di Oncologia Medica (AIOM). *Neoplasia della Mammella*; Linee Guida; Associazione Italiana di Oncologia Medica (AIOM): Milano, Italy, 2020.
21. Gradishar, W.J.; Anderson, B.O.; Abraham, J.; Aft, R.; Agnese, D.; Allison, K.H.; Blair, S.L.; Burstein, H.J.; Dang, C.; Elias, A.; et al. *NCCN Clinical Practice Guidelines in Oncology—Breast Cancer*; National Comprehensive Cancer NetworkNCCN: Plymouth Meeting, PA, USA, 2020.
22. Christian, N.; Zabor, E.C.; Cassidy, M.; Flynn, J.; Morrow, M.; Gemignani, M.L. Contralateral prophylactic mastectomy use after neoadjuvant chemotherapy. *Ann. Surg. Oncol.* **2020**, *27*, 743–749. [CrossRef] [PubMed]
23. Terkelsen, T.; Rønning, H.; Skytte, A.B. Impact of genetic counseling on the uptake of contralateral prophylactic mastectomy among younger women with breast cancer. *Acta Oncol.* **2020**, *59*, 60–65. [CrossRef]
24. Okonji, D.O.; Sinha, R.; Phillips, I.; Fatz, D.; Ring, A. Comprehensive geriatric assessment in 326 older women with early breast cancer. *Br. J. Cancer* **2017**, *117*, 925–931. [CrossRef]
25. Halfter, K.; Ditsch, N.; Kolberg, H.C.; Fischer, H.; Hauzenberger, T.; von Koch, F.E.; Bauerfeind, I.; von Minckwitz, G.; Funke, I.; Crispin, A.; et al. Prospective cohort study using the breast cancer spheroid model as a predictor for response to neoadjuvant therapy—The SpheroNEO study. *BMC Cancer* **2015**, *15*, 519. [CrossRef]
26. von Waldenfels, G.; Loibl, S.; Furlanetto, J.; Machlei, A.; Lederer, B.; Denkert, C.; Hanusch, C.; Kümmel, S.; von Minckwitz, G.; Schneeweiss, A.; et al. Outcome after neoadjuvant chemotherapy in elderly breast cancer patients—A pooled analysis of individual patient data from eight prospectively randomized controlled trials. *Oncotarget* **2018**, *9*, 15168–15179. [CrossRef] [PubMed]
27. Hurria, A.; Togawa, K.; Mohile, S.G.; Owusu, C.; Klepin, H.D.; Gross, C.P.; Lichtman, S.M.; Gajra, A.; Bhatia, S.; Katheria, V.; et al. Predicting chemotherapy toxicity in older adults with cancer: A prospective multicenter study. *J. Clin. Oncol.* **2011**, *29*, 3457–3465. [CrossRef] [PubMed]
28. Arecco, L.; Perachino, M.; Damassi, A.; Latocca, M.M.; Soldato, D.; Vallome, G.; Parisi, F.; Razeti, M.G.; Solinas, C.; Tagliamento, M.; et al. Burning questions in the oncofertility counseling of young breast cancer patients. *Breast Cancer Basic Clin. Res.* **2020**, *14*. [CrossRef]

29. Peccatori, F.A.; Azim, H.A.; Orecchia, R.; Hoekstra, H.J.; Pavlidis, N.; Kesic, V.; Pentheroudakis, G. Pentheroudakis, Cancer, pregnancy and fertility: ESMO Clinical practice guidelines for diagnosis, treatment and follow-up. *Ann. Oncol.* **2013**, *24* (Suppl. 6), vi160–vi170. [CrossRef] [PubMed]
30. Oktay, K.; Harvey, B.E.; Partridge, A.H.; Quinn, G.P.; Reinecke, J.; Taylor, H.S.; Wallace, W.H.; Wang, E.T.; Loren, A.W. Fertility preservation in patients with cancer: ASCO clinical practice guideline update. *J. Clin. Oncol.* **2018**, *36*, 1994–2001. [CrossRef] [PubMed]
31. Magno, S.; Alessio, F.; Scaldaferri, A.; Sacchini, V.; Chiesa, F. Integrative approaches in breast cancer patients: A mini-review. *Integr. Cancer Sci. Ther.* **2016**, *3*, 460–464. [CrossRef]
32. Bozzetti, F.; Arends, J.; Lundholm, K.; Micklewright, A.; Zurcher, G.; Muscaritoli, M. ESPEN guidelines on parenteral nutrition: Non-Surgical oncology. *Clin. Nutr.* **2009**, *28*, 445–454. [CrossRef]
33. Kondrup, J.E.; Allison, S.P.; Elia, M.; Vellas, B.; Plauth, M. ESPEN guidelines for nutrition screening 2002. *Clin. Nutr.* **2003**, *22*, 415–421. [CrossRef]
34. Ryan, A.M.; Power, D.G.; Daly, L.; Cushen, S.J.; Ní Bhuachalla, E.; Prado, C.M. Cancer-Associated malnutrition, cachexia and sarcopenia: The skeleton in the hospital closet 40 years later. *Proc. Nutr. Soc.* **2016**, *75*, 199–211. [CrossRef]
35. World Cancer Research Fund/American Institute for Cancer Research. *World Cancer Research Fund/American Institute for Cancer Research Continous Update Project Report: Diet, Nutrition, Physical Activity and Breast Cancer*; World Cancer Research Fund International: London, UK, 2018; Available online: https://www.wcrf.org/dietandcancer (accessed on 1 April 2021).
36. Prado, C.M.M.; Baracos, V.E.; McCargar, L.J.; Reiman, T.; Mourtzakis, M.; Tonkin, K.; Mackey, J.R.; Koski, S.; Pituskin, E.; Sawyer, M.B. Sarcopenia as a determinant of chemotherapy toxicity and time to tumor progression in metastatic breast cancer patients receiving capecitabine treatment. *Clin. Cancer Res.* **2009**, *15*, 2920–2926. [CrossRef]
37. Carbognin, L.; Trestini, I.; Sperduti, I.; Bonaiuto, C.; Zambonin, V.; Fiorio, E.; Tregnago, D.; Parolin, V.; Pilotto, S.; Scambia, G.; et al. Prospective trial in early-stage breast cancer (EBC) patients (pts) submitted to nutrition evidence-based educational intervention: Early results of adherence to dietary guidelines (ADG) and body weight change (BWC). *J. Clin. Oncol.* **2019**, *37* (Suppl. 15), 11575. [CrossRef]
38. Iyengar, N.M.; Zhou, X.K.; Gucalp, A.; Morris, P.G.; Howe, L.R.; Giri, D.D.; Morrow, M.; Wang, H.; Pollak, M.; Jones, L.W.; et al. Systemic correlates of white adipose tissue inflammation in early-stage breast cancer. *Clin. Cancer Res.* **2016**, *22*, 2283–2289. [CrossRef]
39. Pierce, J.P.; Stefanick, M.L.; Flatt, S.W.; Natarajan, L.; Sternfeld, B.; Madlensky, L.; Al-Delaimy, W.K.; Thomson, C.A.; Kealey, S.; Hajek, R.; et al. Greater survival after breast cancer in physically active women with high vegetable-fruit intake regardless of obesity. *J. Clin. Oncol.* **2007**, *25*, 2345–2351. [CrossRef]
40. Rock, C.L.; Thomson, C.; Gansler, T.; Gapstur, S.M.; McCullough, M.L.; Patel, A.V.; Andrews, K.S.; Bandera, E.V.; Spees, C.K.; Robien, K.; et al. American Cancer Society guideline for diet and physical activity for cancer prevention. *CA Cancer J. Clin.* **2020**, *70*, 245–271. [CrossRef]
41. Lohse, T.; Faeh, D.; Bopp, M.; Rohrmann, S. Adherence to the cancer prevention recommendations of the World Cancer Research Fund/American Institute for Cancer Research and mortality: A census-linked cohort. *Am. J. Clin. Nutr.* **2016**, *104*, 678–685. [CrossRef]
42. Courneya, K.S.; McKenzie, D.C.; Mackey, J.R.; Gelmon, K.; Friedenreich, C.M.; Yasui, Y.; Reid, R.D.; Cook, D.; Jespersen, D.; Proulx, C.; et al. Effects of exercise dose and type during breast cancer chemotherapy: Multicenter randomized trial. *J. Natl. Cancer Inst.* **2013**, *105*, 1821–1832. [CrossRef]
43. Irwin, M.L.; Cartmel, B.; Gross, C.P.; Ercolano, E.; Li, F.; Yao, X.; Fiellin, M.; Capozza, S.; Rothbard, M.; Zhou, Y.; et al. Randomized exercise trial of aromatase inhibitor-induced arthralgia in breast cancer survivors. *J. Clin. Oncol.* **2015**, *33*, 1104–1111. [CrossRef]
44. Lee, A.; Chiu, C.H.; Cho, M.W.A.; Gomersall, C.D.; Lee, K.F.; Cheung, Y.S.; Lai, P.B.S. Factors associated with failure of enhanced recovery protocol in patients undergoing major hepatobiliary and pancreatic surgery: A retrospective cohort study. *BMJ Open* **2014**, *4*, e005330. [CrossRef]
45. Velthuis, M.J.; Agasi-Idenburg, S.C.; Aufdemkampe, G.; Wittink, H.M. The effect of physical exercise on cancer-related fatigue during cancer treatment: A meta-analysis of randomised controlled trials. *Clin. Oncol.* **2010**, *22*, 208–221. [CrossRef]
46. Knols, R.; Aaronson, N.K.; Uebelhart, D.; Fransen, J.; Aufdemkampe, G. Physical exercise in cancer patients during and after medical treatment: A systematic review of randomized and controlled clinical trials. *J. Clin. Oncol.* **2005**, *23*, 3830–3842. [CrossRef]
47. Beaver, K.; Williamson, S.; Briggs, J. Exploring patient experiences of neo-adjuvant chemotherapy for breast cancer. *Eur. J. Oncol. Nurs.* **2015**, *20*, 77–86. [CrossRef]
48. Ganz, P.A.; Desmond, K.A.; Leedham, B.; Rowland, J.H.; Meyerowitz, B.E.; Belin, T.R. Quality of life in long-term, disease-free survivors of breast cancer: A follow-up study. *J. Natl. Cancer Inst.* **2002**, *94*, 39–49. [CrossRef]
49. Magno, S.; Carnevale, S.; Dentale, F.; Belella, D.; Linardos, M.; Masetti, R. Neo-Adjuvant chemotherapy and distress in breast cancer patients: The moderating role of generalized self-efficacy. *J. Clin. Oncol.* **2017**, *35* (Suppl. 15), e21570. [CrossRef]
50. Gil, F.; Grassi, L.; Travado, L.; Tomamichel, M.; Gonzalez, J.R.; Zanotti, P.; Lluch, P.; Hollenstein, M.F.; Maté, J.; Magnani, K.; et al. Use of distress and depression thermometers to measure psychosocial morbidity among southern European cancer patients. *Support Care Cancer* **2005**, *13*, 600–606. [CrossRef]
51. Zigmond, A.S.; Snaith, R.P. The hospital anxiety and depression scale. *Acta Psychiatr. Scand.* **1983**, *67*, 361–370. [CrossRef] [PubMed]

52. Luszczynska, A.; Scholz, U.; Schwarzer, R. The general self-efficacy scale: Multicultural validation studie. *J. Psychol. Interdiscip. Appl.* **2005**, *139*, 439–457. [CrossRef]
53. Magno, S.; Filippone, A.; Scaldaferri, A. Evidence-Based usefulness of integrative therapies in breast cancer. *Transl. Cancer Res.* **2018**, *7*, S379–S389. [CrossRef]
54. Maunsell, E.; Drolet, M.; Brisson, J.; Robert, J.; Deschênes, L. Dietary change after breast cancer: Extent, predictors, and relation with psychological distress. *J. Clin. Oncol.* **2002**, *20*, 1017–1025. [CrossRef]
55. Ozier, A.D.; Kendrick, O.W.; Leeper, J.D.; Knol, L.L.; Perko, M.; Burnham, J. Overweight and obesity are associated with emotion and stress—Related eating as measured by the eating and appraisal due to emotions and stress questionnaire. *J. Am. Diet. Assoc.* **2008**, *108*, 49–56. [CrossRef]
56. Greenlee, H.; DuPont-Reyes, M.J.; Balneaves, L.G.; Carlson, L.E.; Cohen, M.R.; Deng, G.; Johnson, J.A.; Mumber, M.; Seely, D.; Zick, S.M.; et al. Clinical practice guidelines on the evidence-based use of integrative therapies during and after breast cancer treatment. *CA Cancer J. Clin.* **2017**, *67*, 194–232. [CrossRef]
57. Zia, F.Z.; Olaku, O.; Bao, T.; Berger, A.; Deng, G.; Fan, A.Y.; Garcia, M.K.; Herman, P.M.; Kaptchuk, T.J.; Ladas, E.J.; et al. The national cancer institute's conference on acupuncture for symptom management in oncology: State of the science, evidence, and research gaps. *J. Natl. Cancer Inst. Monogr.* **2017**, *2017*, 68–73. [CrossRef]
58. Mao, J.J.; Bowman, M.A.; Xie, S.X.; Bruner, D.; De Michele, A.; Farrar, J.T. Electroacupuncture versus gabapentin for hot flashes among breast cancer survivors: A randomized placebo-controlled trial. *J. Clin. Oncol.* **2015**, *33*, 3615–3620. [CrossRef]
59. Lesi, G.; Razzini, G.; Musti, M.A.; Stivanello, E.; Petrucci, C.; Benedetti, B.; Rondini, E.; Ligabue, M.B.; Scaltriti, L.; Botti, A.; et al. Acupuncture as an integrative approach for the treatment of hot flashes in women with breast cancer: A prospective multicenter randomized controlled trial (AcCliMaT). *J. Clin. Oncol.* **2016**, *34*, 1795–1802. [CrossRef]
60. Ju, Z.Y.; Wang, K.; Cui, H.S.; Yao, Y.; Liu, S.M.; Zhou, J.; Chen, T.Y.; Xia, J. Acupuncture for neuropathic pain in adults. *Cochrane Database Syst. Rev.* **2017**, *2017*, CD012057. [CrossRef]
61. Wardley, A.M.; Ryder, D.; Misra, V.; Hall, P.S.; Mackereth, P.; Stringer, J. ACUFOCIN: Randomized clinical trial of ACUpuncture plus standard care versus standard care alone FOr chemotherapy induced peripheral neuropathy (CIPN). *J. Clin. Oncol.* **2020**, *38* (Suppl. 15), 12003. [CrossRef]
62. Molassiotis, A.; Suen, L.K.P.; Cheng, H.L.; Mok, T.S.K.; Lee, S.C.Y.; Wang, C.H.; Lee, P.; Leung, H.; Chan, V.; Lau, T.K.H.; et al. A randomized assessor-blinded wait-list-controlled trial to assess the effectiveness of acupuncture in the management of chemotherapy-induced peripheral neuropathy. *Integr. Cancer Ther.* **2019**, *18*. [CrossRef]
63. Bao, T.; Patil, S.; Chen, C.; Zhi, I.W.; Li, Q.S.; Piulson, L.; Mao, J.J. Effect of acupuncture vs sham procedure on chemotherapy—Induced peripheral neuropathy symptoms: A randomized clinical trial. *JAMA Netw. Open* **2020**, *3*, e200681. [CrossRef]
64. Jordan, B.; Margulies, A.; Cardoso, F.; Cavaletti, G.; Haugnes, H.S.; Jahn, P.; Le Rhun, E.; Preusser, M.; Scotté, F.; Taphoorn, M.J.B.; et al. Systemic anticancer therapy-induced peripheral and central neurotoxicity: ESMO–EONS–EANO clinical practice guidelines for diagnosis, prevention, treatment and follow-up. *Ann. Oncol.* **2020**, *31*, 1306–1319. [CrossRef]
65. Hoffman, C.J.; Ersser, S.J.; Hopkinson, J.B.; Nicholls, P.G.; Harrington, J.E.; Thomas, P.W. Effectiveness of mindfulness-based stress reduction in mood, breast-and endocrine-related quality of life, and well-being in stage 0 to III breast cancer: A randomized, controlled trial. *J. Clin. Oncol.* **2012**, *30*, 1335–1342. [CrossRef]
66. Henderson, V.P.; Clemow, L.; Massion, A.O.; Hurley, T.G.; Druker, S.; Hébert, J.R. The effects of mindfulness-based stress reduction on psychosocial outcomes and quality of life in early-stage breast cancer patients: A randomized trial. *Breast Cancer Res. Treat.* **2012**, *131*, 99–109. [CrossRef]
67. Lerman, R.; Jarski, R.; Rea, H.; Gellish, R.; Vicini, F. Improving symptoms and quality of life of female cancer survivors: A randomized controlled study. *Ann. Surg. Oncol.* **2012**, *19*, 373–378. [CrossRef]
68. Gross, C.R.; Kreitzer, M.J.; Reilly-Spong, M.; Wall, M.; Winbush, N.Y.; Patterson, R.; Mahowald, M.; Cramer-Bornemann, M. Mindfulness-Based stress reduction versus pharmacotherapy for chronic primary insomnia: A randomized controlled clinical trial. *Explor. J. Sci. Heal.* **2011**, *7*, 76–87. [CrossRef]
69. Shapiro, S.L.; Bootzin, R.R.; Figueredo, A.J.; Lopez, A.M.; Schwartz, G.E. The efficacy of mindfulness-based stress reduction in the treatment of sleep disturbance in women with breast cancer. An exploratory study. *J. Psychosom. Res.* **2003**, *54*, 85–91. [CrossRef]
70. Carlson, L.E.; Garland, S.N. Impact of mindfulness-based stress reduction (MBSR) on sleep, mood, stress and fatigue symptoms in cancer outpatients. *Int. J. Behav. Med.* **2005**, *12*, 278–285. [CrossRef]
71. Carlson, L.E.; Speca, M.; Patel, K.D.; Goodey, E. Mindfulness-Based stress reduction in relation to quality of life, mood, symptoms of stress, and immune parameters in breast and prostate cancer outpatients. *Psychosom. Med.* **2003**, *65*, 571–581. [CrossRef]
72. Würtzen, H.; Dalton, S.O.; Elsass, P.; Sumbundu, A.D.; Steding-Jensen, M.; Karlsen, R.V.; Andersen, K.K.; Flyger, H.L.; Pedersen, A.E.; Johansen, C. Mindfulness significantly reduces self-reported levels of anxiety and depression: Results of a randomised controlled trial among 336 Danish women treated for stage I–III breast cancer. *Eur. J. Cancer* **2013**, *49*, 1365–1373. [CrossRef]

73. Lengacher, C.A.; Reich, R.R.; Paterson, C.L.; Ramesar, S.; Park, J.Y.; Alinat, C.; Johnson-Mallard, V.; Moscoso, M.; Budhrani-Shani, P.; Miladinovic, B.; et al. Examination of broad symptom improvement resulting from mindfulness-based stress reduction in breast cancer survivors: A randomized controlled trial. *J. Clin. Oncol.* **2016**, *34*, 2827–2834. [CrossRef]
74. Andersen, S.R.; Würtzen, H.; Steding-Jessen, M.; Christensen, J.; Andersen, K.K.; Flyger, H.; Mitchelmore, C.; Johansen, C.; Dalton, S.O. Effect of mindfulness-based stress reduction on sleep quality: Results of a randomized trial among Danish breast cancer patients. *Acta Oncol.* **2013**, *52*, 336–344. [CrossRef] [PubMed]

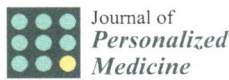

Article

Conventional CT versus Dedicated CT Angiography in DIEP Flap Planning: A Feasibility Study

Anna D'Angelo [1,*,†], Alessandro Cina [1,†], Giulia Macrì [2], Paolo Belli [1], Sara Mercogliano [1], Pierluigi Barbieri [1], Cristina Grippo [3], Gianluca Franceschini [4], Sabatino D'Archi [4], Elena Jane Mason [4], Giuseppe Visconti [2], Liliana Barone Adesi [2], Marzia Salgarello [2] and Riccardo Manfredi [1]

1. Dipartimento di Diagnostica per Immagini, Radioterapia Oncologica ed Ematologia, Fondazione Policlinico Universitario Agostino Gemelli IRCCS, 00168 Rome, Italy; alessandro.cina@policlinicogemelli.it (A.C.); paolo.belli@policlinicogemelli.it (P.B.); saramercogliano90@gmail.com (S.M.); pierluigi.barb@gmail.com (P.B.); riccardo.manfredi@policlinicogemelli.it (R.M.)
2. Divisione di Chirurgia Plastica, Dipartimento di Scienze della Salute della Donna e del Bambino e di Sanità Pubblica, Fondazione Policlinico Universitario Agostino Gemelli IRCCS, 00168 Rome, Italy; giulia.macri@live.com (G.M.); joevisconti@hotmail.com (G.V.); lbaroneadesi@libero.it (L.B.A.); marzia.salgarello@gmail.com (M.S.)
3. Dipartimento di Diagnostica per Immagini, Radiologia Terapeutica ed Interventistica, Azienda Ospedaliera Santa Maria Terni, 05100 Terni, Italy; cris.grippo@gmail.com
4. Centro Integrato di Senologia, Dipartimento di Scienze della Salute della Donna e del Bambino e di Sanità Pubblica, Fondazione Policlinico Universitario Agostino Gemelli IRCCS, 00168 Rome, Italy; gianlucafranceschini70@gmail.com (G.F.); sabatinodarchi@gmail.com (S.D.); elenajanemason@gmail.com (E.J.M.)
* Correspondence: anna.dangelo05@gmail.com; Tel.: +39-393-287-314-720
† These authors have contributed equally to this work.

Citation: D'Angelo, A.; Cina, A.; Macrì, G.; Belli, P.; Mercogliano, S.; Barbieri, P.; Grippo, C.; Franceschini, G.; D'Archi, S.; Mason, E.J.; et al. Conventional CT versus Dedicated CT Angiography in DIEP Flap Planning: A Feasibility Study. *J. Pers. Med.* **2021**, *11*, 277. https://doi.org/10.3390/jpm11040277

Academic Editor: Hisham Fansa

Received: 22 February 2021
Accepted: 31 March 2021
Published: 7 April 2021

Publisher's Note: MDPI stays neutral with regard to jurisdictional claims in published maps and institutional affiliations.

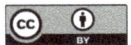

Copyright: © 2021 by the authors. Licensee MDPI, Basel, Switzerland. This article is an open access article distributed under the terms and conditions of the Creative Commons Attribution (CC BY) license (https://creativecommons.org/licenses/by/4.0/).

Abstract: The deep inferior epigastric perforator (DIEP) flap is used with increasing frequency in post-mastectomy breast reconstruction. Preoperative mapping with CT angiography (CTa) is crucial in reducing surgical complications and optimizing surgical techniques. Our study's goal was to investigate the accuracy of conventional CT (cCT), performed during disease staging, compared to CTa in preoperative DIEP flap planning. In this retrospective, single-center study, we enrolled patients scheduled for mastectomy and DIEP flap breast reconstruction, subjected to cCT within 24 months after CTa. We included 35 patients in the study. cCT accuracy was 95% (CI 0.80–0.98) in assessing the three largest perforators, 100% (CI 0.89–100) in assessing the dominant perforator, 93% (CI 0.71–0.94) in assessing the perforator intramuscular course, and 90.6% (CI 0.79–0.98) in assessing superficial venous communications. Superficial inferior epigastric artery (SIEA) caliber was recognized in 90% of cases (CI 0.84–0.99), with an excellent assessment of superficial inferior epigastric vein (SIEV) integrity (96% of cases, CI 0.84–0.99), and a lower accuracy in the evaluation of deep inferior epigastric artery (DIEA) branching type (85% of cases, CI 0.69–0.93). The mean X-ray dose spared would have been 788 ± 255 mGy/cm. Our study shows that cCT is as accurate as CTa in DIEP flap surgery planning.

Keywords: breast cancer; conventional CT and CT angiography; DIEP flap planning

1. Introduction

The deep inferior epigastric perforator (DIEP) flap is, nowadays, considered the "gold standard" in autologous breast reconstruction [1]. Subcutaneous tissue and skin are transferred from the abdomen to the thorax in order to guarantee a more natural appearance of the reconstructed breast, compared to heterologous approach [2,3] (Figures 1 and 2). A low donor site morbidity with an aesthetical abdomen improvement is an important factor for choosing DIEP flap in autologous breast reconstruction. The inconsistent anatomy of the abdominal perforators leads to a more challenging and time-consuming technique compared to a (muscle sparing) Transverse Rectus Abdominis Muscle (TRAM) flap [4,5].

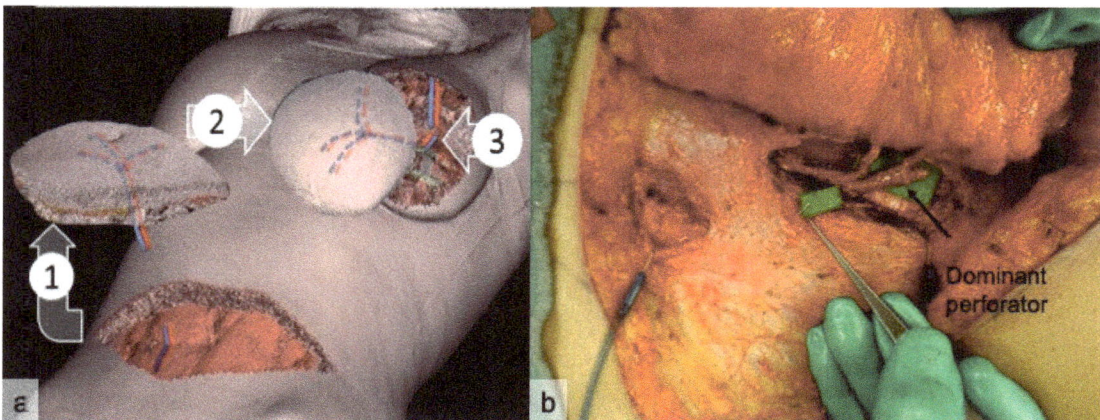

Figure 1. Three-dimensional graphic illustration of a DIEP (deep inferior epigastric perforator) flap procedure (**a**). In 1, skin and fat, with the perforating vascular pedicle from the deep inferior epigastric artery, are dissected from the abdominal wall; in 2 the flap is sized to reconstruct the breast; in 3 the internal mammary vessels are anastomosed to the vascular pedicle of the flap. (**b**) A surgical view of a DIEP dissection. The rectus abdominis is dissected with its fascia to isolate the inferior epigastric pedicle with its dominant perforator (arrow). Microgrid was employed to measure perforator caliber.

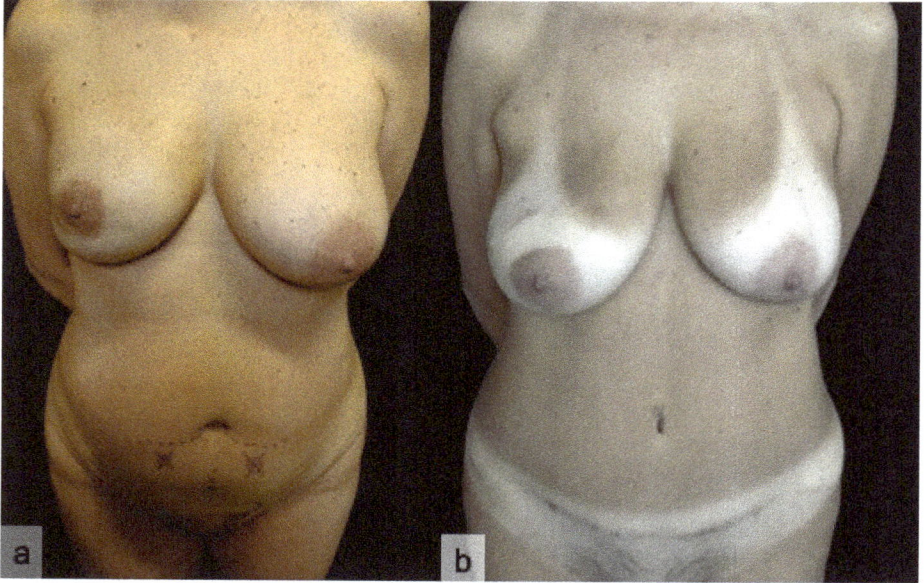

Figure 2. Preoperative planning (**a**) of a DIEP flap reconstruction for right breast carcinoma, requiring nipple-sparing mastectomy. Eight-month postoperative result (**b**).

Preoperative planning is crucial [6] in order to identify perforator vessels originating from the deep inferior epigastric vascular system, and to evaluate superficial inferior epigastric vessels. DIEP flap survival depends on adequate blood supply, which is guaranteed by perforator vessels that are amply variable in terms of number, anatomical location, intramuscular course, caliber, and tortuosity. Preoperative assessment includes visualization of the deep inferior epigastric artery (DIEA) and evaluation of its intramuscular course and branching pattern. The latter is described by Taylor's classification, which defines three types of DIEA branching above the arcuate line: in type I the artery ascends as a single intramuscular vessel; in type II, the artery divides, at the arcuate line, into two vessels with an intramuscular course; in type III, the artery divides, at the arcuate line, into three vessels with an intramuscular course [7].

The DIEA originates from the external iliac artery, above the inguinal ligament, and crosses the lateral margin of the rectus abdominis muscle 3–4 cm below the arcuate line, with an average pedicle length of 10.3 cm and an average vessel diameter of 3.6 mm [8]. It then normally divides into two branches, lateral and medial; in case of a central course (28%), multiple small branches with centrally located perforators can be detected [9].

Perforators arise on each side of the midline from the anterior rectus fascia in a central rectangular area, which extends craniocaudally from 2 cm above to 6 cm below the umbilicus, and laterally between 1 cm and 6 cm from the midline. A thorough preoperative anatomical study also allows an assessment of the communications between the superficial and deep systems. The caliber of the superficial inferior epigastric artery (SIEA) should be compared to that of the dominant perforator, in order to select the best pedicle for the flap. In addition, assessing the integrity of the superficial inferior epigastric veins (SIEVs) could be helpful, in case of a flap additional venous discharge requirement [8].

Different perforator locations are associated with a harder or easier dissection, and sometimes lead to extensive splitting of the muscle; compared to lateral vessels, medial perforators offer better flap perfusion but a harder dissection due to a long intramuscular course. Perforator dissection is carried out along the deep inferior epigastric pedicle up to its origin from the external iliac artery. The DIEP flap should be adapted and shaped to the single patient and type of breast reconstruction, with an optimized anatomical preoperative study that allows the identification of personal anatomical characteristics in order to accelerate dissection and flap harvesting, as well as to avoid vascularization deficiencies. An accurate preoperative planning with evaluation of single anatomical variants allows a decrease in decrease operating time and theatre utilization, with a consequent benefit in terms of surgical waiting lists and staff optimization.

Among the available imaging techniques, which include Magnetic Resonance Imaging (MRI) and color-Doppler ultrasound (US) [3,10], Computed Tomography Angiography (CTa), with the injection of contrast medium, has become the gold standard in planning surgery [11,12] thanks to its ability to map out the vascular anatomy and, consequently, select the best DIEP flap to harvest. Its high accuracy has been proved in studies performed, both on cadavers [8] and post-surgery. CTa also allows 3D surface and vascular tree-rendering [9], which can bring huge benefits to cross-sectional imaging and represents a valid visual tool for surgeons. The primary role of CTa in preoperative assessment is, therefore, motivated by its wide availability, fast acquisition time, high reproducibility, and great sensitivity in the identification of perforator vessels with calibers larger than 1mm. Still, CTa is associated with possible complications, such as allergic reactions to contrast medium, nephrotoxicity in patients with impaired renal function, and exposure to ionizing radiation in patients often already subjected to multiple CT scans to stage primary breast cancer [13].

Our goal was to investigate the accuracy of conventional CT (cCT), performed during breast cancer disease staging, compared to CTa in obtaining information required for DIEP flap surgical planning. We evaluated the accuracy of both techniques in identifying "dominant" perforator arteries, measuring their caliber and intramuscular course length, assessing superficial venous communications (SVC) and DIEA branching type according to Taylor's classification, identifying the caliber of SIEA, and assessing SIEV integrity. In addition, the total X-ray dose that could have been potentially spared by avoiding CTa was evaluated.

2. Materials and Methods

From January 2010 to February 2019, 344 patients programmed to receive mastectomies with immediate or delayed DIEP flap reconstruction, referred to our Institute, were enrolled in the study. Inclusion criteria were: cCT performed during disease staging with standardized technique (slice thickness of 1.25 mm in the portal venous-phase) in our Institution within 24 months after CTa. Exclusion criteria were: abdominal surgery between the two examinations or cCT performed in other Institutions.

This retrospective single-center study was conducted according to the guidelines of the Declaration of Helsinki, and approved by the Institutional Review Board and Ethics Committee of Fondazione Policlinico Universitario Agostino Gemelli IRCCS on 11 June 2020. Anyone involved in the research agreed to participate and agreed to have the results of the research about them published.

2.1. CTa and cCT Technique

CTa and cCT were performed using a 64-slice multidetector CT (LightSpeed VCT, GE Healthcare, Waukeska, WI, USA), table travel per rotation was 23 mm (gantry rotation time 0.4 s) and field of view (FOV) was 40 cm in order to match patient width, matrix side 512 × 512. Tube voltage was 120 kVp, with Smart mAs (GE Healthcare) dose enabled (noise index set to 22). For CTa, the arterial-phase images were acquired at a 0.65 mm slice thickness; to minimize radiation exposure, a small field of view (FOV), which only includes the area of interest, is scanned: from the origin of the inferior epigastric artery at the level of the groin to a level approximately 3 cm above the umbilicus in a caudal-cranial direction. We administered, intravenously, 100 mL of iodinated contrast medium (Ultravist, Bayer Schering Pharma AG, Berlin, Germany) with a concentration of 370 mgL/mL (18-G cannula) at 4 mL/s flow rate, followed by 60 mL saline flush. A large-gauge (18 G) peripheral intravenous line was preferred to allow rapid infusion of contrast (4–5 mL/s) and, thus, an optimal opacification of small epigastric vessels. The arterial peak of enhancement was captured using bolus tracking (Smart Prep, GE Healthcare, Wuakuesha, WI, USA), so as to begin image acquisition upon the contrast medium arrival in the region of interest (ROI) on the common femoral artery; acquisition should be obtained with a minimum possible delay after contrast arrival is detected, with blood attenuation within ROI of 100–120 Hounsfield units (HU). During the exam, since a whole scan can be accomplished in one held breath, and the effect of breathing motion on the abdomen and pelvis may be relevant, patients are required to hold their breath and are supine, with their arms placed according to the programmed sugery (upwards for immediate breast reconstruction, downwards in case of delayed reconstruction).

For cCT, the venous-phase images were acquired at a 1.25 mm slice thickness, in cranio-caudal direction, with patients in a supine position with their arms lying upwards. Following our department's routine for oncologic staging cCT, 1.6 mL/kg of contrast medium (Ultravist 370 mgL/mL) was administered to patients at a rate of 3 mL/s, followed by 40 mL of saline solution at the same injection rate. The scan delay was empirically chosen at 70 s.

2.2. Image Analysis

Two radiologists with specific experience in flap surgery imaging reviewed, respectively, the cCT and aCT exams to assess the diagnostic accuracy of cCT in identifying: the main perforators, the "dominant" perforator, and the perforation site of the rectus abdominal fascia using volumetric reconstructions. The errors on x and y virtual coordinates were then calculated (Figure 3). The reader also evaluated the course of the dominant perforator, assigning a value from 1 to 4 ("1" extramuscular, "2" intramuscular for a length <2 cm, "3" <4 cm and "4" >4 cm); the branching of the DIEA according to Taylor's classification (Figure 4); the caliber of the SIEA compared to the dominant perforator (from 1 to 3, "1" <dominant, "2" =dominant, "3" >dominant) (Figure 5); the integrity of the SIEV (from 1 to 3, "1" intact, "2" attracted, "3" interrupted); and the presence of superficial venous communications between the right and left hemi-abdomen ("0" if absent, "1" scarce, "2" moderate, "3" clearly evident) (Figure 6).

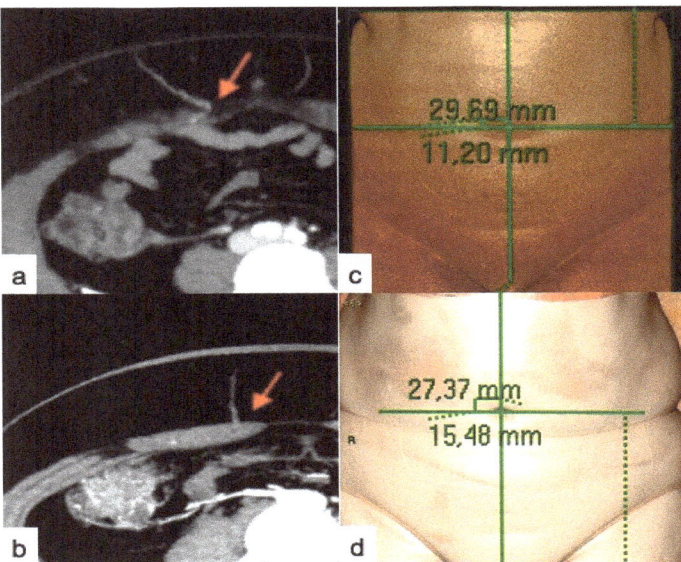

Figure 3. Dominant perforator's emergence from the anterior rectus abdominis fascia (red arrows) in cCT (**a**) and CTa (**b**) axial sub-volume maximum intensity projection (MIP) reconstructions. Images (**c**,**d**) show mapping of the dominant perforator on a VR reconstruction of the abdominal surface via a virtual coordinate system centered on a zero point, corresponding to the umbilicus in cCT (**c**) and CTa (**d**).

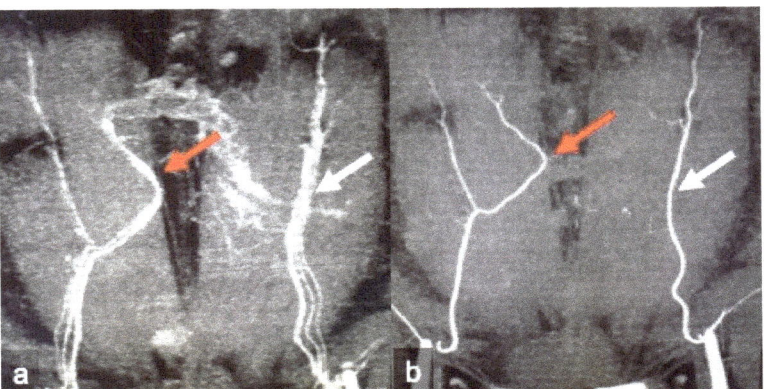

Figure 4. Identification of the deep inferior epigastric artery branching according to Taylor's classification. cCT (**a**) and CTa (**b**) oblique-coronal sub-volume maximum intensity projection reconstruction (MIP) of the superficial abdominal wall revealed a bifurcated artery on the right hemi-abdomen (red arrows) and a single on the left (white arrows).

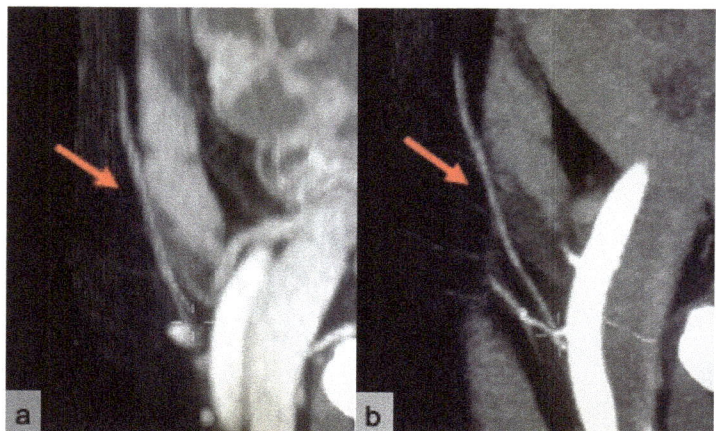

Figure 5. Assessment of the SIEA caliber compared to the dominant perforator. cCT (**a**) and CTa (**b**) sub-volume sagittal MIP reconstructions show a SIEA (red arrows) with a 2 score (equal to the dominant perforator).

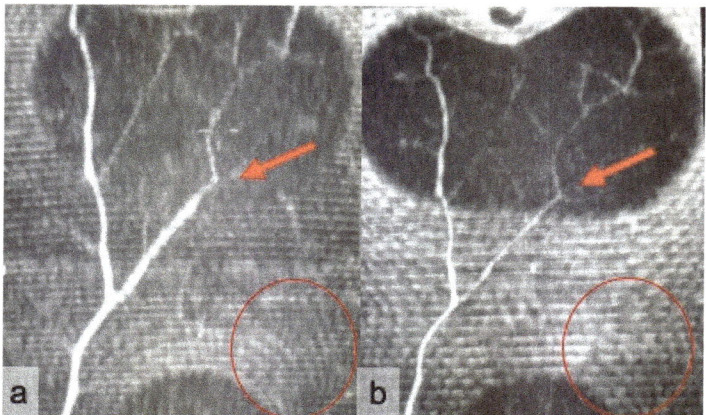

Figure 6. Assessment of superficial venous communications running between the right and left portion of the abdomen. Coronal sub-volume maximum intensity projection (MIP) reconstructions of the superficial abdominal wall for cCT (**a**) and CTa (**b**) show a large venous trunk on the right hemi-abdomen (red arrows), with a 3 score. Superficial inferior epigastric vein integrity was absent on the left (red circles).

2.3. Statistical Analysis

A Shapiro–Wilk test was employed to assess the parametric vs nonparametric distribution of variables. Continuous variables were described by mean and standard deviation. The accuracy of cCT was tested, with CTa employed as a standard of reference. Confidence intervals were reported at 95%. For inferential statistics, a Student t-test and Wilcoxon rank–sum test were employed, respectively, for parametric and nonparametric variables. Setting a type II error $(1 - \beta)$ of 0.9 and a Type I error rate of 0.05, and assuming as clinically relevant a 0.9 accuracy of the cCT vs. CTa, a sample size of 35 patients was needed.

3. Results

We enrolled 35 patients with a mean age of 40 years (range 27–73 years) and a mean BMI of 25,2 kg/m² (range 21.2–32.3). No statistically significant differences were observed in patient characteristics. The accuracy of cCT in assessing the three largest perforators was 95% (CI 0.80–0.98). The dominant perforator was identified by cCT in all cases (100%, CI 0.89–100). cCT correctly identified the perforator intramuscular course in 93% of cases (CI 0.71–0.94) and the superficial venous communications in 90.6% of patients (CI 0.79–0.98). The SIEA caliber was correctly assessed by cCT in 90% of cases (CI 0.84–0.99). cCT was less accurate in the evaluation of DIEA branching type (85% of cases, CI 0.69–0.93), but had an excellent assessment of the integrity of SIEV (96% of cases, CI 0.84–0.99). The mean error in topographic localization was 4.8 ± 3.8 mm along the Y axis and 2.6 ± 3.8 mm along the X axis. If CTa had been spared before surgery, relying on cCT for DIEP planning, the mean X-ray dose potentially avoided would have been 788 ± 255 mGy/cm. Data reported are shown in Table 1.

Table 1. Performance of cCT versus CTa.

Items	%	CI
3 largest perforators	95%	0.80–0.98
Dominant perforator	100%	0.89–100
Perforator intramuscular course	93%	0.71–0.94
Superficial venous communications	90.6%	0.79–0.98
DIEA branching type	85%	0.69–0.93
SIEA calibre	90%	0.84–0.99
Integrity of SIEV	96%	0.84–0.99

4. Discussion

The results of our study show that cCT, performed routinely during breast cancer disease staging, is as accurate as CTa in obtaining information required for DIEP flap planning. CTa, first described by Rozen in 2008 [8], has been suggested as the gold standard in preoperative assessment of perforating vessels. Other modalities, such as MRI [14] and color-Doppler US, have been compared to CTa. Preoperative breast MRI performed for breast malignancy characterization can be extended to the lower abdomen, but still allows visualization and localization of only some of the perforator vessels, as it possesses a lower spatial resolution compared to CT angiography [15]. The prone position required to perform breast MRI modifies the natural anatomy of the abdomen, and, together with artefacts due to respiratory movements and enhanced vascular assessment, constitutes a limitation to using MRI, as reported in our previous study [11]. Color-Doppler US, though it offers a more accurate spatial resolution than CTa, is an operator dependent procedure and requires advanced training to obtain a satisfying mapping of perforators [16]. To our knowledge, no previous studies investigated the role of CTa versus cCT. Our results show an excellent diagnostic accuracy of cCT in identifying the three largest perforators, the perforator intramuscular course, SCVs, the dominant perforator, SIEA caliber, and SIEV integrity. cCT was less accurate in the evaluation of DIEA branching type, probably because of lower contrast resolution during the venous phase, different contrast medium injection speed, and the cranial-caudal direction of acquisition. The mean error in topographic localization of the dominant perforator was 4.8 ± 3.8 mm along the Y axis and 2.6 ± 3.8 mm along the X axis, probably because of the different arm position in delayed surgical reconstruction and the presence of clothes (knickers) when the cCT is performed. Results from both techniques were compared with intraoperative findings: all preoperatively assessed dominant perforators were confirmed intraoperatively, without significant differences in terms of expected position.

Our study suggests that performing cCT alone, in the preoperative assessment of DIEP-flap candidates, is safe and feasible. Furthermore, everyday clinical practice could benefit from the adoption of this technique in several ways: preoperative assessment is faster without the necessity of programming a CTa exam; there is also the matter of reduced healthcare costs and patient discomfort, both in terms of psychological stress and x-ray or contrast medium exposure. This evidence is particularly significant when dealing with patients who are already exposed, because of their underlying disease, to multiple CT examinations. If CTa had been withheld before surgery, relying on cCT alone for DIEP planning, the patient would have been spared a mean X-ray dose of 788 ± 255 mGy/cm. Furthermore, this technique is easily applicable to most centers around the world, including facilities without access to CTa, as it does not require a dedicated acquisition protocol or a radiologist specialized in vascular anatomy.

Our study has some limitations, the major of which being that we could not assess interobserver variability between CTa and cCT because only one experienced radiologist was present for each method. Furthermore, DIEP flap procedure total surgical time was not taken into account in this study, although it was widely analyzed in our previous manuscript [3].

5. Conclusions

We found that cCT, although not intentionally performed for preoperative surgical assessment, nonetheless provided an accurate visualization of the best perforator and of the main abdominal vessels involved in DIEP planning, thus, overcoming the limits of US in terms of reproducibility and operator dependence, and of MRI in terms of spatial resolution, costs, and artifacts related to the prone position. In this way, patients scheduled for DIEP flap surgery with a recent cCT could avoid further assessment with CTa. In conclusion, in order to strongly reduce radiation exposure, time, and costs in DIEP flap planning, a previous recent cCT may be a valuable option due to high concordance with CTa findings.

Author Contributions: Conceptualization, A.C., A.D. and G.M.; methodology, P.B. (Paolo Belli); software, S.D.; validation, R.M., M.S. and G.F.; formal analysis, E.J.M. and C.G.; investigation, S.M.; resources, P.B. (Pierluigi Barbieri); data curation, L.B.A. and G.V.; writing—original draft preparation, A.D., G.M., C.G. and A.C.; writing—review and editing, E.J.M., S.D.; visualization, S.M.; supervision, A.C.; project administration, R.M. All authors have read and agreed to the published version of the manuscript.

Funding: This research received no external funding.

Institutional Review Board Statement: The study was conducted according to the guidelines of the Declaration of Helsinki, and approved by the Institutional Review Board and Ethics Committee of Fondazione Policlinico Universitario Agostino Gemelli IRCCS; Università Cattolica del Sacro Cuore, Rome, Italy.

Informed Consent Statement: Informed consent was obtained from all subjects involved in the study.

Data Availability Statement: The data presented in the study are available on request from the corresponding author.

Conflicts of Interest: The authors declare no conflict of interest.

References

1. Munhoz, A.M.; Arruda, E.; Montag, E.; Aldrighi, C.; Aldrighi, J.M.; Gemperli, R.; Ferreira, M.C. Immediate skin-sparing mastectomy reconstruction with deep inferior epigastric perforator (DIEP) flap: Technical aspects and outcome. *Breast J.* **2007**, *13*, 470–478. [CrossRef] [PubMed]
2. Ireton, J.E.; Lakhiani, C.; Saint-Cyr, M. Vascular anatomy of the deep inferior epigastric artery perforator flap: A systematic review. *Plast. Reconstr. Surg.* **2014**, *134*, 810e–821e. [CrossRef] [PubMed]
3. Cina, A.; Salgarello, M.; Barone-Adesi, L.; Rinaldi, P.; Bonomo, L. Planning breast reconstruction with deep inferior epigastric artery perforating vessels: Multidetector CT angiography versus color Doppler US. *Radiology* **2010**, *255*, 979–987. [CrossRef] [PubMed]
4. Allen, R.J. Comparison of the costs of DIEP and TRAM flaps. *Plast. Reconstr. Surg.* **2001**, *108*, 2165. [CrossRef] [PubMed]
5. Kaplan, J.L.; Allen, R.J. Cost-based comparison between perforator flaps and TRAM flaps for breast reconstruction. *Plast. Reconstr. Surg.* **2000**, *105*, 943–948. [CrossRef] [PubMed]

6. Tønseth, K.A.; Hokland, B.M.; Tindholdt, T.T.; Abyholm, F.E.; Stavem, K. Quality of life, patient satisfaction and cosmetic outcome after breast reconstruction using DIEP flap or expandable breast implant. *J. Plast. Reconstr. Aesthet. Surg.* **2008**, *61*, 1188–1194. [CrossRef] [PubMed]
7. Taylor, G.I.; Hamdy, H.; El-Mrakby, H.H.; Milner, R.H. Vascular anatomy of the lower anterior abdominal wall: A microdissection study on the deep inferior epigastric vessels and the perforator branches. *Plast. Reconstr. Surg.* **2002**, *109*, 544.
8. Rozen, W.M.; Ashton, M.W.; Stella, D.L.; Phillips, T.J.; Taylor, G.I. The accuracy of computed tomographic angiography for mapping the perforators of the DIEA: A cadaveric study. *Plast. Reconstr. Surg.* **2008**, *122*, 363–369. [CrossRef] [PubMed]
9. Gacto-Sánchez, P.; Sicilia-Castro, D.; Gómez-Cía, T.; Lagares, A.; Collell, T.; Suárez, C.; Parra, C.; Infante-Cossío, P.; De La Higuera, J.M. Use of a Three-Dimensional Virtual Reality Model for Preoperative Imaging in DIEP Flap Breast Reconstruction. *J. Surg. Res.* **2010**, *162*, 140–147. [CrossRef] [PubMed]
10. Giunta, R.E.; Geisweid, A.; Feller, A.M. The value of preoperative doppler sonography for planning free perforator flaps. *Plast. Reconstr. Surg.* **2000**, *105*, 2381–2386. [CrossRef] [PubMed]
11. Cina, A.; Barone-Adesi, L.; Rinaldi, P.; Cipriani, A.; Salgarello, M.; Masetti, R.; Bonomo, L. Planning deep inferior epigastric perforator flaps for breast reconstruction: A comparison between multidetector computed tomography and magnetic resonance angiography. *Eur. Radiol.* **2013**, *23*, 2333–2343. [CrossRef] [PubMed]
12. Casey, W.J., III; Chew, R.T.; Rebecca, A.M.; Smith, A.A.; Collins, J.M.; Pockaj, B.A. Advantages of preoperative computed tomography in deep inferior epigastric artery perforator flap breast reconstruction. *Plast. Reconstr. Surg.* **2009**, *123*, 1148–1155. [CrossRef] [PubMed]
13. McMillan, K.; Bostani, M.; Cagnon, C.H.; Yu, L.; Leng, S.; McCollough, C.H.; McNitt-Gray, M.F. Estimating patient dose from CT exams that use automatic exposure control: Development and validation of methods to accurately estimate tube current values. *Med. Phys.* **2017**, *44*, 4262–4275. [CrossRef] [PubMed]
14. Schaverien, M.; Ludman, C.; Neil-Dwyer, J.; Perks, G.B.; Akhtar, N.; Rodrigues, J.N.; Benetatos, K.; Raurell, A.; Rasheed, T.; McCulley, S.J.; et al. Contrast-Enhanced magnetic resonance angiography for preoperative imaging in DIEP flap breast reconstruction. *Plast. Reconstr. Surg.* **2011**, *128*, 56–62. [CrossRef] [PubMed]
15. Rozen, W.M.; Stella, D.L.; Bowden, J.; Taylor, G.I.; Ashton, M.W. Advances in the pre-operative planning of deep inferior epigastric artery perforator flaps: Magnetic resonance angiography. *Microsurgery* **2009**, *29*, 119–123. [CrossRef] [PubMed]
16. Klasson, S.; Svensson, H.; Malm, K.; Wassélius, J.; Velander, P. Preoperative CT angiography versus Doppler ultrasound mapping of abdominal perforator in DIEP breast reconstructions: A randomized prospective study. *J. Plast. Reconstr. Aesthet. Surg.* **2015**, *68*, 782–786. [CrossRef] [PubMed]

Article

Development of a Digital Research Assistant for the Management of Patients' Enrollment in Oncology Clinical Trials within a Research Hospital

Alfredo Cesario [1], Irene Simone [1], Ida Paris [2], Luca Boldrini [3], Armando Orlandi [4], Gianluca Franceschini [5], Filippo Lococo [6], Emilio Bria [4], Stefano Magno [7], Antonino Mulè [5], Angela Santoro [5], Andrea Damiani [3], Daniele Bianchi [8], Daniele Picchi [8,9], Guido Rasi [10], Gennaro Daniele [10,11], Alessandra Fabi [12], Paolo Sergi [8], Giampaolo Tortora [4], Riccardo Masetti [5,13], Vincenzo Valentini [3], Marika D'Oria [1,*] and Giovanni Scambia [2,14]

1. Open Innovation Unit, Scientific Directorate, Fondazione Policlinico Universitario A. Gemelli IRCCS, 00168 Roma, Italy; alfredo.cesario@policlinicogemelli.it (A.C.); irene.simone@guest.policlinicogemelli.it (I.S.)
2. Division of Gynecologic Oncology, Department of Woman and Child Health and Public Health, Fondazione Policlinico Universitario A. Gemelli IRCCS, 00168 Roma, Italy; ida.paris@policlinicogemelli.it (I.P.); giovanni.scambia@policlinicogemelli.it (G.S.)
3. Department of Imaging, Oncological Radiotherapy, and Hematology, Fondazione Policlinico Universitario A. Gemelli IRCCS, 00168 Roma, Italy; luca.boldrini@policlinicogemelli.it (L.B.); andrea.damiani@policlinicogemelli.it (A.D.); vincenzo.valentini@policlinicogemelli.it (V.V.)
4. Comprehensive Cancer Center, Fondazione Policlinico Universitario A. Gemelli IRCCS, 00168 Roma, Italy; armando.orlandi@policlinicogemelli.it (A.O.); emilio.bria@policlinicogemelli.it (E.B.); giampaolo.tortora@policlinicogemelli.it (G.T.)
5. Department of Woman and Child Health and Public Health, Fondazione Policlinico Universitario A. Gemelli IRCCS, 00168 Roma, Italy; gianluca.franceschini@policlinicogemelli.it (G.F.); antonino.mule@policlinicogemelli.it (A.M.); angela.santoro@policlinicogemelli.it (A.S.); riccardo.masetti@policlinicogemelli.it (R.M.)
6. Thoracic Surgery Unit, Fondazione Policlinico Universitario A. Gemelli IRCCS, 00168 Roma, Italy; filippo.lococo@policlinicogemelli.it
7. Center for Integrative Oncology, Fondazione Policlinico Universitario A. Gemelli IRCCS, 00168 Roma, Italy; stefano.magno@policlinicogemelli.it
8. Information and Communication Technology Unit, Fondazione Policlinico Universitario A. Gemelli IRCCS, 00168 Roma, Italy; daniele.bianchi@policlinicogemelli.it (D.B.); daniele.picchi@unikey.it (D.P.); paolo.sergi@policlinicogemelli.it (P.S.)
9. Unikey srl, 00168 Roma, Italy
10. Clinical Trial Center S.p.A., 00168 Roma, Italy; guido.rasi@policlinicogemelli.it (G.R.); gennaro.daniele@policlinicogemelli.it (G.D.)
11. Phase I Unit, Fondazione Policlinico Universitario A. Gemelli IRCCS, 00168 Roma, Italy
12. Precision Medicine in Senology Unit, Scientific Directorate, Fondazione Policlinico Universitario A. Gemelli IRCCS, 00168 Roma, Italy; alessandra.fabi@policlinicogemelli.it
13. Dipartimento di Medicina e Chirurgia Traslazionale, Università Cattolica del Sacro Cuore, 00168 Roma, Italy
14. Scientific Directorate, Fondazione Policlinico Universitario A. Gemelli IRCCS, 00168 Roma, Italy
* Correspondence: marika.doria@policlinicogemelli.it; Tel.: +39-06-3015-6263

Abstract: Clinical trials in cancer treatment are imperative in enhancing patients' survival and quality of life outcomes. The lack of communication among professionals may produce a non-optimization of patients' accrual in clinical trials. We developed a specific platform, called "Digital Research Assistant" (DRA), to report real-time every available clinical trial and support clinician. Healthcare professionals involved in breast cancer working group agreed nine minimal fields of interest to preliminarily classify the characteristics of patients' records (including omic data, such as genomic mutations). A progressive web app (PWA) was developed to implement a cross-platform software that was scalable on several electronic devices to share the patients' records and clinical trials. A specialist is able to use and populate the platform. An AI algorithm helps in the matchmaking between patient's data and clinical trial's inclusion criteria to personalize patient enrollment. At the same time, an easy configuration allows the application of the DRA in different oncology working groups (from breast cancer to lung cancer). The DRA might represent a valid research tool supporting clinicians and scientists, in order to optimize the enrollment of patients in clinical trials. User Experience and Technology The acceptance of participants using the DRA is topic of a future analysis.

Keywords: clinical trial; patient enrollment; artificial intelligence; machine learning; breast cancer; lung cancer; oncology; web app; personalized medicine

1. Introduction

Cancer care is a complex pathway that is based on a multidisciplinary collaboration among professionals who share the latest evidence and pool their expertise and information through regular communication flows [1]. Multidisciplinary data sharing is an essential approach for tracing patients' pathways, optimizing therapeutic opportunities, and improving healthcare quality. This approach increases evidence-based practice and avoids treating patients outside standardized protocols and recommended guidelines [2,3].

Clinical trials are imperative for testing novel cancer treatments, advancing the knowledge of care, and determining the best strategies to enhance patients' survival and quality of life outcomes [4,5]. Nevertheless, the possible lack of communication and real-time synchronization among professionals may produce a fragmentation of services and practices, potentially resulting in the non-optimization of patients' accrual in clinical trials and the limitation of their access to innovative therapeutic solutions [4–6].

One possible solution can be represented by data sharing approaches, facilitating the enrollment of patients in clinical trials that allow for increasing the chances of recovery, testing novel treatments, and improving knowledge of disease. Less than 5% of the patients are currently enrolled in clinical trials due to logistical issues, a lack of resources, and difficulty in data sharing [4,7–9].

Our research hospital has a notable oncological vocation, with nearly 60,000 patients annually accessing our facility with its complex organization in clinical, surgical, and service departments that welcome and manage all of the needs of the cancer patients. Specifically, the Comprehensive Cancer Center coordinates and optimizes all of the cancer related activities, guaranteeing the functionality of specific multidisciplinary working groups and the access to innovative therapies through enrollment in clinical trials or comprehensive interpretation of big data at the institutional and network levels [9–11]. In order to reduce daily communication inconveniences [12,13], a specific platform, called "Digital Research Assistant" (DRA), was developed to report real-time every available clinical trial active within our research hospital and assist clinicians in properly matching patients with the more appropriate studies.

The aim of this paper is to show how the DRA was implemented for breast cancer clinical trials to map all of the active studies on this specific disease and encouraging proper patients' enrollment. Its scalability was also evaluated presenting the lung cancer case study.

2. Materials and Methods

2.1. Ideation

A project manager and two Information and Communication Technology (ICT) professionals started a pilot project with the Breast and Lung Cancer institutional Working Groups, following a user-centered designed approach [14] (Figure 1).

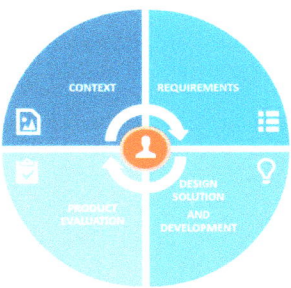

Figure 1. User-centered designed approach. Context: the program manager identifies who are the primary users of the product, how and why they will use it, what are their needs, and which environment they will use the tool. Requirements: when the context is defined, the program manager identifies the detailed requirements of the product, according to the needs of the user. Design solutions and development: once goals and requirements are settled, the ICT professionals and the project manager design and develop the tool for its usability. Evaluate Product: product designers (in this case, ICT professionals) run usability tests to obtain users' feedback on the product.

Healthcare professionals of the involved working groups agreed on nine minimal fields of interest to preliminarily classify the characteristics of patients' records in the platform (Table 1) and obtain a quick evaluation of the patients and its possible link to the active and open clinical trials, using breast cancer as a case study.

Table 1. Fields chosen by the professionals of the Breast Cancer Working Group, in order to classify the patients inserted in the platform.

Field	Value Type	Values	Notes
TNM	Text	T (1,2,3,4, IS) N (0,1,2,3) M (0,1)	
TNM stage	Numerical	From 0 to 4	If 1,2,3 specify the TNM
Age	Numerical	Range	
Immunophenotype	Text	Luminal A Luminal B Triple Negative HER 2 +	
Histological examination	Bit	Internal External	
BMI	Numerical	Mathematic formula	Specify if ≥25
Therapy stage	Text	Neoadjuvant Adjuvant First line metastatic After the first line	
Genetic test	Ternary	Positive Negative Not applicable	Possibility to specify the test
Mutated PI3K	Ternary	Yes No Not applicable	

- TNM classification and corresponding stage were obtained through the input of numerical values according to the 8th edition of TNM classification of malignant tumor [15];
- age is a continuous numerical value;
- immunophenotype consists on the classification into 4 subtypes of breast cancer according to the cellular expression of estrogen (ER: positive or negative) and pro-

gesterone (PgR: positive or negative) receptors, epidermal growth factor receptor 2 (HER2: positive or negative) and the proliferation index (Ki67: from 1% to 100%):
- Luminal A: ER positive and/or PgR positive, HER2 negative, Ki 67 < 25%;
- Luminal B: ER positive and/or PgR positive, HER2 negative, Ki 67 > 25%;
- HER2 positive: any expression of ER, PgR and Ki67, but HER2 positive;
- triple negative: negativity of ER, PgR and HER2 and any expression of Ki67;
- histological examination allows to acquire the information of whether the tumor tissue sample is available at our institution or not (internal or external);
- BMI is calculated automatically, underlining when value is greater than 25 which represents a general risk factor;
- the stage of therapy indicates the type of systemic treatment that the patient is undergoing: neoadjuvant, adjuvant, first line, and beyond the first line in metastatic setting;
- genetic test indicates patient's BRCA1/BRCA2 or multigenic panel mutational status; and,
- PI3Kmutation indicates the mutational status of this specific gene.

Particularly, prognosis and treatment are determined by the stage (TNM classification) of the tumor at the time of diagnosis, but also by the histological/molecular subtype that is obtained with biopsies or in the definitive pathological examination.

2.2. Implementation

The DRA was created with the aim to meet several essential clinical and research points:
- define an operational app that allows to update data informing all users in real-time;
- ensure GDPR-compliant data security;
- allow access to both authorized internal and external users (i.e., for multicentric studies);
- implement a scalable infrastructure manageable by various specialists (i.e., medical doctors, data managers, research nurses, etc.); and,
- develop a matchmaking algorithm between eligible patients and clinical trials.

The infrastructure was designed and developed by separating the front-end (i.e., the exposed services) from the back-end (information content) in order to ensure data protection and security (Figure 2).

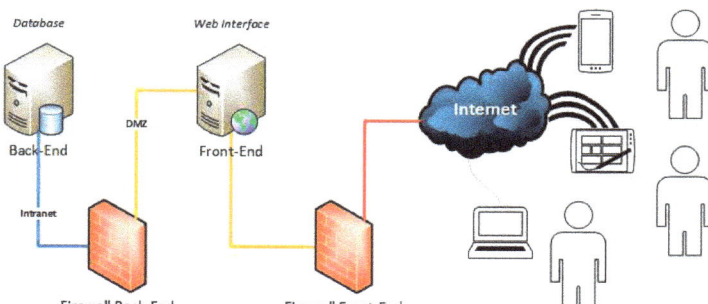

Figure 2. Hardware infrastructure.

Infrastructure versatility was then tested using a different case study (lung cancer), to confirm the possibility to easily adapt the platform for indications other than the one used for the first development.

2.2.1. Technologies and Software

A progressive web app (PWA) was developed to implement a cross-platform software scalable on several electronic devices (i.e., PC, tablet, smartphone). Differently from classic web apps, a PWA that is installed on mobile devices acts as if it was a native app of the device itself, allowing:

- to use its functionalities with all the browser through a reference URL, without installation;
- to adapt the display according to the screen size of the device; and,
- to access its functionalities off-line, guaranteeing data loading by using micro service technologies (APIs).

Business logic was developed using the Microsoft, NetCore 3.1 Framework. This software was structured with APIs that make access to data in secure mode with a https protocol scalable and decoupled from the front-end. The app is scalable in terms of the evolution and reutilization of the code, as well as maximization of loading information on the network.

The angular open source framework version 9.07 was used to develop the front-end, directly running from the browser after being downloaded from the web server. This choice was taken to have an advance in terms of efficiency, saving the exchange of information between client and server every time that there is a request for action by the user.

The SignalR open source framework was used to guarantee a real-time update of data, even when the app is open on a browser. This technology automatically updates information modified by other users, using a two-way channel between the client (browser) and the server (web app). In order to ensure the communication of changes in information to clients, even when they are not connected to the web app, neither it is open, push notifications have been activated using the Google Firebase engine. This open source service allows for sending messages through a web service that transmits notifications to the users of the service. Finally, Microsoft Sql Server 2016 Enterprise Edition was the DBMS used to define the relational model related to this architecture.

2.2.2. Accessibility

System access is possible through a hybrid authentication architecture (Figure 3) that allows specialists and healthcare professionals located in various research centers to use the platform:

- internal users, through access with personal domain credentials; and,
- external users from other research centers (after compiling a standard registration form), through authentication managed internally by the application.

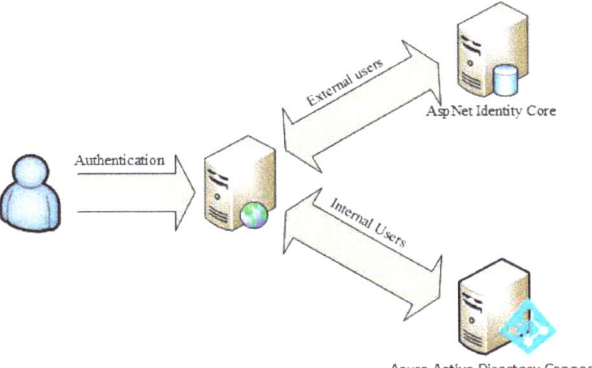

Figure 3. Authentication architecture.

The app admits three profiles:

- System Administrator: enabled to manage configuration features of the app, as described in the "Functionalities" section;
- User: enabled to input information about a patient, to enroll and to ask for patients enrollment; and,

- Study Manager: enabled to use the same functions of the "User" profile, as well as to manage the creation and modification of trials.

"System Administrators" manage the access of internal users (with "User" and "Study Manager" profiles) enabling them to use the app. An HR representative of the research hospital supervises the list of users.

3. Results

3.1. Functionalities and Configuration

From the side menu, the following functionalities are available:

- List of Patients
- List of Clinical Trials
- My Requests
- My Interests
- My Clinical Trials (or Studies)
- Pending Requests
- Configuration
  - Users
  - Clinical Trial (or Study)
  - Type of Clinical Trial (or Study)
  - Phase
  - Settings
- Enable notifications

Other functionalities include system management and configurations, which are dedicated to "System Administrator" profiles.

3.1.1. Patients' Management and Enrollment (Matching) to Clinical Trials

Under the operational functions, it is possible to see a real-time updated patients list from the activated module to:

- check their status with a color legend (enrolled, pending, etc.) (Figure 4);
- select the relevant specialist if the user has access to more than one;
- add a new patient and/or modify data related to a specific one;
- add a patient to a study (for "Study Manager" profiles) or send a request to the Study Manager of the selected trial to insert him (for "User" profiles);
- add a patient in your interests; and,

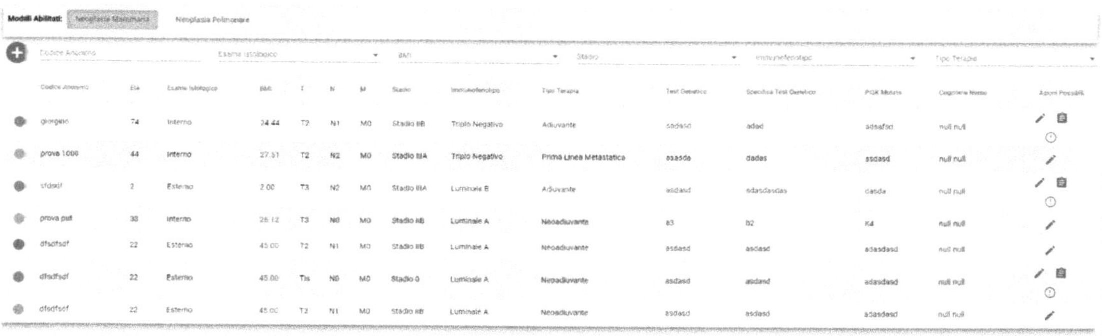

Figure 4. List of patients uploaded in the system (in Italian). Names are examples and do not correspond to real cases.

Search filters are available for a better user experience.
In particular, the legend includes four entries:

- Free (green): the patient can be enrolled in a trial;
- Enrolled (red): the patient is currently enrolled in a trial;
- Requested Enrollment (yellow): the patient has already been requested for a trial. The "Study Manager" will be able to deny the request or allow the patient in the study; and,
- Selected for Possible Enrollment: the patient has been selected from a "User" to be evaluated for possible enrollment.

Patient enrollment changes according to the logged profile. If the profile is "Study Manager", then the enrollment occurs immediately, otherwise a "User" sends a request to the "Study Manager" of the selected trial, which allows or denies access to the patient in the study. When a patient is accepted, or directly recruited, the "Study Manager" inserts the starting and ending date of the trial.

3.1.2. Clinical Trial Configuration

A list of Clinical Trials with their status (i.e., active, suspended, closed) is displayed for all of the profiles (Figure 5). To configure a Clinical Trial, the "User", or the "Study Manager" can enter the information related to the study in which patients can be enrolled (Figure 6). These information are shared with other users, especially those that are interested in the same pathology.

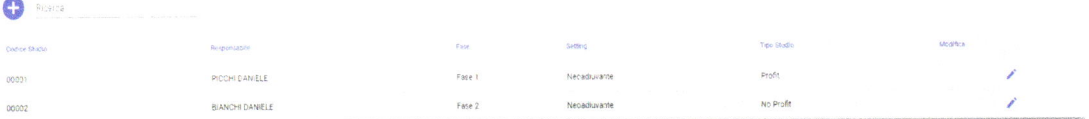

Figure 5. List of Clinical Trials (in Italian). Names are examples and do not correspond to real cases.

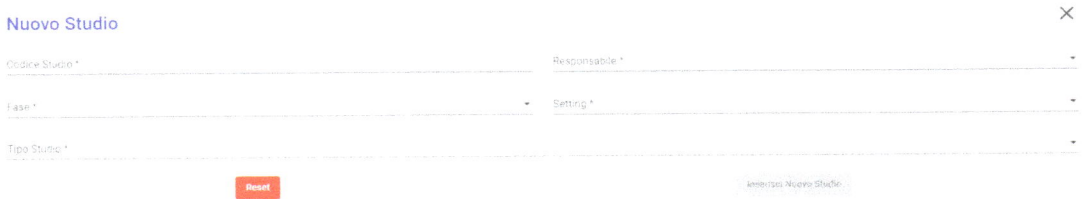

Figure 6. New Clinical Trial form (in Italian).

3.1.3. Phase of the Clinical Trial Configuration

"User" and "Study Manager" profiles can input and modify the Phase of the clinical trial, visible on the selection menu while configuring a trial (Figures 7 and 8).

Figure 7. List of Phases (in Italian).

Figure 8. New Phase insert form (in Italian).

Matchmaking option. An algorithm then configures the clinical trial. By defining the inclusion-exclusion criteria of a patient in a trial enrollment, these criteria become the rules of the algorithm that allows matchmaking between an eligible patient and a trial. When the "User" inserts a new patient, it is possible to click on the action "assign the patient to a study". This action shows the list of clinical trials for which the patient is eligible. If the patient has characteristics that are coherent with the study, he/she can be enrolled. In particular, omic characteristics (such as genomic mutations) may help achieve a Personalized Medicine approach in oncological clinical trial enrollment.

As an enrichment of the services offered by the platform, a connection with the GEmelli NEtwoRk for Analysis and Tests in Oncology and medical Research "Generator"—Real World Data facility is offered to the clinician. Gemelli Generator Real-World Data is a research facility whose aim is the integration of the vast amount of patient data that are available in the Gemelli Data warehouse (about 700 million data items as measured at the end of December 2020). The generator takes care of the integration of these data items, in anonymized form, into specific datamarts, based on appropriate terminological systems, quality-checked and normalized with regard to the information originated from different, heterogeneous data sources, like traditional electronic health records (EHRs), omics data, Patient-Reported Experience Measures (PREMS), and Patient-Reported Outcome Measures (PROMS).

Machine Learning and Artificial Intelligence-based methods are at the heart of the Generator infrastructure, allowing for researchers to develop state of the art models, clustering, and decision support systems [16]. After the patient selection phase of the DRA, a simple user interface will give clinicians the opportunity to query the Generator datamarts for the availability of further covariates, referred to the selected patients, that can add more information to what is already present in the DRA core. Full integration between the two systems, at the ICT level, will guarantee an automatic and swift response in a privacy protected environment.

In this way, researchers can have a deeper view of the available data and formulate more study hypotheses, based on the large variety of information coming from heterogeneous data sources.

3.1.4. Settings Configuration

"System Administrators" can insert or modify the characteristics of the setting attributes (that are chosen by the WG) related to the clinical trials (Figures 9 and 10), while "User" and "Study Manager" profiles can select them directly.

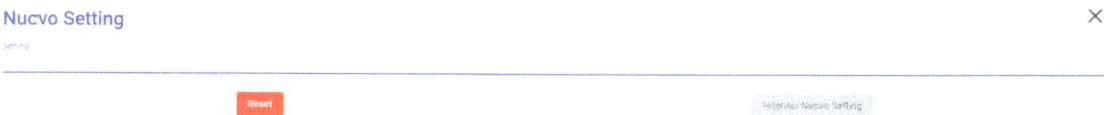

Figure 9. New Setting form (in Italian).

Figure 10. List of Settings descriptions (in Italian).

3.1.5. User Requests

In the "User Requests" section, all of the requests and their status (accepted, refused, and pending for evaluation) are displayed as well as other users' information requests about a patient or a trial (Figure 11).

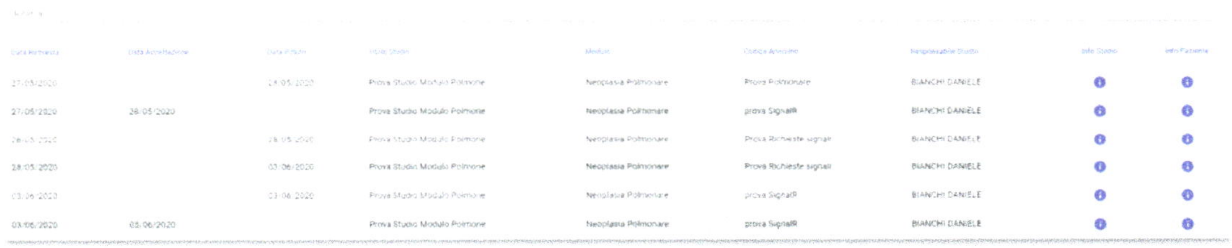

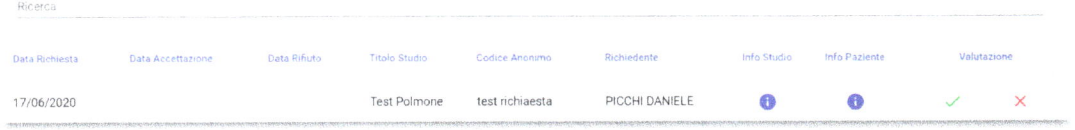

Figure 11. User Requests (in Italian). Names are examples and do not correspond to real cases.

3.1.6. Requests Management

This section is only accessible to "Study Manager" profiles and allows accepting or declining a request (Figure 12). Each row shows a single request with the possibility of examining patient or trial information.

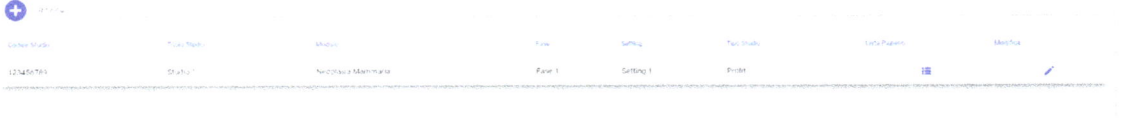

Figure 12. Requests Management (in Italian). Names are examples and do not correspond to real cases.

3.1.7. Clinical Trials List

This section shows a list of all the clinical trials that the logged profile is responsible for. The "Study Manager" profile also allows editing information about the trials and examining the enrolled patients' full list (Figure 13).

Figure 13. Trials list (in Italian). Names are examples and do not correspond to real cases.

3.1.8. Possible Enrollment List

This section shows all of the patients preferred by "User" profiles, and preference can be deselected. It is possible to send or accept requests of admission in a trial (Figure 14).

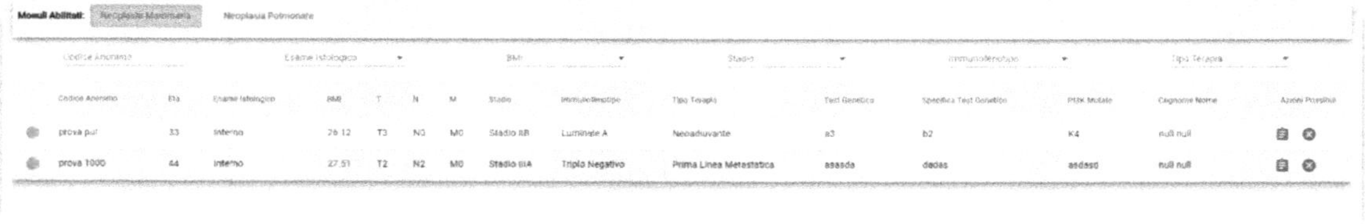

Figure 14. Possible enrollment list (in Italian). Names are examples and do not correspond to real cases.

4. Customization

In this paper, we described the scale-up customization of the first DRA model on breast cancer to lung cancer thought for a high volume cancer care center. Table 2 shows all the varied characteristics of the patient, except for the "Age" field.

Table 2. Fields chosen by the professionals of the Lung Cancer Working Group, in order to classify patients inserted in the platform.

Field	Value Type	Values	Notes
Patient Code (Social Security Number)	Text	Alphanumeric	
Pathological TNM	Text	pT (X, 0, 1a, 1b, 1c, 2a, 2b, 3, 4) pN (X, 0, 1, 2, 3) pM (X, 0, 1a, 1b, 1c)	Only for complete oncological interventions Information not mandatory, only if available
Clinical TNM descriptors	Numerical	cT (X; 0; 1a; 1b; 1c; 2a; 2b; 3; 4) cN (X; 0; 1; 2; 3) cM (X; 0; 1a; 1b; 1c)	
Clinical Stage	Numerical	Occult, 0, IA1, IA2, IA3, IB, IIA, IIB, IIIA, IIIB, IIIC, IVA, IVB	
Age	Numerical	Range	
ECOG performance status	Numerical	0; 1; 2; 3; 4	
Surgery	Binary	Yes; No	
Histology	Text	small cells carcinoma; adenocarcinoma; squamous cell carcinoma; other	
Grading	Text	G1; G2; G3	If applicable
Residual disease	Text	R0; R1	
Molecular characteristics	Text	Re-arrangement of ALK and ROS genes; EGFR and KRAS gene mutation; PDL1 expression	Information not mandatory, only if available
Therapy type	Text	Surgery; Chemotherapy; Immunotherapy; Radiotherapy; Other	

The parameters included in the "Minimum Fields" (Table 2) were selected while considering the main characteristics of lung cancer patients that can guide the accrual in clinical trials.

- TNM descriptors and the relative stage have been reported according to the criteria illustrated in the 8th edition of TNM classification of lung malignant tumor [17], where the clinical stage is determined according to radiological or radiometabolic assessment, while pathological staging is determined on the basis of pathological confirmations;
- age is a continuous numerical value;
- performance status was described according to the Eastern Cooperative Oncology Group (ECOG) criteria [18];
- surgery is considered only if performed with curative intent:

- histology: we indicated the most common histological subtypes among lung tumors;
- grading has been reported according to 2015 WHO Classification [19];
- resection margin status, indicating the pathological report of the specimen margin;
- genetic test indicates whether the patient has carried out genetic testing for ALK and ROS1 genes, EGFR and KRAS gene mutation and PDL1 expression; and,
- therapy type indicates which strategy of care has been adopted.

Prognosis and treatment are determined by disease stage (TNM classification), as identified by preliminary diagnostic investigations and histology. Surgery remains the main prognostic factor in the early-stage tumors and the completeness of resection (negative margin status) is a widely recognized factor influencing the long-term results in this setting. Otherwise, in locally advanced and metastatic stages, the molecular characterization represents the main determinant of long-term outcomes, based on the dramatic predictive role of featured biomarkers of activity/efficacy for molecular targeted agents and immunotherapy.

Table 3 shows the numerical data from a pilot test of the DRA database.

Table 3. Number of patients available in the Digital Research Assistant.

Pathology	N. Patients in the Database	N. Patients Requested for a Trial	N. Enrolled Patients
Breast Cancer	62	1	0
Lung Cancer	34	6	0

5. Discussion and Conclusions

Our solution exploited communication among professionals that are involved in oncological care and cancer research. The DRA we developed allows them to know all of the running clinical trials, guaranteeing all patients the best access to cure and research protocols, reducing the fragmentation of patients' access to the oncological care-path with the multiple therapeutic intersections available in high volume centers (radiotherapy, surgery, and new lines of systemic therapy managed by multiple specialists).

This digital tool appeared to be well performing for patients' data sharing within the single institution, but also in setting up networks with other cancer centers facilitating patients' enrollment also for peripheral centers. In fact, in high-patient volume centers, such as our institution, the DRA seems a possible efficient resource to face this issue [20–26]. At the same time, the platform is easily moldable to the needs of different oncology work groups, as evidenced by the easy customization starting from the model for breast cancer to arrive at that for lung cancer.

Taking these considerations together, the platform might represent a valid research tool supporting clinicians and scientists, working in both high- and low-volume centers and the enrollment success rates for each matchmaking run is currently the object of in depth analysis and it will be a topic of future publications. User Experience and Technology Acceptance of participants using the DRA is topic of a second dedicated analysis.

Author Contributions: Conceptualization, all authors; methodology, A.C., I.S., M.D., P.S., D.B., and D.P.; software, P.S., D.B., and D.P.; validation, A.C., I.S., I.P., L.B., A.O., G.F., F.L., E.B., S.M., A.M., G.T., R.M., V.V., G.S.; formal analysis, A.C., M.D.; investigation, A.C., I.S., M.D., and G.S.; writing—original draft preparation, D.B., M.D., L.B., I.P., A.O., G.F., F.L., E.B., S.M., A.D., A.S., and A.M.; writing—review and editing, D.B., M.D., L.B., I.P., A.O., G.F., F.L., E.B., S.M., A.D., A.S., R.M., G.D., A.F., G.R., and A.M.; visualization, all authors. supervision, G.S.; project administration, I.S. All authors have read and agreed to the published version of the manuscript.

Funding: This research received no external funding.

Institutional Review Board Statement: Not applicable.

Informed Consent Statement: Not applicable.

Data Availability Statement: Data sharing not applicable.

Conflicts of Interest: The authors declare no conflict of interest.

References

1. Specchia, M.L.; Frisicale, E.M.; Carini, E.; Di Pilla, A.; Cappa, D.; Barbara, A.; Ricciardi, W.; Damiani, G. The impact of tumor board on cancer care: Evidence from an umbrella review. *BMC Health Serv. Res.* **2020**, *20*, 1–14. [CrossRef]
2. Pillay, B.; Wootten, A.C.; Crowe, H.; Corcoran, N.; Tran, B.; Bowden, P.; Crowe, J.; Costello, A.J. The impact of multidisciplinary team meetings on patient assessment, management and outcomes in oncology settings: A systematic review of the literature. *Cancer Treat. Rev.* **2016**, *42*, 56–72. [CrossRef]
3. Savage, N. Collaboration is the key to cancer research. *Nat. Cell Biol.* **2018**, *556*, S1–S3. [CrossRef] [PubMed]
4. Lara, P.N.; Higdon, R.; Lim, N.; Kwan, K.; Tanaka, M.; Lau, D.H.; Wun, T.; Welborn, J.; Meyers, F.J.; Christensen, S.; et al. Prospective Evaluation of Cancer Clinical Trial Accrual Patterns: Identifying Potential Barriers to Enrollment. *J. Clin. Oncol.* **2001**, *19*, 1728–1733. [CrossRef] [PubMed]
5. Barger, S.; Sullivan, S.D.; Bell-Brown, A.; Bott, B.; Ciccarella, A.M.; Golenski, J.; Gorman, M.; Johnson, J.; Kreizenbeck, K.; Kurttila, F.; et al. Effective stakeholder engagement: Design and implementation of a clinical trial (SWOG S1415CD) to improve cancer care. *BMC Med. Res. Methodol.* **2019**, *19*, 119. [CrossRef] [PubMed]
6. Salamone, J.M.; Lucas, W.; Brundage, S.B.; Holloway, J.N.; Stahl, S.M.; Carbine, N.E.; London, M.; Greenwood, N.; Goyes, R.; Chisholm, D.C.; et al. Promoting Scientist-Advocate Collaborations in Cancer Research: Why and How. *Cancer Res.* **2018**, *78*, 5723–5728. [CrossRef]
7. Murthy, V.H.; Krumholz, H.M.; Gross, C.P. Participation in Cancer Clinical Trials. *JAMA* **2004**, *291*, 2720–2726. [CrossRef]
8. Unger, J.M.; Cook, E.; Tai, E.; Bleyer, A. The Role of Clinical Trial Participation in Cancer Research: Barriers, Evidence, and Strategies. *Am. Soc. Clin. Oncol. Educ. Book* **2016**, *35*, 185–198. [CrossRef]
9. Meldolesi, E.; Van Soest, J.; Damiani, A.; Dekker, A.; Alitto, A.R.; Campitelli, M.; DiNapoli, N.; Gatta, R.; Gambacorta, M.A.; Lanzotti, V.; et al. Standardized data collection to build prediction models in oncology: A prototype for rectal cancer. *Future Oncol.* **2016**, *12*, 119–136. [CrossRef]
10. Deist, T.M.; Dankers, F.J.; Ojha, P.; Marshall, M.S.; Janssen, T.; Faivre-Finn, C.; Masciocchi, C.; Valentini, V.; Wang, J.; Chen, J.; et al. Distributed learning on 20 000+ lung cancer patients—The Personal Health Train. *Radiother. Oncol.* **2020**, *144*, 189–200. [CrossRef]
11. Quinn, M.; Forman, J.; Harrod, M.; Winter, S.; Fowler, K.E.; Krein, S.L.; Gupta, A.; Saint, S.; Singh, H.; Chopra, V. Electronic health records, communication, and data sharing: Challenges and opportunities for improving the diagnostic process. *Diagnosis* **2018**, *6*, 241–248. [CrossRef] [PubMed]
12. Post, D.M.; Shapiro, C.L.; Cegala, N.J.; David, P.; Katz, M.L.; Krok, J.L.; Phillips, G.S.; McAlearney, A.S.; Lehman, J.S.; Hicks, W.; et al. Improving symptom communication through personal digital assistants: The CHAT (Communicating Health Assisted by Technology) project. *J. Natl. Cancer Inst. Monogr.* **2013**, *2013*, 153–161. [CrossRef]
13. Richards, R.; Kinnersley, P.; Brain, K.; McCutchan, G.; Staffurth, J.; Wood, F. Use of Mobile Devices to Help Cancer Patients Meet Their Information Needs in Non-Inpatient Settings: Systematic Review. *JMIR mHealth uHealth* **2018**, *6*, e10026. [CrossRef]
14. Norman, D. *The Design of Everyday Things*; Verlag Franz Vahlen GmbH: München, Germany, 2016.
15. Cserni, G.; Chmielik, E.; Cserni, B.; Tot, T. The new TNM-based staging of breast cancer. *Virchows Arch. Pathol. Anat. Physiol. Klin. Med.* **2018**, *472*, 697–703. [CrossRef]
16. Marchiano, R.D.M.; Di Sante, G.; Piro, G.; Carbone, C.; Tortora, G.; Boldrini, L.; Pietragalla, A.; Daniele, G.; Tredicine, M.; Cesario, A.; et al. Translational Research in the Era of Precision Medicine: Where We Are and Where We Will Go. *J. Pers. Med.* **2021**, *11*, 216. [CrossRef]
17. Goldstraw, P.; Chansky, K.; Crowley, J.; Rami-Porta, R.; Asamura, H.; Eberhardt, W.E.; Nicholson, A.G.; Groome, P.; Mitchell, A.; Bolejack, V.; et al. The IASLC Lung Cancer Staging Project: Proposals for Revision of the TNM Stage Groupings in the Forthcoming (Eighth) Edition of the TNM Classification for Lung Cancer. *J. Thorac. Oncol.* **2016**, *11*, 39–51. [CrossRef]
18. Oken, M.M.; Creech, R.H.; Tormey, D.C.; Horton, J.; Davis, T.E.; McFadden, E.T.; Carbone, P.P. Toxicity and response criteria of the Eastern Cooperative Oncology Group. *Am. J. Clin. Oncol.* **1982**, *5*, 649–655. [CrossRef] [PubMed]
19. Geisinger, K.; Rami-Porta, R.; Moreira, A.L.; Travis, W.D.; Nicholson, A.G. Lung cancer staging and grading. In *World Health Organization Clas-sification of Tumors. Pathology and Genetics of the Lung, Pleura, Thymus and Heart*; Travis, W.D., Brambilla, E., Burke, A.P., Marx, A., Nicholson, A.G., Eds.; IARC Press: Lyon, France, 2015; pp. 14–15.
20. Cesario, A.; Auffray, C.; Agusti, A.; Apolone, G.; Balling, R.; Barbanti, P.; Bellia, A.; Boccia, S.; Bousquet, J.; Cardaci, V.; et al. A Systems Medicine Clinical Platform for Understanding and Managing Non- Communicable Diseases. *Curr. Pharm. Des.* **2014**, *20*, 5945–5956. [CrossRef]
21. Gartner, D.; Padman, R. E-HOSPITAL–A Digital Workbench for Hospital Operations and Services Planning Using Information Technology and Algebraic Languages. *Stud. Health Technol. Inform.* **2017**, *245*, 84–88. [PubMed]
22. Anderberg, P.; Barnestein-Fonseca, P.; Guzman-Parra, J.; Garolera, M.; Quintana, M.; Mayoral-Cleries, F.; Lemmens, E.; Berglund, J.S. The Effects of the Digital Platform Support Monitoring and Reminder Technology for Mild Dementia (SMART4MD) for People With Mild Cognitive Impairment and Their Informal Carers: Protocol for a Pilot Randomized Controlled Trial. *JMIR Res. Protoc.* **2019**, *8*, e13711. [CrossRef] [PubMed]

23. Mira, J.J.; Vicente, M.A.; Lopez-Pineda, A.; Carrillo, I.; Guilabert, M.; Fernández, C.; Pérez-Jover, V.; Delgado, J.M.; Pérez-Pérez, P.; Vargas, A.C.; et al. Preventing and Addressing the Stress Reactions of Health Care Workers Caring for Patients With COVID-19: Development of a Digital Platform (Be + Against COVID). *JMIR mHealth uHealth* **2020**, *8*, e21692. [CrossRef] [PubMed]
24. Baumel, A.; Tinkelman, A.; Mathur, N.; Kane, J.M. Digital Peer-Support Platform (7Cups) as an Adjunct Treatment for Women With Postpartum Depression: Feasibility, Acceptability, and Preliminary Efficacy Study. *JMIR mHealth uHealth* **2018**, *6*, e38. [CrossRef] [PubMed]
25. Semakula-Katende, N.S.; Andronikou, S.; Lucas, S. Digital platform for improving non-radiologists' and radiologists' interpretation of chest radiographs for suspected tuberculosis—A method for supporting task-shifting in developing countries. *Pediatr. Radiol.* **2016**, *46*, 1384–1391. [CrossRef]
26. Jalalabadi, F.; Shultz, K.P.; Sussman, N.L.; Fisher, W.E.; Reece, E.M. Initiating Telehealth in a Complex Organization. *Semin. Plast. Surg.* **2018**, *32*, 159–161. [CrossRef] [PubMed]

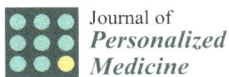

Article

Different Impact of Definitions of Sarcopenia in Defining Frailty Status in a Population of Older Women with Early Breast Cancer

Andrea Bellieni [1], Domenico Fusco [1,*], Alejandro Martin Sanchez [2], Gianluca Franceschini [2], Beatrice Di Capua [1], Elena Allocca [3], Enrico Di Stasio [4], Fabio Marazzi [5], Luca Tagliaferri [5], Riccardo Masetti [2], Roberto Bernabei [6] and Giuseppe Ferdinando Colloca [5]

1. Dipartimento di Scienze dell'Invecchiamento, Neurologiche, Ortopediche e della Testa-Collo, Fondazione Policlinico Universitario "A. Gemelli" IRCCS, 00168 Rome, Italy; andrea.bellieni@gmail.com (A.B.); beatricedicapua@gmail.com (B.D.C.)
2. Multidisciplinary Breast Center, Dipartimento Scienze della Salute della Donna, del Bambino e di Sanità Pubblica, Fondazione Policlinico Universitario "A. Gemelli" IRCCS, 00168 Rome, Italy; martin.sanchez@policlinicogemelli.it (A.M.S.); gianluca.franceschini@policlinicogemelli.it (G.F.); riccardo.masetti@policlinicogemelli.it (R.M.)
3. Istituto per la Sicurezza Sociale, 47890 Cailungo, Città di San Marino, San Marino; el.allocca@gmail.com
4. Dipartimento di Scienze Biotecnologiche di Base, Cliniche Intensivologiche e Perioperatorie, Università Cattolica del Sacro Cuore, 00168 Rome, Italy; enrico.distasio@unicatt.it
5. Dipartimento di Diagnostica per Immagini, Radioterapia Oncologica ed Ematologia, Fondazione Policlinico Universitario "A. Gemelli" IRCCS, 00168 Rome, Italy; fabio.marazzi@policlinicogemelli.it (F.M.); luca.tagliarri@policlinicogemelli.it (L.T.); giuseppeferdinando.colloca@policlinicogemelli.it (G.F.C.)
6. Università Cattolica del Sacro Cuore, 00168 Rome, Italy; roberto.bernabei@unicatt.it
* Correspondence: domenico.fusco@policlinicogemelli.it; Tel.: +39-063-0151

Citation: Bellieni, A.; Fusco, D.; Sanchez, A.M.; Franceschini, G.; Di Capua, B.; Allocca, E.; Di Stasio, E.; Marazzi, F.; Tagliaferri, L.; Masetti, R.; et al. Different Impact of Definitions of Sarcopenia in Defining Frailty Status in a Population of Older Women with Early Breast Cancer. *J. Pers. Med.* 2021, 11, 243. https://doi.org/10.3390/jpm11040243

Academic Editor: Anguraj Sadanandam

Received: 23 February 2021
Accepted: 22 March 2021
Published: 26 March 2021

Publisher's Note: MDPI stays neutral with regard to jurisdictional claims in published maps and institutional affiliations.

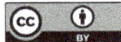

Copyright: © 2021 by the authors. Licensee MDPI, Basel, Switzerland. This article is an open access article distributed under the terms and conditions of the Creative Commons Attribution (CC BY) license (https://creativecommons.org/licenses/by/4.0/).

Abstract: Sarcopenia is a geriatric syndrome characterized by losses of quantity and quality of skeletal muscle, which is associated with negative outcomes in older adults and in cancer patients. Different definitions of sarcopenia have been used, with quantitative data more frequently used in oncology, while functional measures have been advocated in the geriatric literature. Little is known about the correlation between frailty status as assessed by comprehensive geriatric assessment (CGA) and sarcopenia in cancer patients. We retrospectively analyzed data from 96 older women with early breast cancer who underwent CGAs and Dual X-ray Absorptiometry (DXA) scans for muscle mass assessment before cancer treatment at a single cancer center from 2016 to 2019 to explore the correlation between frailty status as assessed by CGA and sarcopenia using different definitions. Based on the results of the CGA, 35 patients (36.5%) were defined as frail. Using DXA Appendicular Skeletal Mass (ASM) or the Skeletal Muscle Index (SMI=ASM/height^2), 41 patients were found to be sarcopenic (42.7%), with no significant difference in prevalence between frail and nonfrail subjects. Using the European Working Group on Sarcopenia in Older People (EWGSOP2) definition of sarcopenia (where both muscle function and mass are required), 58 patients were classified as "probably" sarcopenic; among these, 25 were sarcopenic and 17 "severely" sarcopenic. Only 13 patients satisfied both the requirements for being defined as sarcopenic and frail. Grade 3-4 treatment-related toxicities (according to Common Terminology Criteria for Adverse Events) were more common in sarcopenic and frail sarcopenic patients. Our data support the use of a definition of sarcopenia that includes both quantitative and functional data in order to identify frail patients who need tailored treatment.

Keywords: sarcopenia; physical performance; frailty; older cancer patients

1. Introduction

Breast cancer is the most frequent cancer diagnosed in women and the leading cause of cancer death among women [1]. About 60% of these new diagnoses involve patients > 65 years of age and about 40% of patients are >70 [2].

Chronological age per se is a misleading criterion when deciding the best treatment for older women with breast cancer. A group of older patients with the same cancer of identical chronologic age can demonstrate wide heterogeneity concerning vitality, comorbidity, functional status, physiologic reserve, and psychosocial functioning [3–5]. Nonetheless, the accrual of older adults in cancer trials has been poor and undermined by several barriers through the years [6]. This is a severe matter of concern when evidence-based guidelines are applied to older populations, with negative consequences on survival [7]. Thus, a personalized approach based on individual patients' clinical conditions and functionality rather than age [8–11] should be considered the standard of care for older women with breast cancer.

To help guide treatment decisions, two geriatric medicine features have been incorporated in geriatric oncology: the concept of frailty and the comprehensive geriatric assessment. The Comprehensive Geriatric Assessment (CGA) represents the most efficient evaluation instrument, as recommended by the International Society of Oncological Geriatrics (SIOG) [12] and recently by the American Society of Clinical Oncology (ASCO) [13], to identify and define the frailty of the patient and his/her functional reserve [14]. Despite accumulating evidence regarding the value of the geriatric assessment in terms of encompassing older patients' diversity, a full CGA is considered rather time-consuming. Its effectiveness is far limited without interdepartment collaborative care and frailty-targeted optimized intervention programs to implement daily oncology practices [15–21]. CGA is the only method capable of assessing older cancer patients' frailty, predicting the risk of toxicity related to the treatments and the risk of mortality [22]. The CGA approach is considered essential to identify problems that are not immediately evident. Several studies have demonstrated the ability of CGA to identify otherwise unrecognized conditions of vulnerability to support the decision-making of the specialist (oncologist, radiotherapist, surgeon) when estimating the risk of toxicity to prevent said toxicity and preserve the functional performance of patients [23–26].

CGA can help to identify several geriatric syndromes [27]. Among all of them, sarcopenia has played an increasing role [28]. Sarcopenia is now considered one of the biological mechanisms underlying the concept of frailty. A reduction, compared to physiological criteria, in skeletal muscle mass characterizes this, with essential structural changes in muscle quality, and typically manifests itself with an alteration in function and/or a reduction in strength [29,30]. Several studies have shown the association between sarcopenia and functional decline, disability, frailty, falls, risk of fractures, multiple hospitalizations, and death [31,32]. A high prevalence of sarcopenia has been described in cancer patients, and its occurrence is associated with an increased risk of treatment toxicity, increased postoperative complications, increased sensitivity to antiblastic treatments, and a higher mortality rate, regardless of cancer stage [33]. It should also be stressed that cancer and cancer treatments may themselves be responsible for increasing disability, thereby accelerating the functional decline trajectory.

Several definitions of sarcopenia have been proposed. Initially, low muscle mass was considered the only criterion for diagnosis [34]. This is also the case for the vast majority of reports on cancer populations, with different indexes and cut-offs proposed. By contrast, in the geriatric field, the role of physical performance and muscle strength has been stressed as a necessary complement to the definition. The original operational definition of sarcopenia by the European Working Group on Sarcopenia in Older People (EWGSOP) [35] in 2010 was a significant change at the time, adding the muscle function to the former definitions, which were based only on detection of low muscle mass [28,29,31,32]. In its 2018 definition (Table 1), EWGSOP2 uses low muscle strength as a primary parameter of sarcopenia. It is considered a more reliable measure of muscle function and a better predictor of adverse outcomes [36,37]. Specifically, sarcopenia is probable when low muscle strength is detected. A sarcopenia diagnosis is confirmed by the presence of low muscle quantity or quality. When low muscle strength, low muscle quantity/quality, and low physical performance are all detected, sarcopenia is considered severe (Table 1). Techniques for evaluating muscle quantity are available in many but not all clinical settings. As instruments and methods for assessing muscle quality are developed and refined in the future, this parameter is expected to grow in importance as a defining feature of sarcopenia. Physical performance was formerly considered part of the core definition of sarcopenia. In the revised guidelines, it is used to categorize the severity of sarcopenia.

Table 1. Definition of sarcopenia by European Working Group on Sarcopenia in Older People (EWGSOP2) guidelines [1].

Criteria:	Suggested Measures and Cut-offs (for Women)
(1) Low muscle strength	Grip strength, <16 kg Chair standing, >15 s for five rises
(2) Low muscle quantity or quality	ASM (appendicular skeletal muscle mass), <15 kg SMI (Skeletal Muscle Index): ASM/height^2, <5.5 kg/m^2
(3) Low physical performance	Gait speed, $\leq$0.8 m/s Short Physical Performance Battery (SPPB), $\leq$8 points score Timed Up-and-Go Test, $\geq$20 s 400 m walk test, noncompletion or $\geq$6 min for completion

Definitions:
Probable sarcopenia is identified by Criterion 1.
Confirmed sarcopenia: both Criterion 1 and Criterion 2 are satisfied.
Severe sarcopenia: if Criteria 1, 2 and 3 are all met.

[1] Cruz-Jentoft et al., (2019). Sarcopenia: revised European consensus on definition and diagnosis. Age and Ageing, 48(1):16–31.

The present study aimed to assess sarcopenia's prevalence using different definitions in a population of older women with breast cancer and investigate possible correlations between sarcopenia and frailty status and the impact of these conditions on toxicities from oncological treatments.

2. Materials and Methods

We retrospectively analyzed data on the comprehensive geriatric evaluation of older women admitted at the Breast Surgery Unit of the Fondazione Policlinico Universitario A. Gemelli IRCCS, starting in January 2016 and ending in December 2019. All breast cancer patients aged $\geq$ 70 with a histological confirmed early breast cancer (stage 0–III, according to TNM) underwent CGA. The patients were selected weekly during the multidisciplinary tumor board (TBM), based on the registry criteria, and sent for geriatric evaluation. The only exclusion criteria were: life expectancy less than six months and refusal to participate in the study. Anthropometric measures (weight, height, BMI), the socio-family context, and support of all the patients were recorded and investigated. The patients underwent a medical examination, including medical history and physical examination. The primary socio-demographic data, the comorbidities, and the information on the oncological history and the anatomo-pathological and cancer immunohistochemical features, in accordance with the data present in the patients' medical records, were detected. Anthropometric measures (weight, height, body mass index) were collected for all patients. The comprehensive geriatric assessment (CGA) was based on recommendations from SIOG and national clinical guidelines [38]. The following areas were evaluated: performance status by Eastern Cooperative Oncology Group (ECOG) [39,40], comorbidity burden by the Charlson Comorbidity Index [41], functional status by Activity of Daily Living (Katz ADL) [42] and by Instrumental Activities of Daily Living (Lawton IADL) [43], cognition by Mini-Mental State Examination (MMSE) [44], nutritional status by Mini Nutritional Assessment (MNA) [45], mood by Geriatric Depression Scale (GDS) [46], physical performance by Short Physical Performance Battery (SPPB), gait speed and time up-and-go test (TUGT) [47–49], muscular strength by handgrip (Jamar dynamometer) [50] and chair stand test [51]. Patients were asked about the presence of common geriatric syndromes, such as falls or incontinence. Only patients who completed a Dual X-ray Absorptiometry (DXA) scan for muscle mass evaluation were included for the present study.

2.1. Sarcopenia and Frailty Definitions

The definition of sarcopenia by EWGSOP2 [28] was applied, using cut-offs proposed by the guidelines mentioned above (Table 1). Muscle mass was measured by (DXA) total body (Hologic Horizon) Appendicular Skeletal Mass (ASM), calculated as the sum of arm and limb lean mass measured through DXA and expressed in kg. Frailty was defined by Balducci's criteria [52,53] considered as the detection of deficits in two or more domains of the CGA.

2.2. Toxicities

We retrospectively analyzed hospital electronic medical records of the patients included in the present study after a 12-month follow-up period in order to detect toxicities as they were reported by treating clinicians. Toxicities were evaluated using Common Terminology Criteria for Adverse Events (CTCAE) v5.0.

2.3. Analysis

All evaluations were performed by geriatricians belonging to the geriatric oncology team of the Fondazione Policlinico Universitario A. Gemelli IRCCS and who were specialized in the field of geriatric oncology and appropriately trained within the training courses of the International Society of Oncological Geriatrics (SIOG) [54]. Once the data collection was completed, all analyses were carried out using IBM SPSS 23. The collected data were synthesized using means and standard deviations for continuous variables and absolute and percentage frequencies for categorical variables. Statistical significance was conventionally set at $p < 0.05$.

3. Results

From January 2016 to December 2019, over 300 elderly patients aged ≥ 70 years belonging to the Breast Surgery Unit of Fondazione Policlinico Universitario A. Gemelli IRCCS (Rome), were evaluated.

Using the inclusion criteria, 96 patients were enrolled. The medium age of the examined sample was 76.9 (70 ÷ 89; SD 4.586), with an average level of comorbidity measured by the Charlson Comorbidity Index (CCI) of 6.7 (5 ÷ 13; SD—1.904), while ECOG performance status was mainly between 0 and 1 (89.6% of patients). Invasive ductal carcinoma was the most common histotype (75%), followed by lobular carcinoma (14.6%) (Table 2).

All patients underwent surgery: 84.38% (81) received a conservative treatment (quadrantectomy), representing 12.3% of cases (10 patients) with total lymphadenectomy, while 41.9% of cases (34 patients) received the removal of the sentinel lymph node. A total of 14.58% (14) received a full mastectomy, of whom three also underwent total lymphadenectomy. Less than 20% of patients received adjuvant chemotherapy, while almost two-thirds received adjuvant radiotherapy. In total, 85.4% of the patients were prescribed hormone suppressive therapy (with an aromatase inhibitor), based on hormone receptor status.

Table 2. Characteristics of the study population.

	N. of Patients	%
Histotype	96	100
Invasive Ductal Carcinoma	72	75
Invasive Lobular Carcinoma	14	14.6
other	10	9.6
STAGE		
0	1	1
I	45	46.9
II	37	38.5
IIIa	10	10.4
IIIb	3	3.1
ECOG Performance status		
0–1	86	89.6
≥2	9	9.4
Breast Surgery		
Conservative	82	85.4
Mastectomy	14	14.58
Axillary Surgery		
None	17	17.7
Sentinel Lymph Node	38	39.6
Lymph Node Sampling	21	21.9
Lymphadenectomy	13	13.5
Adjuvant Treatments		
Chemotherapy	19	19.8
Radiotherapy	62	64.6
Hormone therapy	82	85.4
Toxicities	52	100
Grade 1–2	42	81
Grade 3–4	10	19

ECOG: Eastern Cooperative Oncology Group.

Based on CGA results, 35 patients (36.5% of the sample) were defined as frail, according to Balducci's criteria, and 61 (63.5) as nonfrail (Table 3).

Table 3. Characteristics of frail and nonfrail patients (based on comprehensive geriatric assessment (CGA) results).

Parameters	N	Nonfrail Patients			Frail Patients			$p < 0.05$
		N	Mean	Std. Dev.	N	Mean	Std. Dev.	
AGE	96	61	75.6	3.88	35	79	4.994	0.000
CCI	96	61	6.11	1.462	35	7.71	2.163	0.01
FRIED criteria	96	61	1.13	1.049	35	2.88	1.066	0.000
ADL	96	61	5.72	0.488	35	5	0.97	0.000
IADL	96	61	7.64	0.895	35	5.4	2.316	0.000
MMSE	96	61	27.88	2.345	35	25.09	3.76	0.001
MNA	93	60	25.87	2.262	33	23.12	3.517	0.001
GDS	85	58	3.47	2.617	27	6.19	3.903	0.000
SPPB	96	61	9.38	1.823	35	4.66	2.3	0.000
TUGT	75	49	10.29	2.227	26	16.76	6.018	0.000
SPEEDs	90	58	4.27	1.099	32	7.32	3.532	0.000
HANDGRIP	66	40	17.51	4.695	26	11.77	5.279	0.002
BMI	96	61	28.18	4.598	35	28.71	5.723	0.01
POLYPHARMACY Mean number of drugs	96	61	4.79	2.583	35	6.34	2.449	0.001
SMI	96	61	6.46	0.73	35	6.51	1.134	0.959
ASM	96	61	15.7	2.1	35	15.7	3	0.988

CCI = Charlson Comorbidity Index; ADL = Activities of Daily Living; IADL = Instrumental Activities of Daily Living; MMSE = Mini-Mental State Examination; MNA = Mini Nutritional Assessment; GDS = Geriatric Depression Scale; SPPB = Short Physical Performance Battery; TUGT = Time Up and Go Test; BMI = Body Mass Index; SMI = Skeletal Muscle Index; ASM = Appendicular Skeletal Muscle mass.

Frail patients were older compared to nonfrail ones (79 years, SD 4.994; 75.67, SD 3.88; $p = 0.000$) and had a slightly higher burden of comorbidities (mean CCI of frail patients was 7.71 against 6.11 for nonfrail patients, $p = 0.10$) and a higher level of disability (ADL mean 5 vs. 5.72 for nonfrail; IADL mean 5.4 vs. 7.64 for nonfrail; $p = 0.000$), and were at higher risk of malnutrition (MNA mean 23.12 vs. 25.87; $p = 0.001$).

The cognitive level of frail patients assessed by the MMSE screening test was almost 2 points lower than the other patients (25.09 frail patients; 27.88 nonfrail patients; $p = 0.001$) and they had a higher frequency of depressive symptoms than the nonfrail ones (average GDS 6.19 vs. 3.47 for nonfrail; $p = 0.000$). Polypharmacy, defined as taking five or more medications daily, was the case for 74.3% of frail patients and 49.2% of nonfrail patients.

Using the DXA parameters (either appendicular skeletal mass (ASM) or Skeletal Muscle Index {SMI = ASM/height^2}), 41 of 96 patients undergoing evaluation by DXA were found to be sarcopenic (42.7% of the sample examined) and 55 nonsarcopenic (57.3%). The average SMI of the sample was 6.47 (4.91 ÷ 9.73; SD 0.893). There were no significant differences in the prevalence of sarcopenia between frail and nonfrail patients (see Table 3)

According to the revised EWGSOP2 [28] criteria, 58 patients could be classified as "probably" sarcopenic with low muscle strength, defined as a chair stand test > 15 s for five rises (average value 17.09 s; 15.07 ÷ 26.7; SD 4.175). Among them, only 25 (out of 58) had a confirmed diagnosis of sarcopenia (either ASM < 15 kg or SMI DXA < 5.5 kg/m^2) with an average ASM of 13.46 kg and an average SMI value of 5.6 kg/m^2. In total, 17 (out of 25) patients could be defined as severely sarcopenic with an SPPB score ≤ 8 (mean value 4.7) (Figure 1).

Frail sarcopenic patients had a mean ASM of 12.89 kg (SD 1.087) and a mean SMI value of 5.49 kg/m^2 (SD 0.376). Frail nonsarcopenic patients had a mean ASM of 17.39 kg (SD 2.47) and a mean SMI value of 7.11 kg/m^2 (SD 0.991).

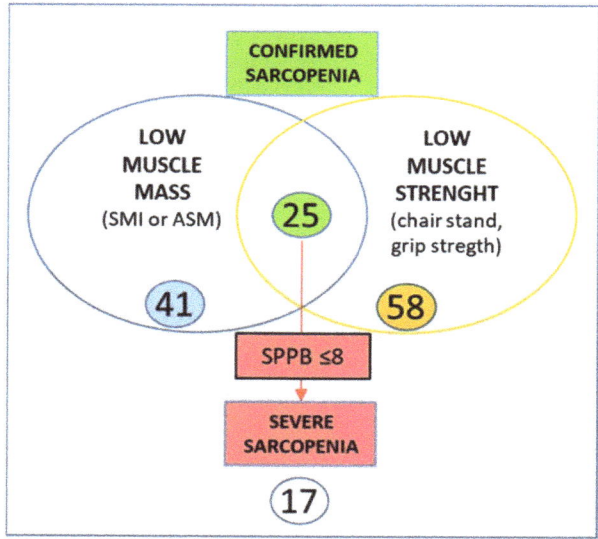

Figure 1. Prevalence of sarcopenia according EWGSOP2 definition [16]. SMI = =Skeletal Muscle Index; ASM = Appendicular Skeletal Muscle mass; SPPB = Short Physical Performance Battery

Figure 2 shows the overlap between sarcopenia and frailty (as assessed by the results of CGA). Only 13 patients satisfied both the requirements for being defined sarcopenic ("confirmed" sarcopenia along to EWGSOP2) and frail (using modified Balducci's criteria derived from CGA). Among the sarcopenic population, the proportion of patients that are also frail increases, moving from "probable" sarcopenia to "severe" sarcopenia (proportion of frail patients is 55.2% for "probable", 56.5% for "confirmed", and 72.2% for "severe" sarcopenia).

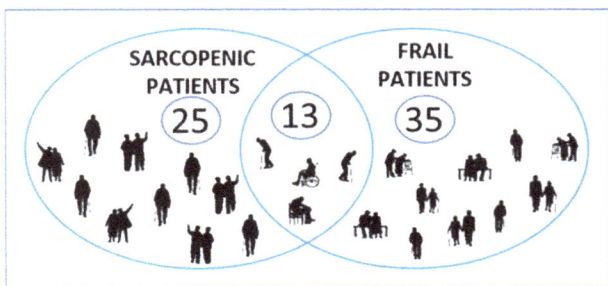

Figure 2. Prevalence of frailty and sarcopenia in the study sample.

In a one-year follow-up, the whole sample reported 52 cases of treatment toxicities (54.16%). According to the Common Terminology Criteria for Adverse Events (CTCAE), in the frail group 17 out of 35 patients developed toxicities of any types: five patients had grade 3–4 toxicities (14%). Among sarcopenic patients, 12 out of 23 patients developed toxicities of any types; five patients experienced grade 3–4 toxicities (22%).

Among patients reporting toxicities, frail patients reported Grade 3–4 toxicities (according to CTCAE) more frequently than nonfrail (29% vs. 14%) ones, while sarcopenic patients reported G3–G4 toxicities more than nonsarcopenic patients (42% vs. 13%) (Figure 3).

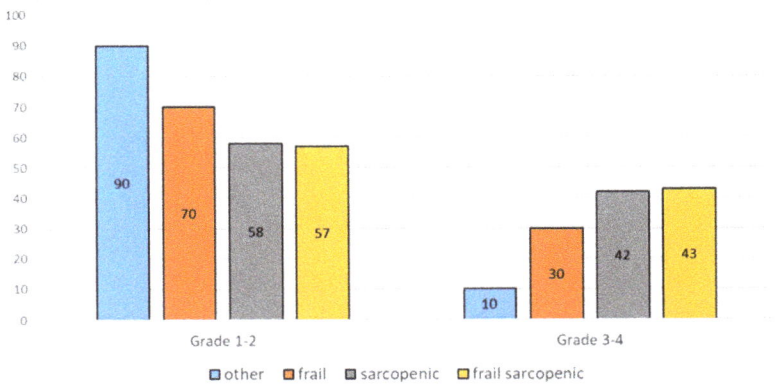

Figure 3. Percentage of patients who experienced Grade 1–2 and Grade 3–4 toxicities (according to Common Terminology Criteria for Adverse Events, CTCAE) in our population.

4. Discussion

In the aging scenario of the general population and the increasing number of diagnosed and treated cancers in older adults, it has become critical to identify, understand, and assess the so-called geriatric syndromes. Among these, more attention is being placed on sarcopenia. For this reason, it has become essential to know the differences between sarcopenia and the loss of muscle mass related to the normal process of muscle aging or other pathological conditions such as cachexia [30].

In our sample, we identified different frequencies of sarcopenia depending on the definition used. Sarcopenia can be defined as a pathological loss of skeletal muscle mass characterized by essential structural changes in muscle quality, which occurs in older adults and shows functional impairment and/or strength reduction [55]. Aging is related to a decline in muscle mass and strength [56] but only when this decline becomes pathological (sarcopenia) does this process lead to adverse health outcomes [57].

In patients with cancer, many studies showed how the loss of muscle mass is a prevalent condition independent of disease stage and body mass [58]. This is due to many factors leading to the deterioration of muscles: inflammation, cancer-derived catabolic factors, malnutrition, reduced physical activity, and the effect of cytotoxic and targeted treatments on muscle mass and quality [10,59].

Loss of muscle mass can precede the cancer and further complicate its course, predisposing patients to a shorter time of tumor progression, increased chemotherapy-related toxicity, postoperative complications, poor functional status, hospitalization, increased length of hospital stay, high 30-day readmission rate, and mortality [60]. While the loss of muscle mass has been proven to be an independent predictor of adverse outcomes at all ages and for several cancers, such as breast cancer, hepatocellular carcinoma, and advanced urothelial cancer [60,61], the presence of sarcopenia in older cancer patients, who could be at higher risk for this condition, has been associated with therapy-related toxicities and increased adverse outcomes [33], [61–63].

In oncology, the skeletal muscle index (SMI) is the main parameter used to evaluate sarcopenia. Several epidemiologic studies have determined the prevalence of sarcopenia using cut-off values determined by CT scans or DXA when muscle mass is normalized for height [64,65]. Muscle function has rarely been taken into consideration. This is mainly due to most existing studies' retrospective natures, relying on large CT scan datasets for oncological reasons (disease staging or surgical evaluation). At the same time, physical function tests are seldom conducted in routine clinical practice.

In recent years, first in the geriatric field and then in other settings, the definition of sarcopenia has shifted from an evaluation of muscle mass to a qualitative assessment of muscle function. Physical performance is a powerful predictor of adverse outcomes. This concept has been an integral part of the "physical frailty phenotype" construct [32]. Indeed, sarcopenia can be considered the most relevant biological determinant of physical frailty. Moreover, measurement of muscle mass and quality has many technological limitations, while the selection of specific cut-offs is a matter of debate [66], while muscle function is much easier to measure, at least in geriatric clinics (where hang grip or chair standing tests are routinely conducted). This new definition of sarcopenia correlates with many adverse outcomes (institutionalization risk, toxicity, mortality). This aspect has meant that sarcopenia, from a simple geriatric syndrome, has become one of the fundamental bases of modern geriatrics.

Still, in the nongeriatric setting, there is often confusion between frailty and sarcopenia, so we designed this study to try to identify those factors that can identify patients at greater risk of adverse outcomes.

Our study shows different ways to define sarcopenia and that the quantitative data (i.e., muscle mass measurement) alone is not sufficient. We detected a high prevalence of low muscle mass in the whole sample (almost 42.7%), almost equally distributed in frail and nonfrail patients. The proportion of patients with reduced muscle mass is in line with what has been reported in the literature [67]. However, when more stringent criteria that incorporate muscle function (such as EWGSOP 2) were used, only a limited proportion of patients (26%) could still be defined as "sarcopenic". Indeed, severely sarcopenic patients were almost always classified as frail on the results of CGA.

Even though sarcopenia has been regarded as a key component of the frailty status in older adults, it should be kept in mind that frailty is a multidimensional concept that goes beyond each of its features. Relying solely on what is usually defined as "sarcopenia" in oncological research (that is, low muscle mass) can be misleading, resulting in classifying many more patients as frail and possibly omitting valuable treatments. On the contrary, a stricter definition, where muscle loss is coupled with reduced muscle function (both strength and performance), could enable a better selection of patients.

In this study, 13.5% of patients have a correspondence between sarcopenia and frailty; this group has a very high probability of experiencing adverse outcomes. Identifying this subgroup will allow a real personalization of treatments in the near future and the identification of the risk of adverse events for apparently fit patients.

DXA is a noninvasive instrument for body composition assessments. Information on muscle and adipose tissue can also be gathered by other tools such as CT scans. Identifying reduced muscle mass should be promoted in oncology to avoid the adverse outcomes associated with this condition [28]. For example, chemotherapy could be personalized based on body composition, with doses adapted to the individual patient to limit toxicities [68]. Frailty is better identified by CGA which allows the detection of unidentified problems and the correct malignancy prognosis estimation [69]. Thus, CGA avoids over- and undertreatments in a scenario focus on tailored treatments.

In our sample, both frailty and sarcopenia are associated with treatment-related toxicities, especially with more severe (G3–G4) ones. However, this association is stronger for sarcopenic or sarcopenic-frail patients than it is for frail patients, although these differences are not statistically significant. It should be kept in mind that treating clinicians were aware of frailty status, so that more potentially toxic treatments were spared to frailer patients. On the other side, it is also possible that sarcopenia was not routinely considered when planning surgery or adjuvant therapies. This could have resulted in more adverse effects both in sarcopenic nonfrail patients and in sarcopenic frail patients, which indeed showed a comparable frequency of high-grade treatment-related toxicities.

The novelty of this study is in having identified for the first time in the same group of breast cancer patients the various degrees of sarcopenia and frailty through the available gold standards and a subgroup at high risk of adverse events (toxicity, reduced compliance, etc.) between the two.

Some limitations of our study have to be acknowledged. Firstly, given the cross-sectional nature of our data, it was not possible to make inferences on otherwise clinically significant outcomes associated with frailty and sarcopenia, such as survival or loss of functional independence. Secondly, the small sample size prevents us from generalizing our results to other clinical situations. Indeed, we believe that these data should prompt further research on the association between frailty, sarcopenia, and body composition, hopefully with a longer follow patients report to identify which parameter constitutes the best clinical deterioration predictor. More research is also needed on possible interventions to counteract sarcopenia, restoring muscle mass, and function. Physical exercise is a promising intervention that could prevent functional decline in older adults [70]. More data on the effect of structured physical activity in older adults with cancer are needed.

5. Conclusions

Our data support the use of a comprehensive definition of sarcopenia that takes into account both physical performance and muscle mass in order to identify older women with breast cancer at higher risk of clinical deterioration and treatment-related toxicities. A multidimensional geriatric assessment in this population is strongly recommended and evaluation of muscle mass and function should be regarded as an essential part of it, with the aim of offering patients the best personalized treatment.

Author Contributions: Conceptualization, A.B., D.F. and G.F.C.; methodology, A.B., D.F., A.M.S., B.D.C. and E.A.; data curation, A.B., D.F. and E.D.S.; writing—original draft preparation, A.B., D.F., B.D.C. and E.A.; writing—review and editing, A.M.S., G.F., F.M., L.T., R.M., R.B. and G.F.C.; supervision, D.F. and G.F.C.; project administration, R.B. All authors have read and agreed to the published version of the manuscript.

Funding: This research received no external funding.

Informed Consent Statement: Informed consent was obtained from all subjects involved in the study.

Conflicts of Interest: The authors declare no conflict of interest.

References

1. Ferlay, J.; Ervik, M.; Lam, F.; Colombet, M.; Mery, L.; Piñeros, M.; Znaor, A.; Soerjomataram, I.; Bray, F. *Global Cancer Observatory: Cancer Today*; International Agency for Research on Cancer: Lyon, France, 2020. Available online: https://gco.iarc.fr/today (accessed on February 2021).
2. Siegel, R.L.; Miller, K.D.; Jemal, A. Cancer statistics, 2019. *CA Cancer J. Clin.* **2019**, *69*, 7–34. [CrossRef] [PubMed]
3. Jolly, T.A.; Deal, A.M.; Nyrop, K.A.; Williams, G.R.; Pergolotti, M.; Wood, W.A.; Alston, S.M.; Gordon, B.E.; Dixon, S.A.; Moore, S.G.; et al. Geriatric Assessment-Identified Deficits in Older Cancer Patients with Normal Performance Status. *Oncologist* **2015**, *20*, 379–385. [CrossRef] [PubMed]
4. Paillaud, E.; Caillet, P.; Laurent, M.; Bastuji-Garin, S.; Liuu, E.; Lagrange, J.-L.; Culine, S.; Canoui-Poitrine, F. Optimal management of elderly cancer patients: Usefulness of the Comprehensive Geriatric Assessment. *Clin. Interv. Aging* **2014**, *9*, 1645–1660. [CrossRef] [PubMed]
5. Colloca, G.; Santoro, M.; Gambassi, G. Age-related physiologic changes and perioperative management of elderly patients. *Surg. Oncol.* **2010**, *19*, 124–130. [CrossRef]
6. Sedrak, M.S.; Freedman, R.A.; Cohen, H.J.; Muss, H.B.; Jatoi, A.; Klepin, H.D.; Wildes, T.M.; Le-Rademacher, J.G.; Kimmick, G.G.; Tew, W.P.; et al. Older adult participation in cancer clinical trials: A systematic review of barriers and interventions. *CA Cancer J. Clin.* **2021**, *71*, 78–92. [CrossRef]
7. Singh, R.; Hellman, S.; Heimann, R. The natural history of breast carcinoma in the elderly. *Cancer* **2004**, *100*, 1807–1813. [CrossRef]
8. Wildiers, H.; Kunkler, I.; Biganzoli, L.; Fracheboud, J.; Vlastos, G.; Bernard-Marty, C.; Hurria, A.; Extermann, M.; Girre, V.; Brain, E.; et al. Management of breast cancer in elderly individuals: Recommendations of the International Society of Geriatric Oncology. *Lancet Oncol.* **2007**, *8*, 1101–1115. [CrossRef]
9. NICE. Early and Locally Advanced Breast Cancer: Diagnosis and Treatment. 2018. Available online: https://www.nice.org.uk/guidance/ng101 (accessed on February 2021).
10. Colloca, G.; Di Capua, B.; Bellieni, A.; Fusco, D.; Ciciarello, F.; Tagliaferri, L.; Valentini, V.; Balducci, L. Biological and Functional Biomarkers of Aging: Definition, Characteristics, and How They Can Impact Everyday Cancer Treatment. *Curr. Oncol. Rep.* **2020**, *22*, 1–12. [CrossRef]
11. Fusco, D.; Allocca, E.; Villani, E.R.; Franza, L.; Laudisio, A.; Colloca, G. An update in breast cancer management for elderly patients. *Transl. Cancer Res.* **2018**, *7*, S319–S328. [CrossRef]
12. Extermann, M.; Aapro, M.; Bernabei, R.; Cohen, H.J.; Droz, J.-P.; Lichtman, S.; Mor, V.; Monfardini, S.; Repetto, L.; Sørbye, L.; et al. Use of comprehensive geriatric assessment in older cancer patients. *Crit. Rev. Oncol.* **2005**, *55*, 241–252. [CrossRef] [PubMed]
13. Mohile, S.G.; Dale, W.; Somerfield, M.R.; Schonberg, M.A.; Boyd, C.M.; Burhenn, P.S.; Canin, B.; Cohen, H.J.; Holmes, H.M.; Hopkins, J.O.; et al. Practical Assessment and Management of Vulnerabilities in Older Patients Receiving Chemotherapy: ASCO Guideline for Geriatric Oncology. *J. Clin. Oncol.* **2018**, *36*, 2326–2347. [CrossRef]
14. Colloca, G.; Corsonello, A.; Marzetti, E.; Balducci, L.; Landi, F.; Extermann, M.; Scambia, G.; Cesari, M.; Carreca, I.; Monfardini, S.; et al. Treating Cancer in Older and Oldest Old Patients. *Curr. Pharm. Des.* **2015**, *21*, 1699–1705. [CrossRef] [PubMed]
15. Palumbo, A.; Bringhen, S.; Mateos, M.-V.; LaRocca, A.; Facon, T.; Kumar, S.; Offidani, M.; McCarthy, P.; Evangelista, A.; Lonial, S.; et al. Geriatric assessment predicts survival and toxicities in elderly myeloma patients: An International Myeloma Working Group report. *Blood* **2015**, *125*, 2068–2074. [CrossRef]
16. Corre, R.; Greillier, L.; Le Caër, H.; Audigier-Valette, C.; Baize, N.; Bérard, H.; Falchero, L.; Monnet, I.; Dansin, E.; Vergnenègre, A.; et al. Use of a Comprehensive Geriatric Assessment for the Management of Elderly Patients with Advanced Non–Small-Cell Lung Cancer: The Phase III Randomized ESOGIA-GFPC-GECP 08-02 Study. *J. Clin. Oncol.* **2016**, *34*, 1476–1483. [CrossRef] [PubMed]
17. Goede, V.; Bahlo, J.; Chataline, V.; Eichhorst, B.; Dürig, J.; Stilgenbauer, S.; Kolb, G.; Honecker, F.; Wedding, U.; Hallek, M. Evaluation of geriatric assessment in patients with chronic lymphocytic leukemia: Results of the CLL9 trial of the German CLL study group. *Leuk. Lymphoma* **2015**, *57*, 789–796. [CrossRef] [PubMed]
18. Kroep, J.R.; Van Werkhoven, E.; Polee, M.; Van Groeningen, C.J.; Beeker, A.; Erdkamp, F.; Weijl, N.; Van Bochove, A.; Erjavec, Z.; Kapiteijn, E.; et al. Randomised study of tegafur–uracil plus leucovorin versus capecitabine as first-line therapy in elderly patients with advanced colorectal cancer—TLC study. *J. Geriatr. Oncol.* **2015**, *6*, 307–315. [CrossRef] [PubMed]
19. Wildes, T.M.; O'Donovan, A.; Colloca, G.F.; Cheung, K.-L. Tumour boards in geriatric oncology. *Age Ageing* **2018**, *47*, 168–170. [CrossRef] [PubMed]
20. Garcovich, S.; Colloca, G.; Sollena, P.; Andrea, B.; Balducci, L.; Cho, W.C.; Bernabei, R.; Peris, K. Skin Cancer Epidemics in the Elderly as An Emerging Issue in Geriatric Oncology. *Aging Dis.* **2017**, *8*, 643–661. [CrossRef] [PubMed]
21. Colloca, G.; Lattanzio, F.; Balducci, L.; Onder, G.; Ronconi, G.; Landi, F.; Morlans, G.; Bernabei, R. Treating Cancer and No-Cancer Pain in Older and Oldest Old Patients. *Curr. Pharm. Des.* **2015**, *21*, 1706–1714. [CrossRef]
22. Luciani, A.; Biganzoli, L.; Colloca, G.; Falci, C.; Castagneto, B.; Floriani, I.; Battisti, N.; Dottorini, L.; Ferrari, D.; Fiduccia, P.; et al. Estimating the risk of chemotherapy toxicity in older patients with cancer: The role of the Vulnerable Elders Survey-13 (VES-13). *J. Geriatr. Oncol.* **2015**, *6*, 272–279. [CrossRef] [PubMed]

23. Dale, W.; Mohile, S.G.; Eldadah, B.A.; Trimble, E.L.; Schilsky, R.L.; Cohen, H.J.; Muss, H.B.; Schmader, K.E.; Ferrell, B.; Extermann, M.; et al. Biological, Clinical, and Psychosocial Correlates at the Interface of Cancer and Aging Research. *J. Natl. Cancer Inst.* **2012**, *104*, 581–589. [CrossRef]
24. Extermann, M.; Overcash, J.; Lyman, G.H.; Parr, J.; Balducci, L. Comorbidity and functional status are independent in older cancer patients. *J. Clin. Oncol.* **1998**, *16*, 1582–1587. [CrossRef]
25. Hurria, A.; Togawa, K.; Mohile, S.G.; Owusu, C.; Klepin, H.D.; Gross, C.P.; Lichtman, S.M.; Gajra, A.; Bhatia, S.; Katheria, V.; et al. Predicting Chemotherapy Toxicity in Older Adults with Cancer: A Prospective Multicenter Study. *J. Clin. Oncol.* **2011**, *29*, 3457–3465. [CrossRef] [PubMed]
26. Colloca, G.; Tagliaferri, L.; Di Capua, B.; Gambacorta, M.A.; Lanzotti, V.; Bellieni, A.; Monfardini, S.; Balducci, L.; Bernabei, R.; Cho, W.C.; et al. Management of The Elderly Cancer Patients Complexity: The Radiation Oncology Potential. *Aging Dis.* **2020**, *11*, 649–657. [CrossRef] [PubMed]
27. Repetto, L.; Fratino, L.; Audisio, R.A.; Venturino, A.; Gianni, W.; Vercelli, M.; Parodi, S.; Lago, D.D.; Gioia, F.; Monfardini, S.; et al. Comprehensive Geriatric Assessment Adds Information to Eastern Cooperative Oncology Group Performance Status in Elderly Cancer Patients: An Italian Group for Geriatric Oncology Study. *J. Clin. Oncol.* **2002**, *20*, 494–502. [CrossRef] [PubMed]
28. Cruz-Jentoft, A.J.; Bahat, G.; Bauer, J.; Boirie, Y.; Bruyère, O.; Cederholm, T.; Cooper, C.; Landi, F.; Rolland, Y.; Sayer, A.A.; et al. Sarcopenia: Revised European consensus on definition and diagnosis. *Age Ageing* **2019**, *48*, 16–31. [CrossRef] [PubMed]
29. Janssen, I.; Heymsfield, S.B.; Ross, R. Low Relative Skeletal Muscle Mass (Sarcopenia) in Older Persons Is Associated with Functional Impairment and Physical Disability. *J. Am. Geriatr. Soc.* **2002**, *50*, 889–896. [CrossRef]
30. Colloca, G.; Di Capua, B.; Bellieni, A.; Cesari, M.; Marzetti, E.; Valentini, V.; Calvani, R. Muscoloskeletal aging, sarcopenia and cancer. *J. Geriatr. Oncol.* **2019**, *10*, 504–509. [CrossRef] [PubMed]
31. Pahor, M.; Manini, T.; Cesari, M. Sarcopenia: Clinical evaluation, biological markers and other evaluation tools. *J. Nutr. Health Aging* **2009**, *13*, 724–728. [CrossRef]
32. Landi, F.; Calvani, R.; Cesari, M.; Tosato, M.; Martone, A.M.; Bernabei, R.; Onder, G.; Marzetti, E. Sarcopenia as the Biological Substrate of Physical Frailty. *Clin. Geriatr. Med.* **2015**, *31*, 367–374. [CrossRef] [PubMed]
33. Feliciano, E.M.C.; Kroenke, C.H.; Meyerhardt, J.A.; Prado, C.M.; Bradshaw, P.T.; Dannenberg, A.J.; Kwan, M.L.; Xiao, J.; Quesenberry, C.; Weltzien, E.K.; et al. Metabolic Dysfunction, Obesity, and Survival Among Patients with Early-Stage Colorectal Cancer. *J. Clin. Oncol.* **2016**, *34*, 3664–3671. [CrossRef]
34. Baumgartner, R.N.; Koehler, K.M.; Gallagher, D.; Romero, L.; Heymsfield, S.B.; Ross, R.R.; Garry, P.J.; Lindeman, R.D. Epidemiology of Sarcopenia among the Elderly in New Mexico. *Am. J. Epidemiol.* **1998**, *147*, 755–763. [CrossRef]
35. Cruz-Jentoft, A.J.; Baeyens, J.P.; Bauer, J.M.; Boirie, Y.; Cederholm, T.; Landi, F.; Martin, F.C.; Michel, J.-P.; Rolland, Y.; Schneider, S.M.; et al. Sarcopenia: European consensus on definition and diagnosis: Report of the European Working Group on Sarcopenia in Older People. *Age Ageing* **2010**, *39*, 412–423. [CrossRef] [PubMed]
36. Schaap, L.A.; Van Schoor, N.M.; Lips, P.; Visser, M. Associations of Sarcopenia Definitions, and Their Components, With the Incidence of Recurrent Falling and Fractures: The Longitudinal Aging Study Amsterdam. *J. Gerontol. Ser. A Biol. Sci. Med. Sci.* **2018**, *73*, 1199–1204. [CrossRef]
37. Leong, D.P.; Teo, K.K.; Rangarajan, S.; Lopez-Jaramillo, P.; Avezum, A., Jr.; Orlandini, A.; Seron, P.; Ahmed, S.H.; Rosengren, A.; Kelishadi, R.; et al. Prognostic value of grip strength: Findings from the Prospective Urban Rural Epidemiology (PURE) study. *Lancet* **2015**, *386*, 266–273. [CrossRef]
38. Fusco, D.; Ferrini, A.; Pasqualetti, G.; Giannotti, C.; Cesari, M.; Laudisio, A.; Ballestrero, A.; Scabini, S.; Odetti, P.R.; Colloca, G.F.; et al. Comprehensive geriatric assessment in older adults with cancer: Recommendations by the Italian Society of Geriatrics and Gerontology (SIGG). *Eur. J. Clin. Investig.* **2021**, *51*, e13347. [CrossRef]
39. Sorensen, J.B.; Klee, M.R.; Palshof, T.; Hansen, H.H. Performance status assessment in cancer patients. An inter-observer variability study. *Br. J. Cancer* **1993**, *67*, 773–775. [CrossRef]
40. Oken, M.M.; Creech, R.H.; Tormey, D.C.; Horton, J.; Davis, T.E.; McFadden, E.T.; Carbone, P.P. Toxicity and response criteria of the Eastern Cooperative Oncology Group. *Am. J. Clin. Oncol.* **1982**, *5*, 649–655. [CrossRef]
41. Charlson, M.E.; Pompei, P.; Ales, K.L.; MacKenzie, C. A new method of classifying prognostic comorbidity in longitudinal studies: Development and validation. *J. Chronic Dis.* **1987**, *40*, 373–383. [CrossRef]
42. Katz, S.; Downs, T.D.; Cash, H.R.; Grotz, R.C. Progress in Development of the Index of ADL. *Gerontologist* **1970**, *10*, 20–30. [CrossRef] [PubMed]
43. Lawton, M.P.; Brody, A.E.M. Assessment of Older People: Self-Maintaining and Instrumental Activities of Daily Living. *Gerontologist* **1969**, *9*, 179–186. [CrossRef]
44. Cockrell, J.R.; Folstein, M.F. Mini-Mental State Examination (MMSE). *Psychopharmacol. Bull.* **1988**, *24*, 689–692. [PubMed]
45. Guigoz, P.Y.; Vellas, M.B.; Garry, P.P.J. Assessing the Nutritional Status of the Elderly: The Mini Nutritional Assessment as Part of the Geriatric Evaluation. *Nutr. Rev.* **2009**, *54*, S59–S65. [CrossRef] [PubMed]
46. Conradsson, M.; Rosendahl, E.; Littbrand, H.; Gustafson, Y.; Olofsson, B.; Lövheim, H. Usefulness of the Geriatric Depression Scale 15-item version among very old people with and without cognitive impairment. *Aging Ment. Health* **2013**, *17*, 638–645. [CrossRef] [PubMed]

47. Guralnik, J.M.; Simonsick, E.M.; Ferrucci, L.; Glynn, R.J.; Berkman, L.F.; Blazer, D.G.; Scherr, P.A.; Wallace, R.B. A Short Physical Performance Battery Assessing Lower Extremity Function: Association with Self-Reported Disability and Prediction of Mortality and Nursing Home Admission. *J. Gerontol.* **1994**, *49*, M85–M94. [CrossRef] [PubMed]
48. Pavasini, R.; Guralnik, J.; Brown, J.C.; Di Bari, M.; Cesari, M.; Landi, F.; Vaes, B.; Legrand, D.; Verghese, J.; Wang, C.; et al. Short Physical Performance Battery and all-cause mortality: Systematic review and meta-analysis. *BMC Med.* **2016**, *14*, 215. [CrossRef]
49. Bischoff, H.A.; Stähelin, H.B.; Monsch, A.U.; Iversen, M.D.; Weyh, A.; von Dechend, M.; Akos, R.; Conzelmann, M.; Dick, W.; Theiler, R. Identifying a cut-off point for normal mobility: A comparison of the timed 'up and go' test in community-dwelling and institutionalised elderly women. *Age Ageing* **2003**, *32*, 315–320. [CrossRef]
50. Dodds, R.M.; Syddall, H.E.; Cooper, R.; Benzeval, M.; Deary, I.J.; Dennison, E.M.; Der, G.; Gale, C.R.; Inskip, H.; Jagger, C.; et al. Grip Strength across the Life Course: Normative Data from Twelve British Studies. *PLoS ONE* **2014**, *9*, e113637. [CrossRef]
51. Cesari, M.; Kritchevsky, S.B.; Newman, A.B.; Simonsick, E.M.; Harris, T.B.; Penninx, B.W.; Pt, J.S.B.; Tylavsky, F.A.; Satterfield, S.; Bauer, D.C.; et al. Added Value of Physical Performance Measures in Predicting Adverse Health-Related Events: Results from the Health, Aging and Body Composition Study. *J. Am. Geriatr. Soc.* **2009**, *57*, 251–259. [CrossRef]
52. Balducci, L.; Beghe, C. The application of the principles of geriatrics to the management of the older person with cancer. *Crit. Rev. Oncol.* **2000**, *35*, 147–154. [CrossRef]
53. Balducci, L.; Colloca, G.; Cesari, M.; Gambassi, G. Assessment and treatment of elderly patients with cancer. *Surg. Oncol.* **2010**, *19*, 117–123. [CrossRef] [PubMed]
54. Dubianski, R.; Wildes, T.M.; Wildiers, H. SIOG guidelines-essential for good clinical practice in geriatric oncology. *J. Geriatr. Oncol.* **2019**, *10*, 196–198. [CrossRef]
55. McGregor, R.A.; Cameron-Smith, D.; Poppitt, S.D. It is not just muscle mass: A review of muscle quality, composition and metabolism during ageing as determinants of muscle function and mobility in later life. *Longev. Healthspan* **2014**, *3*, 1–8. [CrossRef] [PubMed]
56. Thomas, D.R. Loss of skeletal muscle mass in aging: Examining the relationship of starvation, sarcopenia and cachexia. *Clin. Nutr.* **2007**, *26*, 389–399. [CrossRef] [PubMed]
57. Ligibel, J.A.; Schmitz, K.H.; Berger, N.A. Sarcopenia in aging, obesity, and cancer. *Transl. Cancer Res.* **2020**, *9*, 5760–5771. [CrossRef] [PubMed]
58. Prado, C.M.; Lieffers, J.R.; McCargar, L.J.; Reiman, T.; Sawyer, M.B.; Martin, L.; Baracos, V.E. Prevalence and clinical implications of sarcopenic obesity in patients with solid tumours of the respiratory and gastrointestinal tracts: A population-based study. *Lancet Oncol.* **2008**, *9*, 629–635. [CrossRef]
59. Damanti, S.; Colloca, G.F.; Ferrini, A.; Consonni, D.; Cesari, M. Sarcopenia (and sarcopenic obesity) in older patients with gynecological malignancies. *J. Geriatr. Oncol.* **2020**. [CrossRef]
60. Prado, C.M.; Baracos, V.E.; McCargar, L.J.; Reiman, T.; Mourtzakis, M.; Tonkin, K.; Mackey, J.R.; Koski, S.; Pituskin, E.; Sawyer, M.B. Sarcopenia as a Determinant of Chemotherapy Toxicity and Time to Tumor Progression in Metastatic Breast Cancer Patients Receiving Capecitabine Treatment. *Clin. Cancer Res.* **2009**, *15*, 2920–2926. [CrossRef] [PubMed]
61. Villaseñor, A.; Ballard-Barbash, R.; Baumgartner, K.B.; Baumgartner, R.N.; Bernstein, L.; McTiernan, A.; Neuhouser, M.L. Prevalence and prognostic effect of sarcopenia in breast cancer survivors: The HEAL Study. *J. Cancer Surviv.* **2012**, *6*, 398–406. [CrossRef] [PubMed]
62. van Vledder, M.G.; Levolger, S.; Ayez, N.; Verhoef, C.; Tran, T.C.K.; Ijzermans, J.N.M. Body composition and outcome in patients undergoing resection of colorectal liver metastases19. *BJS* **2012**, *99*, 550–557. [CrossRef] [PubMed]
63. Kazemi-Bajestani, S.M.R.; Mazurak, V.C.; Baracos, V. Computed tomography-defined muscle and fat wasting are associated with cancer clinical outcomes. *Semin. Cell Dev. Biol.* **2016**, *54*, 2–10. [CrossRef]
64. Kim, Y.-S.; Lee, Y.; Chung, Y.-S.; Lee, D.-J.; Joo, N.-S.; Hong, D.; Song, G.E.; Kim, H.-J.; Choi, Y.J.; Kim, K.-M. Prevalence of Sarcopenia and Sarcopenic Obesity in the Korean Population Based on the Fourth Korean National Health and Nutritional Examination Surveys. *J. Gerontol. Ser. A Biol. Sci. Med. Sci.* **2012**, *67*, 1107–1113. [CrossRef] [PubMed]
65. Baumgartner, R.N. Body Composition in Healthy Aging. *Ann. N. Y. Acad. Sci.* **2006**, *904*, 437–448. [CrossRef] [PubMed]
66. Buckinx, F.; Landi, F.; Cesari, M.; Fielding, R.A.; Visser, M.; Engelke, K.; Maggi, S.; Dennison, E.; Al-Daghri, N.M.; Allepaerts, S.; et al. Pitfalls in the measurement of muscle mass: A need for a reference standard. *J. Cachexia Sarcopenia Muscle* **2018**, *9*, 269–278. [CrossRef] [PubMed]
67. Aleixo, G.F.P.; Williams, G.R.; Nyrop, K.A.; Muss, H.B.; Shachar, S.S. Muscle composition and outcomes in patients with breast cancer: Meta-analysis and systematic review. *Breast Cancer Res. Treat.* **2019**, *177*, 569–579. [CrossRef]
68. Desmedt, C.; Fornili, M.; Clatot, F.; Demicheli, R.; De Bortoli, D.; Di Leo, A.; Viale, G.; De Azambuja, E.; Crown, J.; Francis, P.A.; et al. Differential Benefit of Adjuvant Docetaxel-Based Chemotherapy in Patients with Early Breast Cancer According to Baseline Body Mass Index. *J. Clin. Oncol.* **2020**, *38*, 2883–2891. [CrossRef]
69. Wildiers, H.; Heeren, P.; Puts, M.; Topinkova, E.; Janssen-Heijnen, M.L.G.; Extermann, M.; Falandry, C.; Artz, A.; Brain, E.; Colloca, G.; et al. International Society of Geriatric Oncology Consensus on Geriatric Assessment in Older Patients with Cancer. *J. Clin. Oncol.* **2014**, *32*, 2595–2603. [CrossRef]
70. Pahor, M.; Guralnik, J.M.; Ambrosius, W.T.; Blair, S.; Bonds, D.E.; Church, T.S.; Espeland, M.A.; Fielding, R.A.; Gill, T.M.; Groessl, E.J.; et al. Effect of Structured Physical Activity on Prevention of Major Mobility Disability in Older Adults. *JAMA* **2014**, *311*, 2387–2396. [CrossRef]

Article

Liver Metastasectomy for Metastatic Breast Cancer Patients: A Single Institution Retrospective Analysis

Armando Orlandi [1,*], Letizia Pontolillo [1,2], Caterina Mele [3], Mariangela Pasqualoni [1,2], Sergio Pannunzio [1,2], Maria Chiara Cannizzaro [1,2], Claudia Cutigni [1,2], Antonella Palazzo [1], Giovanna Garufi [1,2], Maria Vellone [2,3], Francesco Ardito [2,3], Gianluca Franceschini [2,4], Alejandro Martin Sanchez [4], Alessandra Cassano [1,2], Felice Giuliante [2,3], Emilio Bria [1,2] and Giampaolo Tortora [1,2]

1. Comprehensive Cancer Center, UOC di Oncologia Medica, Fondazione Policlinico Universitario A. Gemelli IRCCS, 00168 Rome, Italy; letiziapontolillo@gmail.com (L.P.); mariangelapasqualoni@gmail.com (M.P.); sergio.pannunzio90@gmail.com (S.P.); mariachiara.cannizzaro@outlook.com (M.C.C.); claudiacutigni1992@gmail.com (C.C.); antonella.palazzo@policlinicogemelli.it (A.P.); giovanna.garufi@unicatt.it (G.G.); alessandra.cassano@policlinicogemelli.it (A.C.); emilio.bria@policlinicogemelli.it (E.B.); giampaolo.tortora@policlinicogemelli.it (G.T.)
2. Catholic University of Sacred Heart, 00168 Rome, Italy; maria.vellone@policlinicogemelli.it (M.V.); francesco.ardito@policlinicogemelli.it (F.A.); gianluca.franceschini@policlinicogemelli.it (G.F.); felice.giuliante@policlinicogemelli.it (F.G.)
3. Comprehensive Cancer Center, Hepatobiliary Surgery Unit, Fondazione Policlinico Universitario A. Gemelli IRCCS, 00168 Rome, Italy; caterina.mele@policlinicogemelli.it
4. Multidisciplinary Breast Center, Dipartimento Scienze della Salute della donna e del Bambino e di Sanità Pubblica, Fondazione Policlinico Universitario A. Gemelli IRCCS, 00168 Rome, Italy; martin.sanchez@policlinicogemelli.it
* Correspondence: armando.orlandi@policlinicogemelli.it; Tel.: +39-0630-156-318

Abstract: The liver represents the first metastatic site in 5–12% of metastatic breast cancer (MBC) cases. In absence of reliable evidence, liver metastasectomy (LM) could represent a possible therapeutic option for selected MBC patients (patients) in clinical practice. A retrospective analysis including MBC patients who had undergone an LM after a multidisciplinary Tumor Board discussion at the Hepatobiliary Surgery Unit of Fondazione Policlinico Universitario "Agostino Gemelli" IRCCS in Rome, between January 1994 and December 2019 was conducted. The primary endpoint was overall survival (OS) after a MBC-LM; the secondary endpoint was the disease-free interval (DFI) after surgery. Forty-nine MBC patients underwent LM, but clinical data were only available for 22 patients. After a median follow-up of 71 months, median OS and DFI were 67 months (95% CI 45–103) and 15 months (95% CI 11–46), respectively. At univariate analysis, the presence of a negative resection margin (R0) was the only factor that statistically significantly influenced OS (78 months versus 16 months; HR 0.083, $p < 0.0001$) and DFI (16 months versus 5 months; HR 0.17, $p = 0.0058$). A LM for MBC might represent a therapeutic option for selected patients. The radical nature of the surgical procedure performed in a high-flow center and after a multidisciplinary discussion appears essential for this therapeutic option.

Keywords: metastatic breast cancer; liver metastases; hepatic surgery; personalized medicine

1. Introduction

Metastatic breast cancer (MBC) is the first oncological cause of death in women despite the advances in therapeutic strategies, with a 5-year survival of only ~25% [1,2]. The liver represents the first metastatic site in 5–12% of MBC [3] cases. Despite the transient response to chemo or endocrine therapy, most patients experience disease progression after 1–2 years [4]. While current evidence supports a liver metastasectomy (LM) for advanced colorectal cancer in improving survival [5,6] on the basis that hepatic parenchyma filters circulating tumor cells (CTC) from the primary neoplastic site to systemic circulation, LM is considered a possible therapeutic option for selected MBC patients in clinical practice, in the absence of prospective evidence. Several studies reported controversial results about the survival rate after hepatic loco-regional treatment in MBC with liver metastases with a 3-year and 5-year survival rate that ranged between 49–94% and 5–78% respectively [3,7–28]. A recent review of Bale et al. [29] showed that a primary tumor's characteristics such as small tumor size, nodes negativity, low grade, and early-stage may be associated with a better outcome after liver surgery. In addition, they evidenced as an independent positive prognostic factor a long interval between the primary diagnosis and the detection of breast cancer liver metastasis (BCLM) more than 1 year, liver-limited disease (with the exception of isolated pulmonary and bone metastasis), response to preoperative systemic therapy before hepatic surgery, and the BCLM expression of estrogen receptor (ER) and progesterone receptor (PgR). The major limits of the studies in the literature are represented by the small number of patients enrolled and the presence of multiple confounding factors for the heterogeneity of the biology of the primary tumor, the presence of synchronous and metachronous metastases, the presence of extrahepatic disease, and the types of systemic treatments used. However, in all studies, patients with a low burden-disease benefited from R0 resections of BCLM with an improvement in survival rate [7,30]. Therefore, we report data about our experience of MBC patients who underwent liver metastasis surgery.

2. Materials and Methods

2.1. Study Design and Participants

A retrospective analysis including MBC patients who had undergone LM after a multidisciplinary Tumor Board discussion at the Hepatobiliary Surgery Unit of the Fondazione Policlinico Universitario "Agostino Gemelli" IRCCS in Rome, between January 1994 and December 2019, was conducted.

Eligible patients were aged 18 years or older, had a histological diagnosis of invasive BC and synchronous or metachronous LM. All immunophenotype BC were eligible in the study: luminal (ER and/or PgR positive), epidermal growth factor receptor 2 (HER2) positive and triple-negative (TNBC: ER, PgR, and HER2 negative). In all patients, disease assessment was determined by computerized tomography (CT) scan and magnetic resonance imaging (MRI) of the liver. The presence of extrahepatic disease was allowed provided that these sites were stable or in response to previous systemic treatments before hepatic surgery. The evaluation of expression of ER, PgR, and HER2 was done respecting the ASCO-CAP guidelines. Using the pathology report after hepatic surgery, the presence or the absence of disease at the resection margin (R0: no disease at the resected surgical margin, R1: the presence of disease at the resected surgical margin) was determined. For each patient, demographic data were collected including gender and age. Clinicopathological data on menopausal status (defined retrospectively after a woman has experienced 12 months of amenorrhea without any other pathological or physiological cause), metastatic sites, hepatic metastases presentation, number of systemic therapy pre-hepatic surgery, histotype (ductal *versus* lobular), immunophenotype, and resection margins were also collected. The study was approved by the Institutional Review Boards.

2.2. Study Endpoints

The primary endpoint was overall survival (OS) after LM, defined as the time from LM to death; the secondary endpoint was the disease-free interval (DFI) after LM, defined as the time from surgery to recurrence (in patients with liver-only disease) or progression of the disease (in patients with extrahepatic metastases which was stable or in response to previous treatment before LM). An exploratory analysis was performed to evaluate the survival impact of demographic and clinicopathological factors: age (<50 *versus* ≥50 years old), menopausal state (pre-menopausal *versus* menopausal), metastatic sites (only liver *versus* other), hepatic metastases presentation (synchronous *versus* metachronous), number of liver metastases (1 *versus* > 1), number of systemic therapy pre-hepatic surgery (none *versus* $\geq$ 1), histotype (ductal *versus* lobular), immunophenotype (luminal *versus* TNBC *versus* HER2+), and hepatic resection margins (R0 *versus* R1).

2.3. Statistical Analysis

Statistical analyses were performed using MedCalc software version 14 (MedCalc Software Ltd, Ostend, Belgium). Survival curves were calculated according to the Kaplan-Meier method and differences in survival were assessed with the log-rank test. Independent predictors of disease-specific survival and recurrence were identified by Cox proportional hazard analysis. Statistical significance was defined as a p-value < 0.05. As the study was explorative, an estimate of the sample size was not calculated.

3. Results

3.1. Demographic and Clinicopathological Characteristics of Patients

During the study period, a total of 49 patients, all female, underwent LM at our Hospital. Clinical data were available for 22. Patient age at the time of surgery ranged from 34 to 71 years with a median age of 48 years. Ten patients were premenopausal, 12 postmenopausal. Nineteen patients had isolated liver disease, 3 patients had multiorgan metastasis. Among patients with multi-organ metastasis, 2 had bone metastasis and 1 adrenal metastasis. Liver metastasis was metachronous for 17 patients and synchronous for 5 patients. Seven patients underwent surgery upfront, while 15 patients received one line of systemic treatment prior to surgery; the best response to systemic treatment was a partial response (PR) for 11 patients, 3 patients had a stable disease (SD), and only one had a progression disease (PD), with a disease control rate (DCR: PR + SD) of 93%. The histotype was ductal carcinoma for 21 patients, only 1 was lobular; 14 patients had a luminal tumor, 3 patients were HER2+, and 5 patients were TNBC. Nine patients underwent anatomical liver resection (resection of segments in 7 patients and resection of the left hepatic lobes in 2 patients were done) and 13 patients received metastasectomies (not anatomical liver resection). The resection margin was negative (R0) in 20 patients and positive in 2 patients. Among the 11 patients who had obtained a partial response, 4 patients had a pathological complete response (only fibrosis was found in the absence of neoplastic cells). Postoperative mortality (mortality within one month after hepatic surgery) was 0%. Complications occurred only in two patients: 1 patient presented perihepatic abscess and 1 patient with perihepatic abscess and a pulmonary embolism; both cases were resolved with medical therapy. All patients received at least one line of systemic therapy in the post-surgery setting: as maintenance of the previous treatment (hormonal therapy for luminal therapy, trastuzumab +/− hormonal therapy for HER2+ and the same chemotherapy in TNBC) and a new line of therapy after recurrence/progression of the disease.

Demographic and clinicopathological characteristics of patients are listed in Table 1.

Table 1. Demographic and clinicopathological characteristics of patients (n = 22) and correlation with the disease-free interval (DFI) and overall survival (OS).

Characteristics	No. of Patients (n = 22)	DFS (Months)	Long Rank Test (p Value)	OS (Months)	Long Rank Test (p Value)
Age					
<50	12	14	p = 0.7	50	p = 0.22
>50	10	15		103	
Gender					
Male	0	-	-	-	-
Female	22	15		67	
Menopausal Status					
Pre-menopausal	10	14	p = 0.58	50	p = 0.56
Post-menopausal	12	15		78	

Table 1. Cont.

Characteristics	No. of Patients (n = 22)	DFS (Months)	Long Rank Test (p Value)	OS (Months)	Long Rank Test (p Value)
Metastatic sites					
Only liver	19	16	$p = 0.38$	103	$p = 0.14$
Other	3	11		50	
Liver metastases					
Synchronous	5	N.R.	$p = 0.053$	N.R.	$p = 0.2$
Metachronous	17	15		64	
N. of liver metastases					
1	14	15	$p = 0.84$	103	$p = 0.52$
>1	8	11		64	
Systemic therapy pre-liver surgery					
0	7	14	$p = 0.1$	50	$p = 0.89$
≥1	15	46		78	
Histotype					
Ductal	20	15	$p = 0.88$	78	$p = 0.36$
Lobular	2	2		44	
Immunophenotype					
Luminal	14	13		56	
HER2 +	5	17	$p = 0.72$	73	$p = 0.28$
TNBC	3	7		45	
Resection margin					
Negative (R0)	20	16	$p = 0.005$	78	$p < 0.0001$
Positive (R1)	2	5		16	

DFS: disease-free survival after liver resection; OS: overall survival after liver resection. N.: number. N.R.: not reached. Italics and bold: statistical significant p-value.

3.2. Survival Outcomes

At the data cut-off analysis of May 2020, 11 patients were still alive and 7 patients were free of progression disease after hepatic surgery. Of the 15 patients who experienced recurrence, 8 have had disease progression with liver metastases, 3 with liver and bone metastases, 3 with lung metastases, and 1 with brain metastases. After a median follow-up of 71 months, median OS was 67 months (95% CI 45–103) (Figure 1) while median DFI was 15 months (95% CI 11–46) (Figure 2), respectively.

At univariate analysis, the presence of a negative resection margin was the only factor that statistically significantly influenced OS (78 versus 16 months; HR 0.083, $p < 0.0001$) (Figure 3) and the DFI (16 versus 5 months; HR 0.17, $p = 0.0058$) (Figure 4). None of the other factors were significantly associated with OS and the DFI; their association with the DFI and OS is shown in Table 1. A trend toward significance (the boundary of p-value < 0.2) was observed in the OS analysis for metastatic sites (only liver versus other sites, 103 versus 50 months, $p = 0.14$) while a prior systemic therapy showed a trend in favor also for the DFI (none versus ≥ 1, 14 versus 46 months, $p = 0.1$). The multivariate analysis confirmed the negative resection margin as the only factor which statistically significantly influenced OS ($p = 0.0034$) and DFS ($p = 0.024$).

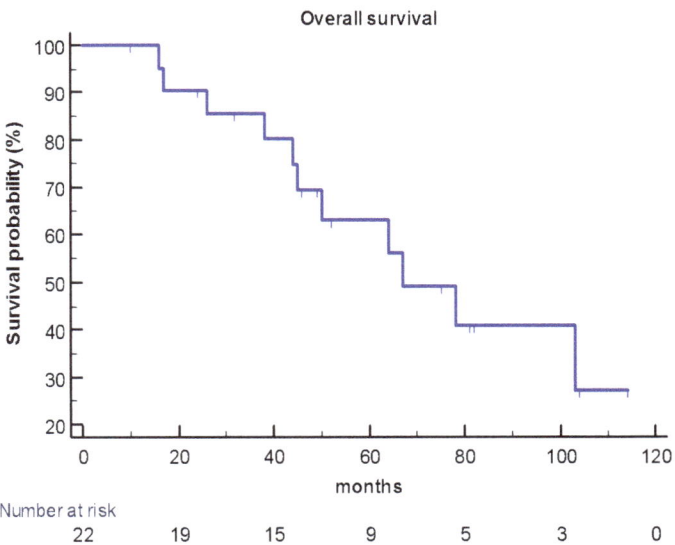

Figure 1. OS in the study population (n = 22): median OS was 67 months (95% CI 45–103).

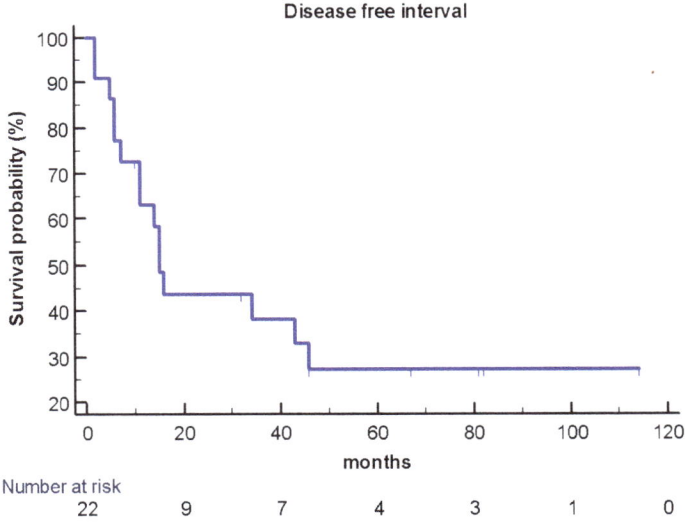

Figure 2. DFS in the study population (n = 22): median DFI was 15 months (95% CI 11–46).

Clinicopathological characteristics of patients with R0 resection are listed in Table 2.

Of the 20 patients with an R0 resection, 13 patients had a single lesion while 7 had two metastases. Radiological dimensions of the liver lesions are available for 13 of the 20 patients and ranged from 9 mm to 80 mm; histological dimensions were available for 15 patients and ranged from 4 to 35 mm. Fourteen patients had received one line of systemic treatment before the surgery: 4 patients had a complete response (CR), 6 patients had a partial response (PR), 3 patients had a stable disease (SD), and one patient experienced a progression of the disease (PD) before hepatic surgery; the DCR was 92.8%. Of about the 20 patients with an R0 resection, 19 had an immunophenotype of liver metastases consistent with primary tumor: 13 patients had a luminal immunophenotype (one of which was HER2 positive at diagnosis), 3 were HER2 positive, and 4 patients were TNBC.

Of the 2 patients with R1 resection, one had multiple (six) liver lesions and one a single metastasis, both were luminal consistent with primary tumor immunophenotype.

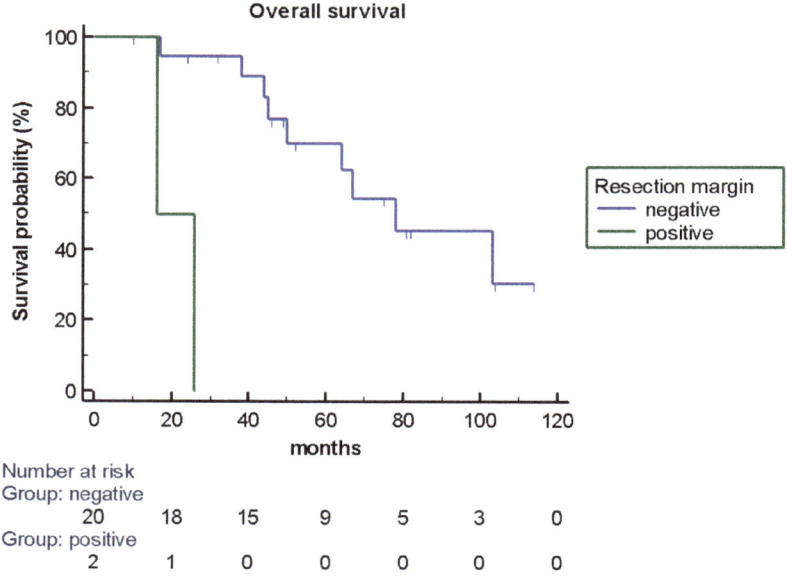

Figure 3. OS according to resection margin of liver metastases (R0 versus R1: 78 *versus* 16 months; HR 0.083, $p < 0.0001$).

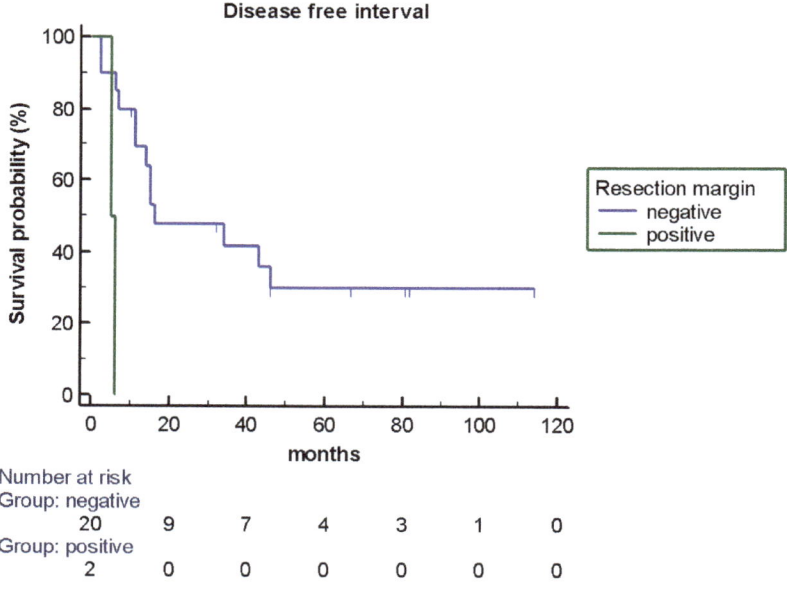

Figure 4. DFI according to resection margin of liver metastases (R0 versus R1: 16 *versus* 5 months; HR 0.17, $p = 0.0058$).

Table 2. Characteristic of patients with liver metastasectomy with negative resection margin (R0).

Characteristics	N. of Patients (n = 20)
Number of liver metastases	
1	13
>1	7
Systemic therapy pre-liver surgery	
0	6
≥1	14
Best response of therapy before surgery	14 *
PR	10
SD	3
PD	1
Immunophenotype	
Luminal	13
HER2+	3
TNBC	4

N.: number. *: number of patients who received treatments before surgery. CR: complete response, PR: partial response, SD: stable disease.

4. Discussion

Despite an improvement in the systemic treatment of MBC, the median survival of patients with metastatic disease is between 18 and 24 months [31]. Resection of breast cancer liver metastasis may represent a therapeutic option for selected patients. The radical nature of the surgical procedure performed in a high-flow center and after a multidisciplinary discussion appears essential for this therapeutic option [32] like in other neoplastic diseases [33].

In a recent systematic review of resection of MBC-LM, the median OS was 35.1 months and the median DFS was 21.5 months [34]. At the same time, in a case-matched analysis, the resection group had an impressive median OS of 82 months versus a median OS of 31 months in the systemic group, so the authors concluded that the combination of surgery with systemic treatment results in an improved OS [7].

The median OS and the DFI in our population were 67 months and 15 months respectively. Thus, our study seems to confirm a possible survival benefit in patients undergoing liver surgery of metastases especially in patients with an R0 resection. In fact, in our study, the presence of a negative resection margin was the only factor that statistically significantly influenced OS (78 versus 16 months; HR 0.083, $p < 0.0001$) and DFI (16 versus 5 months; HR 0.17, $p = 0.0058$). Of the 20 patients with an R0 resection, 13 patients had a single lesion while 7 had two metastases, this implies that a careful selection of patients with limited liver disease is important to obtain an adequate surgical result.

Fourteen patients received one line of treatment before surgery with a DCR of 93%; therefore, it also emerged in this evaluation that the selection of patients with a metastatic disease under control by systemic treatment can allow an important result. However, it is equally important to note that also the patients with PD during systemic therapy before liver surgery achieves an R0 resection, demonstrating how liver resection can also be proposed as a salvage treatment in highly selected cases. Moreover, surgical complications only occurred in two patients in the absence of post-surgery mortality, these data suggest that liver metastasectomy could be a safe procedure. At the same time, in our population, surgical radicality was achieved in almost all patients who were eligible for the study, and the R0 margin was found as the only prognostically relevant factor influencing both the DFI and OS. Taken together, these results confirm the importance of performing LM exclusively in high-flow centers, post a multidisciplinary discussion since, under this condition, the removal of liver metastases from breast cancer can significantly influence the survival of patients without significant side effects.

The main bias of the study is the smallness of the sample, also due to the limited availibility data of all the population of patients with MBC and undergoing liver surgery in our institution (49 versus 22). The sample size might have affected the results, limiting the statistical significance impact for some factors analyzed that appear to have a role in survival. In addition, the DFI and OS may have been influenced by the subsequent systemic therapies, but due to the heterogeneity of the population and the number and characteristics of treatment received post-surgery, it is not possible to evaluate their impact on survival outcomes. The trend benefit of the low tumor burden (only liver *versus* other sites) is in line with other results and with the suggestion of international guidelines to justify a multidisciplinary and more aggressive therapy in patients with limited metastatic disease in order to obtain a greater chance of healing [1]. The correlation with the menopausal state with better prognosis, on the other hand, could be related to a lower biological aggressiveness of the disease. Additionally, the trend benefit of the use of systemic pre-surgery treatment, as it has been shown in previous studies [3,8,18], seems to have a role in the increasing survival eradicating or debulking microscopic lesions. In contrast to other studies [25], in our population, we did not note an improved outcome for patients with luminal disease.

5. Conclusions

Despite the limitations imposed by a retrospective analysis on a small sample, our study confirms the possible positive role of R0 surgical excision of liver metastases from MBC if performed in a high-flow center after multidisciplinary evaluation. The prospective confirmation of this data appears to be increasingly necessary in order to consolidate the use of locoregional treatments in oligometastatic breast cancer disease, in particular, to identify the subgroup of patients who can benefit from surgical treatment.

Author Contributions: Conceptualization, A.O.; methodology, A.O., E.B. and G.T.; Writing—review and editing, all authors; supervision, A.O., E.B. and G.T. All authors have read and agreed to the published version of the manuscript

Funding: This research received no external funding.

Institutional Review Board Statement: The study was conducted according to the guidelines of the Declaration of Helsinki, and approved by the Institutional Review Board (or Ethics Committee) of Fondazione Policlinico Universitario "A. Gemelli" IRCCS Roma (Prot N. 0011515/20-12/03/2020).

Informed Consent Statement: Informed consent was obtained from all subjects involved in the study.

Data Availability Statement: The datasets used and/or analysed during the current study are available from the corresponding author on reasonable request.

Acknowledgments: E.B. is currently supported by the Associazione Italiana per la Ricerca sul Cancro (AIRC) under Investigator Grant (IG) No. IG20583. GT is supported by AIRC, IG18599, AIRC 5 × 1000 21052. E.B. is currently supported by Institutional funds of Università Cattolica del Sacro Cuore (UCSC-project D1-2018/2019).

Conflicts of Interest: The authors declare no conflict of interest.

References

1. Cardoso, F.; Senkus, E.; Costa, A.; Papadopoulos, E.; Aapro, M.; André, F.; Harbeck, N.; Aguilar Lopez, B.; Barrios, C.H.; Bergh, J.; et al. 4th ESO-ESMO international consensus guidelines for advanced breast cancer (ABC 4). *Ann. Oncol.* **2018**, *29*, 1634–1657. [CrossRef] [PubMed]
2. Siegel, R.L.; Miller, K.D.; Jemal, A. Cancer statistics, 2018. *CA Cancer J. Clin.* **2018**, *68*, 7–30. [CrossRef]
3. Adam, R.; Aloia, T.; Krissat, J.; Bralet, M.P.; Paule, B.; Giacchetti, S.; Delvart, V.; Azoulay, D.; Bismuth, H.; Castaing, D. Is liver resection justified for patients with hepatic metastases from breast cancer? *Ann. Surg.* **2006**, *244*, 897–907. [CrossRef]
4. Cristofanilli, M.; Hortobagyi, G.N. New horizons in treating metastatic disease. *Clin. Breast Cancer* **2001**, *1*, 276–287. [CrossRef] [PubMed]
5. Morris, E.J.A.; Forman, D.; Thomas, J.D.; Quirke, P.; Taylor, E.F.; Fairley, L.; Cottier, B.; Poston, G. Surgical management and outcomes of colorectal cancer liver metastases. *Br. J. Surg.* **2010**, *97*, 1110–1118. [CrossRef]

6. House, M.G.; Ito, H.; Gönen, M.; Fong, Y.; Allen, P.J.; DeMatteo, R.P.; Brennan, M.F.; Blumgart, L.H.; Jarnagin, W.R.; D'Angelica, M.I. Survival after Hepatic Resection for Metastatic Colorectal Cancer: Trends in Outcomes for 1,600 Patients during Two Decades at a Single Institution. *J. Am. Coll. Surg.* **2010**, *210*, 744–752. [CrossRef] [PubMed]
7. Ruiz, A.; van Hillegersberg, R.; Siesling, S.; Castro-Benitez, C.; Sebagh, M.; Wicherts, D.A.; de Ligt, K.M.; Goense, L.; Giacchetti, S.; Castaing, D.; et al. Surgical resection versus systemic therapy for breast cancer liver metastases: Results of a European case matched comparison. *Eur. J. Cancer* **2018**, *95*, 1–10. [CrossRef]
8. Kostov, D.V.; Kobakov, G.L.; Yankov, D.V. Prognostic factors related to surgical outcome of liver metastases of breast cancer. *J. Breast Cancer* **2013**, *16*, 184–192. [CrossRef]
9. Lubrano, J.; Roman, H.; Tarrab, S.; Resch, B.; Marpeau, L.; Scotté, M. Liver resection for breast cancer metastasis: Does it improve survival? *Surg. Today* **2008**, *38*, 293–299. [CrossRef]
10. Margonis, G.A.; Buettner, S.; Sasaki, K.; Kim, Y.; Ratti, F.; Russolillo, N.; Ferrero, A.; Berger, N.; Gamblin, T.C.; Poultsides, G.; et al. The role of liver-directed surgery in patients with hepatic metastasis from primary breast cancer: A multi-institutional analysis. *HPB* **2016**, *18*, 700–705. [CrossRef]
11. Mariani, P.; Servois, V.; De Rycke, Y.; Bennett, S.P.; Feron, J.G.; Almubarak, M.M.; Reyal, F.; Baranger, B.; Pierga, J.Y.; Salmon, R.J. Liver metastases from breast cancer: Surgical resection or not? A case-matched control study in highly selected patients. *Eur. J. Surg. Oncol.* **2013**, *39*, 1377–1383. [CrossRef]
12. Martinez, S.R.; Young, S.E.; Giuliano, A.E.; Bilchik, A.J. The utility of estrogen receptor, progesterone receptor, and Her-2/neu status to predict survival in patients undergoing hepatic resection for breast cancer metastases. *Am. J. Surg.* **2006**, *191*, 281–283. [CrossRef]
13. Selzner, M.; Morse, M.A.; Vredenburgh, J.J.; Meyers, W.C.; Clavien, P.A. Liver metastases from breast cancer: Long-term survival after curative resection. *Surgery* **2000**, *127*, 383–389. [CrossRef]
14. Van Walsum, G.A.M.; De Ridder, J.A.M.; Verhoef, C.; Bosscha, K.; Van Gulik, T.M.; Hesselink, E.J.; Ruers, T.J.M.; Van Den Tol, M.P.; Nagtegaal, I.D.; Brouwers, M.; et al. Resection of liver metastases in patients with breast cancer: Survival and prognostic factors. *Eur. J. Surg. Oncol.* **2012**, *38*, 910–917. [CrossRef]
15. Pocard, M.; Pouillart, P.; Asselain, B.; Salmon, R.J. Hepatic resection in metastatic breast cancer: Results and prognostic factors. *Eur. J. Surg. Oncol.* **2000**, *26*, 155–159. [CrossRef]
16. Sabol, M.; Donat, R.; Chvalny, P.; Dyttert, D.; Palaj, J.; Durdik, S. Surgical management of breast cancer liver metastases. *Neoplasma* **2014**, *61*, 601–606. [CrossRef]
17. Sakamoto, Y.; Yamamoto, J.; Yoshimoto, M.; Kasumi, F.; Kosuge, T.; Kokudo, N.; Makuuchi, M. Hepatic resection for metastatic breast cancer: Prognostic analysis of 34 patients. *World J. Surg.* **2005**, *29*, 524–527. [CrossRef]
18. Abbott, D.E.; Brouquet, A.; Mittendorf, E.A.; Andreou, A.; Meric-Bernstam, F.; Valero, V.; Green, M.C.; Kuerer, H.M.; Curley, S.A.; Abdalla, E.K.; et al. Resection of liver metastases from breast cancer: Estrogen receptor status and response to chemotherapy before metastasectomy define outcome. *Surgery* **2012**, *151*, 710–716. [CrossRef]
19. Weinrich, M.; Weiß, C.; Schuld, J.; Rau, B.M. Liver resections of isolated liver metastasis in breast cancer: Results and possible prognostic factors. *HPB Surg.* **2014**, *2014*, 893829. [CrossRef] [PubMed]
20. Vertriest, C.; Berardi, G.; Tomassini, F.; Vanden Broucke, R.; Depypere, H.; Cocquyt, V.; Denys, H.; Van Belle, S.; Troisi, R.I. Resection of single metachronous liver metastases from breast cancer stage I-II yield excellent overall and disease-free survival. Single center experience and review of the literature. *Dig. Surg.* **2015**, *32*, 52–59. [CrossRef]
21. Yoshimoto, M.; Tada, T.; Saito, M.; Takahashi, K.; Makita, M.; Uchida, Y.; Kasumi, F. Surgical treatment of hepatic metastases from breast cancer. *Breast Cancer Res. Treat.* **2000**, *59*, 177–184. [CrossRef]
22. Bacalbasa, N.; Balescu, I.; Ilie, V.; Florea, R.; Sorop, A.; Brasoveanu, V.; Brezean, I.; Vilcu, M.; Dima, S.; Popescu, I. The impact on the long-term outcomes of hormonal status after hepatic resection for breast cancer liver metastases. *In Vivo* **2018**, *32*, 1247–1253. [CrossRef]
23. Dittmar, Y.; Altendorf-Hofmann, A.; Schüle, S.; Ardelt, M.; Dirsch, O.; Runnebaum, I.B.; Settmacher, U. Liver resection in selected patients with metastatic breast cancer: A single-centre analysis and review of literature. *J. Cancer Res. Clin. Oncol.* **2013**, *139*, 1317–1325. [CrossRef] [PubMed]
24. Caralt, M.; Bilbao, I.; Cortés, J.; Escartín, A.; Lázaro, J.L.; Dopazo, C.; Olsina, J.J.; Balsells, J.; Charco, R. Hepatic resection for liver metastases as part of the "oncosurgical" treatment of metastatic breast cancer. *Ann. Surg. Oncol.* **2008**, *15*, 2804–2810. [CrossRef] [PubMed]
25. Elias, D.; Maisonnette, F.; Druet-Cabanac, M.; Ouellet, J.F.; Guinebretiere, J.M.; Spielmann, M.; Delaloge, S. An attempt to clarify indications for hepatectomy for liver metastases from breast cancer. *Am. J. Surg.* **2003**, *185*, 158–164. [CrossRef]
26. Ercolani, G.; Zanello, M.; Serenari, M.; Cescon, M.; Cucchetti, A.; Ravaioli, M.; Del Gaudio, M.; D'Errico, A.; Brandi, G.; Pinna, A.D. Ten-Year Survival after Liver Resection for Breast Metastases: A Single-Center Experience. *Dig. Surg.* **2018**, *35*, 372–380. [CrossRef]
27. He, X.; Zhang, Q.; Feng, Y.; Li, Z.; Pan, Q.; Zhao, Y.; Zhu, W.; Zhang, N.; Zhou, J.; Wang, L.; et al. Resection of liver metastases from breast cancer: A multicentre analysis. *Clin. Transl. Oncol.* **2020**, *22*, 512–521. [CrossRef]
28. Hoffmann, K.; Franz, C.; Hinz, U.; Schirmacher, P.; Herfarth, C.; Eichbaum, M.; Büchler, M.W.; Schemmer, P. Liver resection for multimodal treatment of breast cancer metastases: Identification of prognostic factors. *Ann. Surg. Oncol.* **2010**, *17*, 1546–1554. [CrossRef]

29. Bale, R.; Putzer, D.; Schullian, P. Local treatment of breast cancer liver metastasis. *Cancers* **2019**, *11*, 1–15. [CrossRef]
30. Weichselbaum, R.R.; Hellman, S. Oligometastases revisited. *Nat. Rev. Clin. Oncol.* **2011**, *8*, 378–382. [CrossRef]
31. Eng, L.G.; Dawood, S.; Sopik, V.; Haaland, B.; Tan, P.S.; Bhoo-Pathy, N.; Warner, E.; Iqbal, J.; Narod, S.A.; Dent, R. Ten-year survival in women with primary stage IV breast cancer. *Breast Cancer Res. Treat.* **2016**, *160*, 145–152. [CrossRef] [PubMed]
32. Zegarac, M.; Nikolic, S.; Gavrilovic, D.; Jevric, M.; Kolarevic, D.; Nikolic-Tomasevic, Z.; Kocic, M.; Djurisic, I.; Inic, Z.; Ilic, V.; et al. Prognostic factors for longer disease free survival and overall survival after surgical resection of isolated liver metastasis from breast cancer. *J. BUON* **2013**, *18*, 859–865.
33. Basso, M.; Dadduzio, V.; Ardito, F.; Lombardi, P.; Strippoli, A.; Vellone, M.; Orlandi, A.; Rossi, S.; Cerchiaro, E.; Cassano, A.; et al. Conversion Chemotherapy for Technically Unresectable Colorectal Liver Metastases. *Medicine* **2016**, *95*, 1–6. [CrossRef] [PubMed]
34. Fairhurst, K.; Leopardi, L.; Satyadas, T.; Maddern, G. The safety and effectiveness of liver resection for breast cancer liver metastases: A systematic review. *Breast* **2016**, *30*, 175–184. [CrossRef]

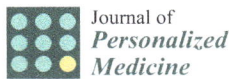

Article

Sentinel Node Biopsy after Neoadjuvant Chemotherapy for Breast Cancer: Preliminary Experience with Clinically Node Negative Patients after Systemic Treatment

Alejandro Martin Sanchez [1,*], Daniela Terribile [1,2], Antonio Franco [1], Annamaria Martullo [1], Armando Orlandi [1,3], Stefano Magno [1], Alba Di Leone [1], Francesca Moschella [1], Maria Natale [1], Sabatino D'Archi [1], Lorenzo Scardina [1], Elena J. Mason [1], Flavia De Lauretis [1], Fabio Marazzi [4], Riccardo Masetti [1,2] and Gianluca Franceschini [1,2]

1 Multidisciplinary Breast Center, Dipartimento Scienze della Salute della donna e del Bambino e di Sanità Pubblica, Fondazione Policlinico Universitario A. Gemelli IRCCS, Largo Agostino Gemelli 8, 00168 Rome, Italy; daniela.terribile@policlinicogemelli.it (D.T.); antonio.franco89@icloud.com (A.F.); annamaria_martullo@virgilio.it (A.M.); armando.orlandi@policlinicogemelli.it (A.O.); stefano.magno@policlinicogemelli.it (S.M.); albadileone@policliunicogemelli.it (A.D.L.); francesca.moschella@policlinicogemelli.it (F.M.); maria.natale@policlinicogemelli.it (M.N.); sabatinodarchi@gmail.com (S.D.); lorenzoscardina@libero.it (L.S.); elenajanemason@gmail.com (E.J.M.); flavia.delauretis@gmail.com (F.D.L.); riccardomasetti@policlinicogemelli.it (R.M.); gianluca.franceschini@policlinicogemelli.it (G.F.)
2 Istituto di Semeiotica Chirurgica, Università Cattolica del Sacro Cuore, 1, 00168 Rome, Italy
3 Division of Medical Oncology, Fondazione Policlinico Universitario A. Gemelli IRCCS, 00168 Rome, Italy
4 Division of Radiotherapy, Dipartimento di Diagnostica per Immagini, Radioterapia Oncologica ed Ematologia, Fondazione Policlinico Universitario A. Gemelli IRCCS, 00168 Rome, Italy; fabio.marazzi@policlinicogemelli.it
* Correspondence: martin.sanchez@hotmail.it; Tel.: +39-06-30156328 or +39-33-93259402

Abstract: Sentinel lymph node biopsy (SLNB) following neoadjuvant treatment (NACT) has been questioned by many studies that reported heterogeneous identification (IR) and false negative rates (FNR). As a result, some patients receive axillary lymph node dissection (ALND) regardless of response to NACT, leading to a potential overtreatment. To better assess reliability and clinical significance of SLNB status on ycN0 patients, we retrospectively analyzed oncological outcomes of 399 patients treated between January 2016 and December 2019 that were either cN0-ycN0 (219 patients) or cN1/2-ycN0 (180 patients). The Endpoints of our study were to assess, furthermore than IR: oncological outcomes as Overall Survival (OS); Distant Disease Free Survival (DDFS); and Regional Disease Free Survival (RDFS) according to SLNB status. SLN identification rate was 96.8% (98.2% in patients cN0-ycN0 and 95.2% in patients cN+-ycN0). A median number of three lymph nodes were identified and removed. Among cN0-ycN0 patients, 149 (68%) were confirmed ypN0(sn), whereas regarding cN1/2-ycN0 cases 86 (47.8%) confirmed an effective downstaging to ypN0. Three year OS, DDFS and RDFS were significantly related to SLNB positivity. Our data seemed to confirm SLNB feasibility following NACT in ycN0 patients, furthermore reinforcing its predictive role in a short observation timing.

Keywords: neoadjuvant chemotherapy; sentinel lymph node; breast cancer; systemic treatment; locally advanced breast cancer; mini-invasive treatment

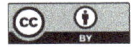

1. Introduction

Sentinel lymph node biopsy (SLNB) is considered the gold standard for axillary staging in early breast cancer patients with clinically negative lymph nodes (cN0), as it reduces potential complications of axillary dissection (ALND) [1–4].

Since many studies have shown a great variation in identification (IR) and false negative rates (FNR), the reliability of SLNB after neoadjuvant chemotherapy (NACT) remains questionable [5–10].

As a result, several patients continue to undergo complete axillary dissection, regardless of axillary staging and response to neoadjuvant chemotherapy, leading to a potential overtreatment of both cN0 and cN1/2 patients who remained or became ycN0 after NACT [3].

For this particular subgroup of patients, recent studies reported acceptable IR and FNR, suggesting that SLNB could be feasible in cN0-ycN0 patients and also in women who are cN1/2 before chemotherapy and achieve an ycN0 status [10–12].

Moreover, for cN0-ycN0 patients, a recently published retrospective study correlates a metastatic SLN with a significant worsening of oncological outcomes, such as Distant Disease Free Survival (DDFS), proving that SLNB is not only feasible after NACT, but that in this setting it could be a good predictive tool to better assess patients at risk [13].

The aim of this analysis, besides reporting our personal workout model for patients receiving neoadjuvant regimens, is to better assess the feasibility and prognostic significance (according to status) of SLNB in ycN0 patients.

With this purpose, we retrospectively analyzed clinical and oncological results obtained from cT1-4 breast cancer patients who were either cN0 or cN1/2 prior to neoadjuvant treatment and became or remained cN0 at the end of the systemic therapy (ycN0).

The endpoints of our study were to evaluate, furthermore than IR: oncological outcomes as Overall Survival (OS); Distant Disease Free Survival (DDFS); and Regional Disease Free Survival (RDFS) according to SLNB status.

2. Materials and Methods

From the prospectively maintained database of the Multidisciplinary Breast Center of the Fondazione Policlinico Universitario Agostino Gemelli IRCCS in Rome, we identified patients with locally advanced breast cancer (cT1-cT4 patients, cN0-cN1/2) who had received neoadjuvant chemotherapy and remained or became ycN0, subsequently undergoing breast surgery and SLNB, between 2016 and 2019.

We excluded from our analysis ycN0 patients in whom a SLN was not identified during surgical procedure, who consequently underwent direct ALND.

Endpoints of our study were:
- "Overall Survival": time from day of surgery to death from any cause or latest follow-up.
- "Distant Disease Free Survival": time from day of surgery to distant recurrence.
- "Regional Disease Free Survival": time from day of surgery to ipsilateral breast and/or axillary recurrence.

3. Clinical Workout

The indication for neoadjuvant treatment (chemotherapy or endocrine therapy) and surgical management of the axilla were discussed during a multidisciplinary meeting (MDM) of breast surgeons, medical oncologists, radiation oncologists, radiologists, pathologists and geneticists.

According to national and international guidelines Associazione Italiana di Oncologia Medica (AIOM) 2019 and National Comprehensive Cancer Network (NCCN) 2020), patients underwent NACT in the following cases:
- Patients with locally advanced breast cancer;
- Patients with operable breast cancer and an unfavorable breast volume/tumor size ratio, in order to reduce the tumor diameter and achieve a conservative treatment instead of mastectomy;
- Patients with operable breast cancer and clinically involved lymph nodes (cN+), with the aim of ensuring a SLNB instead of a direct ALND;
- Young patients with unfavorable risk factors (triple negative tumor, Human Epidermal growth factor—2: HER2+, high Ki-67 rates), to provide prompt systemic treatment.

Pre-neoadjuvant clinical staging: Locoregional staging was assessed by clinical examination, breast and axillary ultrasound, mammography, breast magnetic resonance, or core biopsy of both breast lesion and suspected axillary lymph nodes.

The systemic staging was assessed by total body computed tomography scan or positron emission tomography and bone scintigraphy.

Neoadjuvant regimens: NACT regimen depended on stage and tumor characteristics. We used the following chemotherapy schemes:

- HER2 negative patients:
  - Sequential scheme: Anthracyclines plus Cyclophosphamide on day 1 every 21 days for 4 cycles (4 AC); followed by docetaxel on day 1 every 21 days for 4 cycles or paclitaxel on day 1 every week for 12 cycles.
  - 6 TAC: docetaxel plus Doxorubicin plus Cyclophosphamide on day 1 every 21 days for 6 cycles.
- HER2 positive patients:
  - 6 TCH: docetaxel plus Carboplatin plus Herceptin on day 1 every 21 days for 6 cycles.
  - Sequential scheme: Anthracyclines plus Cyclophosphamide on day 1 every 21 days for 4 cycles (4 AC); followed by docetaxel on day 1 every 21 days for 4 cycles or paclitaxel on day 1 every week for 12 cycles plus Herceptin on day 1 every 21 days for 18 cycles.

Hormone therapy with aromatase inhibitor was delivered to elder and fragile postmenopausal patients with locally advanced breast cancer expressing hormone receptors (ER, PgR) and low Ki-67 (Luminal A and Luminal B). Neoadjuvant protocol was administered for at least six months.

Clinical assessments during and after NACT: Before each cycle of chemotherapy, patients underwent treatment response monitoring with a clinical examination and "in office" breast/axillary ultrasound.

Patients with no evidence of clinical response or with disease progression were the subject of multidisciplinary discussion about a change in NACT scheme or immediate surgery.

One month after NACT finalization, loco-regional staging was repeated (clinical examination, breast and axillary ultrasound, mammography, breast magnetic resonance).

Breast surgical treatment: Surgical management was discussed during a dedicated MDM, taking into account the clinical restaging and patient's preferences.

Patients with a favorable ratio between breast volume and residual lesion were addressed by conservative techniques:

- Level I oncoplastic breast surgery techniques—for resection of <20% of breast volume (peri-areolar, axillary or inframammary fold incisions).
- Level II oncoplastic surgery which involves resection of >20% of breast volume (round block, batwing and reduction mammoplasty techniques) [14].

In case of unfavorable ratio between breast volume and residual tumor size, multicentric cancer, inflammatory cancer and contraindications to adjuvant radiotherapy patients were judged eligible for mastectomy techniques and immediate breast reconstruction (implant or autologous reconstruction):

- "Nipple Sparing Mastectomy" (NSM—removal of all the breast glandular tissue, while the nipple and areola are left in place along with breast skin) if tumor did not involve the nipple or tissue under the areola.
- "Skin Sparing Mastectomy" (removal of breast glandular tissue, nipple and areola while breast skin is kept intact) if tumor involved the nipple–areola complex.
- Simple mastectomy (removal of breast glandular tissue, nipple, areola and breast skin) if tumor involved breast skin.

Axillary assessment: Axillary workout is summarized in Figure 1.

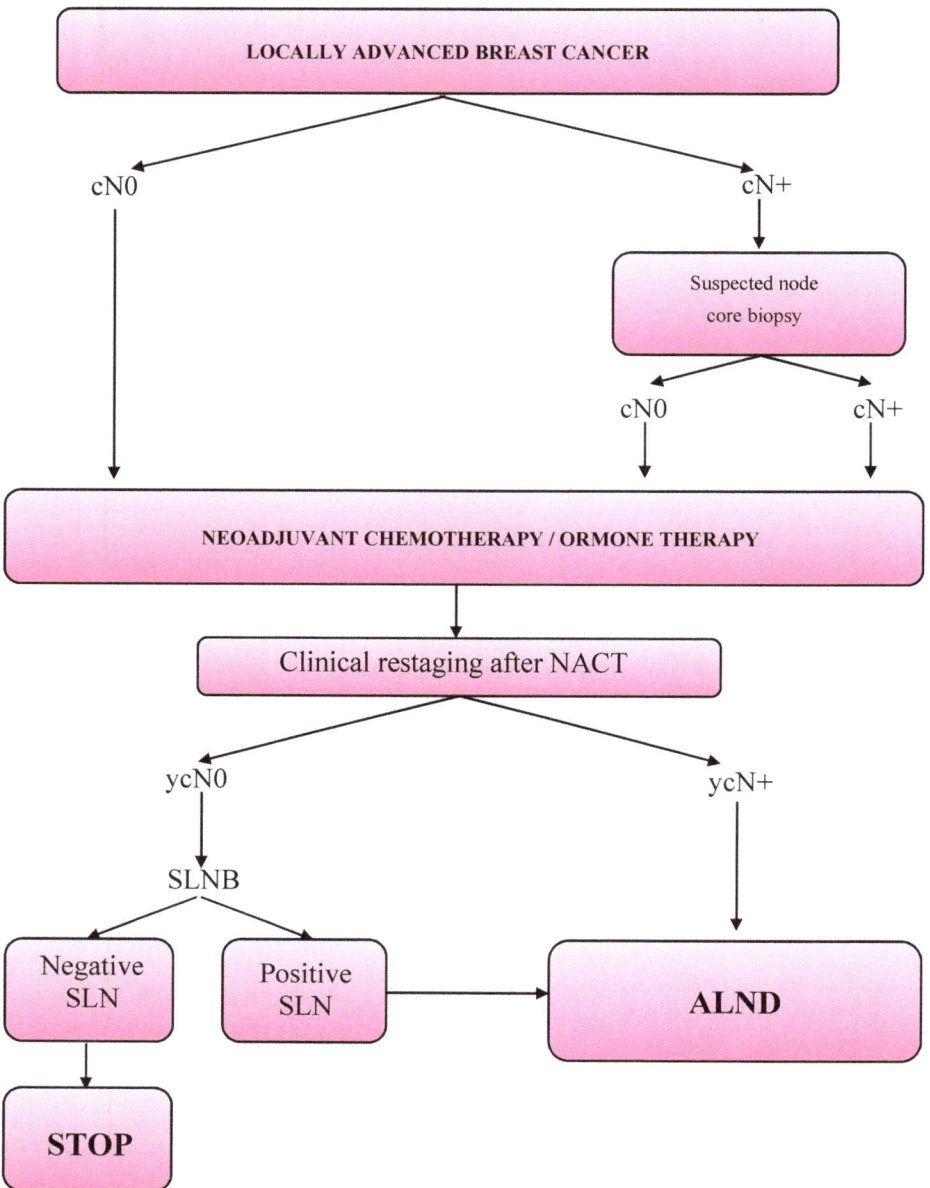

Figure 1. Axillary workout in the neoadjuvant setting.

SLNB was performed using blue dye technique (Patent Blue V or Methylene blue, 2–5 cc) injected sub-dermally, 15–30 min before surgery. Blue-stained axillary lymph nodes were defined as SLNs. Axillary lymph nodes whose consistency and dimension were considered suspicious were also removed and analyzed.

Pathologic examination of the SLN was macroscopic, cytologic and histologic.

The intraoperative cytology examination of the lymph nodes was performed by dissecting them in two parts along the major axis of the capsule if larger than 0.5 cm. After SLN division, a slide was affixed or dragged on the cut surface of both halves and stained with Harris hematoxylin solution.

In case of suspected cytology, lymph node halves were frozen to $-22\ °C$, serially divided in ultrathin sections and stained with Harris hematoxylin solution.

For definitive pathologic assessment, SLN was included and examined along with two consecutive sections stained with Hematoxilyn and Eosin (HE) and, subsequently, with five sequences of three consecutive sections, 200 microns spaced. The middle section of each series was colored with CAM5.2, and those remaining with HE.

All non-sentinel nodes were examined with standard procedure, as mentioned for SLN intraoperative histologic assessment.

For patients with ypN+ (micro or micro-metastatic) disease, axillary dissection was directly performed. I and II level lymph nodes were always removed, while III level lymph nodes were removed only in case of intraoperative detection of clinically suspicious nodes at lower levels.

Patients with isolated tumor cells positivity at SLNB were treated as ypN0 and did not receive ALND.

Adjuvant treatments: were determined on the basis of patient's age, pre-neoadjuvant clinical staging, surgical intervention, pathological staging and tumoral biology.

Adjuvant chemotherapy: Patients who did not make a pathological complete response to neoadjuvant treatment were treated according to different adjuvant regimens.

- Anthracyclines and/or Taxanes were given to patients who did not receive them in the neoadjuvant regimen.
- Triple negative patients were given Capecitabine;
- HER2 positive cancers were treated with Trastuzumab emtansine (TDM-1).
- Cancers expressing hormone receptors (estrogen receptor, progesterone receptor) were treated with selective estrogen receptor modulators (Tamoxifen) or Luteinizing Hormone Release Hormone analogues (Enantone, Decapeptyl) if in premenopausal age while postmenopausal patients were given aromatase inhibitors (Anastrozole, Letrozole, Exemestane).

Adjuvant radiotherapy: was tailored to the type of surgical intervention and pathological staging. Radiation was delivered using 3D conformal schemes and intensity modulated radiotherapy on linear accelerator using 6-10-15 MV photons.

Axillary radiation was considered for patients with pathologically positive lymph nodes and subsequent ALND with less than 10 nodes removed, ypN3 tumor staging, extracapsular invasion or isolated tumor cells (ITC) in SLNs.

4. Statistical Analysis

Statistical analysis was performed with SPSS version 26.0 for Windows. Results are expressed as mean, median and range. Fisher exact test was used for categorical variables. A $p < 0.05$ was considered statistically significant.

Kaplan-Meier curves were used to plot OS, DDFS and RDFS. Oncological outcomes were calculated over a median follow up of 24 months (2–48).

Only factors significantly associated with this outcome in the univariate analyses were included in multivariate models. Multivariate analyses were performed on all patients, and separately for cases cN0 and cN1/2 prior to neoadjuvant treatment.

5. Results

Between January 2016 and December 2019, 4478 patients with invasive breast cancer were treated in our multi-disciplinary center.

From our prospectively maintained database we extracted 412 patients with cT1-cT4 and cN0-cN1/2 diseases, who became or remained ycN0 at the end of neoadjuvant treatment and underwent surgical treatment.

We excluded from this study four cN0–ycN0 patients and nine cN+-ycN0 patients that underwent immediate ALND following a non-identification of a SLN during axillary procedure. The overall SLN identification rate was 96.8% (98.2% in cN0-ycN0 patients and 95.2% in cN+-ycN0 patients).

Regarding the remaining 399 cases that underwent SLNB, in 117 (29.4%) the main indication for NACT was to reduce the tumor diameter and achieve a conservative breast treatment instead of a mastectomy; 104 (26.0%) had the presence of clinically involved lymph nodes (cN+) and 76 cases (19.0%) both concomitant situations.

Furthermore, in 102 cases (25.6%) patients younger than 50 years with unfavorable risk factors received NACT mainly to ensure a prompt systemic treatment, independently of T/N status.

Among patients that underwent NACT, 219 patients that were cN0 at the time of diagnosis remained ycN0, while 180 cN1/2 patients benefit of chemotherapy and down staged to ycN0 status (patients characteristics prior to neoadjuvant chemotherapy, according to axillary clinical status before systemic treatment are summarized in Table 1).

Table 1. Clinical characteristics of 399 patients according to cN status prior to neoadjuvant treatment.

	cN0	cN1/2
All	219 (54.8%)	180 (45.2%)
Age (years)		
<35	21 (9.6%)	12 (6.7%)
35–49	105 (47.9%)	89 (49.4%)
50–69	80 (36.5%)	70 (38.9%)
>70	13 (5.9%)	9 (5%)
Breast Related Cancer Antigens (BRCA) mutations	29 (13.2%)	16 (47.2%)
Menopausal status	103 (47%)	85 (47.2%)
Grading		
G1	3 (1.4%)	2 (1.1%)
G2	78 (35.6%)	66 (36.7%)
G3	118 (53.9%)	96 (53.3%)
Unknown	20 (9.1%)	16 (8.9%)
Tumor subtype		
Luminal A	8 (3.7%)	3 (1.7%)
Luminal B	152 (69.4%)	133 (73.9%)
HER 2 positive	17 (7.8%)	16 (8.9%)
Triple negative	42 (19.2%)	28 (15.6%)
Clinical T		
cT1	28 (12.8%)	27 (15%)
cT2	146 (66.7%)	105 (58.3%)
cT3	29 (13.2%)	33 (18.3%)
cT4	16 (7.3%)	15 (8.3%)
Multifocality/multicentricity	91 (41.6%)	92 (51.1%)

Clinical restaging after NACT: Neoadjuvant regimes and clinical response are summarized in Table 2. Concerning clinical response, we observed an overall complete clinical response in 144 patients (36.1%), a partial response in 228 patients (57.1%) no response in 12 patients (3%) and a progression to T stage, with breast skin or pectoralis major fascia involvement, in 15 patients (3.8%).

Among women treated with hormone-based NACT, we observed four cases of clinical complete response to treatment (16.7%), 15 cases of partial response (62.4%) and five cases of no response (20.9).

Table 2. Schemes of delivered neoadjuvant treatments according to axillary clinical stage at diagnosis and related clinical response.

	cN0	cN1/2
All	219 (54.8%)	180 (45.2%)
Neoadjuvant treatment		
Hormone Therapy	23 (10.5%)	1 (0.6%)
Chemotherapy	196 (89.5%)	179 (99.4%)
Neoadjuvant chemotherapy		
Anthracycline and/or Taxane	5 (2.6%)	4 (2.2%)
Anthracycline + Taxane	159 (81%)	141 (78.8%)
Other	32 (16.4%)	34 (19%)
Herceptin containing regimen	64 (29.2%)	59 (32.8%)
Clinical response		
Complete response	77 (35.2%)	67 (37.2%)
Partial response	125 (57%)	103 (57.3%)
No response	8 (3.7%)	4 (2.2%)
Progression	9 (4.1%)	6 (3.3%)

Breast surgery: 246 patients received conservative OPS and 153 women were given mastectomy (134 patients (87.6%) were treated with conservative mastectomy followed by implant/autologous reconstruction).

Among elderly and fragile patients treated with hormone-based NACT, four patients (16.7%) with initial skin involvement did not experience any response to NACT and were consequently treated with a simple mastectomy (Table 3).

Table 3. Surgical treatment and adjuvant radiotherapy.

	cN0	cN1/2
All	219 (54.8%)	180 (45.2%)
Surgery		
Conservative surgery	142 (64.8%)	104 (57.8%)
Conservative mastectomy	68 (31.1%)	66 (36.7%)
Simple mastectomy	9 (4.1%)	10 (5.6%)
RT after conservative surgery		
No treatment *	6 (4.2%)	3 (2.9%)
Radiotherapy	136 (95.8%)	101 (97.1%)
RT after mastectomy		
No treatment	48 (62.3%)	16 (21.1%)
Radiotherapy	29 (37.7%)	60 (78.9%)

* Patient's refusal or early progression of systemic disease.

Axillary treatment: During SLNB surgical procedure a mean number of 2.7 lymph nodes (3, 1–7) were identified and removed.

Overall, SLNB was negative in 235 cases (58.9%). Among 219 cN0-ycN0 patients, 149 (68%) were confirmed ypN0(sn). Of the 180 cN1/2-ycN0 cases, 86 (47.8%) confirmed an effective downstaging to an ypN0 (sn) status, 76 patients (42.2%) remained macro-metastatic, 10 patients (5.6%) decreased to a micro-metastatic involvement and eight patients (4.4%) patient revealed a residual ITC positivity.

Among patients given ALND, a mean number of 12.8 lymph nodes (11.5, 6–30) were removed. Axillary pathological staging is summarized in Table 4.

Pathological Characteristics: Pathological characteristics are shown in Table 5. Complete breast remission (ypT0) occurred in 132 (33.1%) women. Tumors were luminal A-like, luminal B-like, HER2 positive and triple negative in 75 (18.8%), 121 (30.4%), 10 (2.5%) and 33 (8.2%) cases, respectively. Tumor subtype was not assessable in 160 (40.1%) patients with complete pathological remission in the breast or very limited residual disease.

Table 4. Pathological characteristics according to cN status prior to neoadjuvant treatment.

	cN0	cN1/2
All	219 (54.8%)	180 (45.2%)
ypT		
ypT0	66 (30.2%)	66 (36.7%)
ypTmic	20 (9.1%)	24 (13.3%)
ypT1	92 (42%)	64 (35.5%)
ypT2	36 (16.4%)	21 (11.7%)
ypT3	3 (1.4%)	3 (1.7%)
ypT4	2 (0.9%)	2 (1.1%)
Multifocality/multicentricity	55 (25.1%)	44 (24.4%)
ypN		
ypN0	149 (68%)	86 (47.8%)
ypNi+ *	13 (5.9%)	11 (6.1%)
ypNmic **	18 (8.2%)	10 (5.6%)
ypN1	34 (15.5%)	55 (30.6%)
ypN2	5 (2.3%)	17 (9.4%)
ypN3	0 (0%)	1 (0.6%)
ER		
Positive	112 (51.1%)	80 (44.5%)
Negative	30 (13.7%)	17 (9.4%)
Not evaluable ***	77 (35.2%)	83 (46.1%)
PR		
Positive	83 (37.9%)	50 (27.8%)
Negative	59 (26.9%)	47 (26.1%)
Not evaluable ***	77 (35.2%)	83 (46.1%)
Ki-67		
<24%	94 (42.9%)	64 (35.6%)
≥25%	48 (21.9%)	33 (18.3%)
Not evaluable ***	77 (35.2%)	83 (46.1%)
Tumor subtype		
Luminal A	46 (21%)	29 (16.1%)
Luminal B	70 (32%)	51 (28.4%)
HER2	4 (1.8%)	6 (3.3%)
Triple negative	22 (10%)	11 (6.1%)
Not evaluable ***	77 (35.2%)	83 (46.1%)

* evidence of isolated cancer cells in the lymph node. ** evidence of microscopic residual of tumor (<0.2 mm) in the lymph node. *** ypN0, ypN1mic and ypNi+.

Table 5. Univariate and multivariate analysis for Distant Disease Free Survival.

	All Patients		cN0		cN1/2	
	Univariate Analysis	Multivariate Analysis	Univariate Analysis	Multivariate Analysis	Univariate Analysis	Multivariate Analysis
Clinical Characteristics						
Menopausal status	0.804	/	0.861	/	0.139	/
BRCA1/2 mutation	0.430	/	0.460	/	0.996	/
Multifocality ad the diagnosis	0.288	/	0.430	/	0.811	/
Luminal HER2 +	0.524	/	0.720	/	0.504	/
Triple Negative	1.231 (0.002)	1.879 (0.0001)	1.394 (0.023)	2.606 (0.0001)	1.668 (0.027)	1.888 (0.002)
Pathological Characteristics						
ypT2, ypT3, ypT4	0.873 (0.014)	0.767	0.071	/	0.925 (0.040)	0.417
LS + (ypN+(sn))	2.048 (0.0001)	1.977 (0.0001)	2.502 (0.001)	2.807 (0.001)	1.540 (0.005)	1.213 (0.045)
ypN2, ypN3	1.946 (0.0001)	1.370 (0.003)	2.759 (0.0001)	2.157 (0.004)	1.237 (0.0027)	0.121
pCR on T	−1.815 (0.003)	0.331	−3.704 (0.142)	/	−1.432 (0.020)	0.457

Oncological outcomes: After a median of 35.6 months (2–55), axillary failure (AF) occurred in 2 cN0 patients with a negative SLN and in 4 cN1/2 patients with a negative SLNB.

In our experience, AF occurred in patients that were diagnosed in unfavorable conditions, such as multifocal (two patients; 33%), cT3 (two patients; 33%) and T4b (one patient; 16.5%) tumors. Moreover, we observed an AF in 1 patient with ITC SLN positivity, who refused both ALND and adjuvant axillary radiotherapy.

Furthermore, in 3/6 patients, AF was diagnosed concurrently to a distant relapse (50%).

- Overall survival: During the entire follow-up, we reported the death of 15 (3.8%) women: two in the SN-negative group (OS 97.4%) and 13 in the SN-positive group (OS 82.7%)—$p < 0.0001$. Death was attributed to breast cancer in 92.5% of cases. Three-year OS was 94.3% overall, 95.5% in those initially cN0 and 93% in those initially cN1/N2.
- Distant disease free survival: Overall 36 (9%) patients developed distant metastases (DDFS 83.8%). According to SN-status we report six patients with distant metastasis in SN-negative group (DDFS 95.7%) and 30 patients in the SN-positive group (DDFS 67.9%)—$p < 0.0001$. Three-year DDFS was 92.2% in those initially cN0 and 84.8% in those initially cN1/2.
- Regional Disease Free survival: Overall, 24 patients developed a regional recurrence (RFS 89.4%): eight (2%) women had ipsilateral breast cancer recurrence, two (0.5%) had contralateral breast cancer, and 10 (2.5%) patients developed axillary recurrence. In four (1%) patients we diagnosed a synchronous recurrence in breast and axilla. RDFS was 96.5 % in patients with negative SLNB and 91.3% in those with positive SLNB ($p = 0.007$). Three-year RDFS was 94.2% in those initially cN0 and 87.9% in those initially cN1/2.

OS, DDFS and RDFS were significantly related to SLNB positivity, even overall, and according to axillary staging before NACT (cumulative incidence of regional relapses, as well as OS and DDFS curves, are shown in Figure 2).

At uni- and multivariate analysis (Table 5), positive SLN was confirmed as an independent prognostic factor for DDFS, as well as triple negative immunophenotype and T pathological complete response, even in the cN0-ycN0 and in the c1/2-ycN0 group.

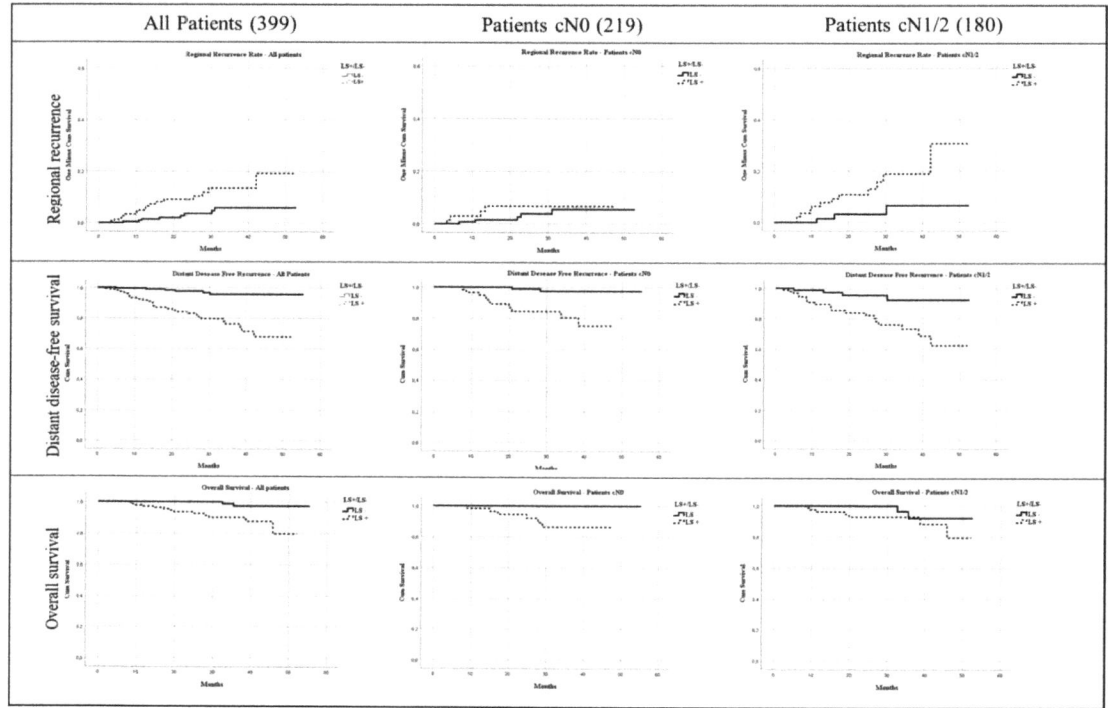

Figure 2. Cumulative Overall Survival, Regional Recurrence and Distant Disease Free Survival.

6. Discussion

In an effort to minimize the clinical impact of breast cancer, several improvements have been made with regards to breast surgical treatment following NACT [14–16].

Conversely, the axillary approach remains a controversial field: SLNB is considered the gold standard for axillary staging in early breast cancer patients with clinically negative lymph nodes, confining ALND to a very limited group of patients.

The purpose of this de-escalation in surgery is to reduce axillary morbidity (seroma formation, loss of arm sensitivity, shoulder dysfunction and lymphedema) by restricting or avoiding axillary dissection without proven oncological advantages.

However, to be reliable SLNB should always be over 90% in identification rate (IR) and below 10% in false negative rate (FNR), conditions that could be easily met in early breast cancer treatment, whereas after NACT initial experiences reported questionable results [17,18].

Despite these initial observations, a progressive set-up of the axillary workout before and after NACT led to metanalysis of retrospective studies that seem to validate SLNB after NACT, reporting acceptable IR and FNR, comparable to those reported for the early breast cancer setting [19–21].

Moreover, recent evidence also seemed to validate SLNB in ycN0 patients, for whom positivity would also play an important role as a significant prognostic factor [13].

We analyzed records regarding 399 consecutively treated patients. We achieved, even with a single agent technique, an acceptable IR for cN0-ycN0 and for cN1/2-ycN0 patients (98.2% and 95.2%, respectively).

These data are in line with previously published results in theoretically more favorable conditions, such as its execution in early breast cancer setting, and obtained with the use of double tracer (radiotracer + blue dye), thus strengthening the observation of Fringuelli et al. [22] that NACT does not influence axillary lymphatic drainage and consequently axillary mapping success, furthermore clearly confirming that identification rate of SLNs actually improves with the surgical experience of the operating team, especially for single tracer technique, as reported by Zhang in the neoadjuvant setting [23].

Regarding prognostic power of SLNB after NACT, the European Institute of Oncology recently published a paper in which Galimberti et al. analyzed 396 cT1-4, cN0/1/2 patients who became or remained cN0 after neoadjuvant treatment and underwent SLNB.

Their data confirmed SLN status as a significant prognostic factor in cN0-ycN0 patients, a finding that seems to be consistent with the known prognostic significance of axillary involvement in the early breast cancer setting. However, at multivariate analysis, SLNB lost its prognostic power in the cN1/2-ycN0 group, suggesting that an axillary involvement before NACT could potentially jeopardize a reliable mini-invasive radiation.

Our data (although a result of limited and preliminary observations) confirm Galimberti's conclusions: in 219 cN0-ycN0 patients SLNB was safely performed. In this subgroup, we observed two cases of axillary failure, and three-year OS, DDFS and RDFS were 95.5%, 92.2% and 94.2%, respectively. Moreover, multivariate analysis showed that strong prognostic factors such as triple negative immunophenotype, persistence of extended involvement of the axilla (ypN2/3) and positivity of SLNB maintain a statistically comparable prognostic role.

In this setting, our observations further reinforce not only the feasibility but also the low risk of false negative rates of SLNB, confirming its predictive role even after NACT.

Among 180 cN1/2-ycN0 patients, a mini-invasive axillary staging by means of SLNB should be taken into account both for the high identification rate and also for the observed axillary complete pathological response rate (in our experience 47.8%).

In such a setting, although there is a higher rate or axillary failure (4.6% versus 1.3% in cN0-ycN0 patients), we registered three-year OS, DDFS and RDFS rates that were comparable to those registered in cN0 patients (93%, 84.8% and 87.9%, respectively).

We also confirmed SLNB's prognostic power at multivariate analysis that, even in a more complex subgroup of patients, resulted in statistical comparability to other strong prognostic factors such as triple negative immunophenotype, and complete pathological response on the breast (ypT0).

This observation differs from Galimberti's conclusions for cN1/2-ycN0 patients, a phenomenon that can be related to our shorter follow up timing, suggesting that in the first three years axillary response could reflect a systemic control of disease, but also to our high rate of patients diagnosed with cN1 axillary status before NACT (144/180 (80%) of cases included in cN1/2 group were cN1).

This particular subset distribution could have influenced uni- and multivariate results, suggesting that SLNB remains a reliable prognostic tool in patients with a lower grade of initial axillary involvement, whereas in patients with a major axillary burden prior to neoadjuvant treatment, the disruption of the lymphatic architecture (caused both by both perinodal infiltration and chemo-therapic agents) could compromise the reliability of SLN in predicting axillary status and therefore compromise its predictive prognostic power.

7. Conclusions

Our results, although from a single institution and being a retrospective experience with a limited follow-up timing, strengthen the possibility of safely performing SLNB after NACT in cN0-ycN0 patients, and reinforce the need for further refinements in the mini-invasive axillary approach for cN1-2 patients who become node-negative after NACT.

Author Contributions: A.M.S., A.F. and A.M.—Designed study, analysis and interpretation of data, drafted paper and revised it critically, approved the submitted version; D.T., A.O., S.M., A.D.L., F.M. (Francesca Moschella), M.N., S.D., L.S., E.J.M., F.D.L., F.M. (Fabio Marazzi): Designed study, analysed and interpretation of data, drafted paper; R.M. and G.F.: Designed study, drafted paper and revised it critically, approved the submitted version. All authors have read and agreed to the published version of the manuscript.

Funding: This research received no external funding.

Institutional Review Board Statement: The study was conducted according to the guidelines of the Declaration of Helsinki, and approved by the Institutional Review Board and Ethics Committee of Fondazione Policlinico Universitario Agostino Gemelli IRCCS; Università Cattolica del Sacro Cuore, Rome, Italy.

Informed Consent Statement: Informed consent was obtained from all subjects involved in the study.

Data Availability Statement: The data presented in this study are available on request from the corresponding author.

Conflicts of Interest: Disclosure of financial interests and potential conflict of interest. All authors submitting this manuscript confirm and attest that they have no conflict of interest. There are no source of support in any form nor funding for this work. There are no financial relationships for this work.

References

1. Franceschini, G.; Sanchez, A.M.; Di Leone, A.; Magno, S.; Moschella, F.; Accetta, C.; Masetti, R. Update on the surgical management of breast cancer. *Ann. Ital. Chir.* **2015**, *86*, 89–99.
2. Classe, J.-M.; Loaec, C.; Alran, S.; Paillocher, N.; Tunon-Lara, C.; Gimbergues, P.; Faure-Virelizier, C.; Chauvet, M.-P.; Lasry, S.; Dupre, P.-F.; et al. Sentinel node detection after neoadjuvant chemotherapy in patient without previous axillary node involvement (GANEA 2 trial): Follow-up of a prospective multi-institutional cohort. *SABCS* **2016**. [CrossRef]
3. Currey, A.; Patten, C.R.; Bergom, C.; Wilson, J.F.; Kong, A.L. Management of the axilla after neo-adjuvant chemotherapy for breast cancer: Sentinel node biopsy and radiotherapy considerations. *Breast J.* **2018**, *24*, 902–910. [CrossRef]
4. Shirzadi, A.; Mahmoodzadeh, H.; Qorbani, M. Assessment of sentinel lymph node biopsy after neoadjuvant chemotherapy for breast cancer in two subgroups: Initially node negative and node positive converted to node negative—A systemic review and meta-analysis. *J. Res. Med. Sci.* **2019**, *24*. [CrossRef]
5. Classe, J.M.; Bordes, V.; Campion, L.; Mignotte, H.; Dravet, F.; Leveque, J.; Sagan, C.; Dupre, P.F.; Body, G.; Giard, S. Sentinel lymph node biopsy after neoadjuvant chemotherapy for advanced breast cancer: Results of Ganglion Sentinelle et Chimiotherapie Neoadjuvante, a French prospective multicentric study. *J. Clin. Oncol.* **2009**, *27*, 726–732. [CrossRef]
6. Hunt, K.K.; Yi, M.; Mittendorf, E.A.; Guerrero, C.; Babiera, G.V.; Bedrosian, I.; Hwang, R.F.; Kuerer, H.M.; Ross, M.I.; Meric-Bernstam, F. Sentinel Lymph Node Surgery After Neoadjuvant Chemotherapy is Accurate and Reduces the Need for Axillary Dissection in Breast Cancer Patients. *Ann. Surg.* **2009**, *250*, 558–566. [CrossRef] [PubMed]
7. Tan, V.K.M.; Goh, B.K.P.; Fook-Cong, S.; Kin, L.W.; Wong, W.-K.; Yong, W.S. The feasibility and Accuracy of Sentinel Lymph Node Biopsy in Clinically Node-Negative Patients after Neoadjuvant Chemotherapy for Breast Cancer—A Systematic Review and Meta-Analysis. *J. Surg. Oncol.* **2011**, *104*, 97–103. [CrossRef] [PubMed]
8. Pilewskie, M.; Morrow, M. Axillary Nodal Management Following Neoadjuvant Chemotherapy. *JAMA Oncol.* **2017**, *3*, 549–555. [CrossRef] [PubMed]
9. Ferrucci, M.; Franceschini, G.; Douek, M. New techniques for sentinel node biopsy in breast cancer. *Transl. Cancer Res.* **2018**, *7*, S405–S417. [CrossRef]
10. Franceschini, G. Sentinel node biopsy after neoadjuvant chemotherapy for breast cancer in patients with pre-treatment node-positive: Recommendations to optimize the performance. *Eur. J. Surg. Oncol.* **2020**, *46*, 216–217. [CrossRef]
11. El Hage, C.; Headon, H.; El Tokhy, O.; Heeney, J.; Kasem, A.; Mokbel, K. Is sentinel lymph node biopsy a viable alternative to complete axillary dissection following neoadjuvant chemotherapy in women with node-positive breast cancer at diagnosis? An updated meta-analysis involving 3,398 patients. *Am. J. Surg.* **2016**, *212*, 969–981. [CrossRef]
12. Kantor, O.; James, T.A. ASO Author Reflections: Improving Patient Selection for Sentinel Lymph Node Biopsy After Neoadjuvant Chemotherapy. *Ann. Surg. Oncol.* **2018**, *25*, 640–641. [CrossRef]
13. Galimberti, V.; Fontana, S.K.R.; Maisonneuve, P.; Steccanella, F.; Vento, A.R.; Intra, M.; Naninato, P.; Caldarella, P.; Iorfida, M.; Colleoni, M.; et al. Sentinel node biopsy after neoadjuvant treatment in breast cancer: Five-year follow-up of patients with clinically node-negative or node-positive disease before treatment. *Eur. J. Surg. Oncol.* **2016**, *42*, 361–368. [CrossRef] [PubMed]
14. Sanchez, A.M.; Franceschini, G.; D'Archi, S.; De Lauretis, F.; Scardina, L.; Di Giorgio, D.; Accetta, C.; Masetti, R. Results obtained with level II oncoplastic surgery spanning 20 years of breast cancer treatment: Do we really need further demonstration of reliability? *Breast J.* **2019**, *26*, 125–132. [CrossRef]

15. Franceschini, G.; Di Leone, A.; Natale, M.; Sanchez, A.M.; Masetti, R. Conservative surgery after neoadjuvant chemotherapy in patients with operable breast cancer. *Ann. Ital. Chir.* **2018**, *89*, 290. [PubMed]
16. Sanchez, A.M.; Franceschini, G.; Orlandi, A.; Di Leone, A.; Masetti, R. New challenges in multimodal workout of locally advanced breast cancer. *Surgeon* **2017**, *15*, 372–378. [CrossRef] [PubMed]
17. Kuehn, T.; Bauerfeind, I.; Fehm, T.; Fleige, B.; Hausschild, M.; Helms, G.; Lebeau, A.; Liedtke, C.; Von Minckwitz, G.; Nekljudova, V.; et al. Sentinel-lymph-node biopsy in patients with breast cancer before and after neoadjuvant chemotherapy (SENTINA): A prospective, multicentre cohort study. *Lancet Oncol.* **2013**, *14*, 609–618. [CrossRef]
18. Boughey, J.C.; Suman, V.J.; Mittendorf, E.A. Alliance for Clinical Trials in Oncology. Sentinel lymph node surgery after neoadjuvant chemotherapy in patients with node-positive breast cancer: The ACOSOG Z1071 (Alliance) clinical trial. *JAMA* **2013**, *310*, 1455–1461. [CrossRef]
19. Simons, J.M.; van Nijnatten, T.J.A.; van der Pol, C.C.; Luiten, E.J.T.; Koppert, L.B.; Smidt, M.L. Diagnostic Accuracy of Different Surgical Procedures for Axillary Staging After Neoadjuvant Systemic Therapy in Node-positive Breast Cancer: A Systematic Review and Meta-analysis. *Ann. Surg.* **2019**, *269*, 432–442. [CrossRef]
20. Geng, C.; Chen, X.; Pan, X.; Li, J. The Feasibility and Accuracy of Sentinel Lymph Node Biopsy in Initially Clinically Node-Negative Breast Cancer after Neoadjuvant Chemotherapy: A Systematic Review and Meta-Analysis. *PLoS ONE* **2016**, *11*, e0162605. [CrossRef]
21. Tee, S.R.; Devane, L.A.; Evoy, D.; Rothwell, J.; Geraghty, J.; Prichard, R.S.; McDermott, E.W. Meta-analysis of sentinel lymph node biopsy after neoadjuvant chemotherapy in patients with initial biopsy-proven node-positive breast cancer. *Br. J. Surg.* **2018**, *105*, 1541–1552. [CrossRef]
22. Fringuelli, F.M.; Lima, G.; Bottini, A.; Aguggini, S.; Allevia, G.; Bonardi, S. Lymphoscintigraphy: The experience of the Cremona breast unit. Internet communication. 2012.
23. Zhang, G.-C.; Liao, N.; Guo, Z.-B.; Qian, X.-K.; Ren, C.-Y.; Yao, M.; Li, X.-R.; Wang, K.; Zu, J. Accuracy and axilla sparing potentials of sentinel lymph node biopsy with methylene blue alone performed before versus after neoadjuvant chemotherapy in breast cancer: A single institution experience. *Clin. Transl. Oncol.* **2012**, *15*, 79–84. [CrossRef]

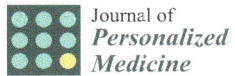

Case Report

Invasive Ductal Breast Cancer with Osteoclast-Like Giant Cells: A Case Report Based on the Gene Expression Profile for Changes in Management

Azzurra Irelli [1], Maria Maddalena Sirufo [2,3], Gina Rosaria Quaglione [4], Francesca De Pietro [2,3], Enrica Maria Bassino [2,3], Carlo D'Ugo [5], Lia Ginaldi [2,3] and Massimo De Martinis [2,3,*]

1. Medical Oncology Unit, Department of Oncology, AUSL 04 Teramo, 64100 Teramo, Italy; azzurra.irelli@hotmail.it
2. Department of Life, Health and Environmental Sciences, University of L'Aquila, 67100 L'Aquila, Italy; maddalena.sirufo@gmail.com (M.M.S.); fra722@hotmail.it (F.D.P.); enricamaria.bassino@gmail.com (E.M.B.); lia.ginaldi@cc.univaq.it (L.G.)
3. Allergy and Clinical Immunology Unit, Center for the diagnosis and treatment of Osteoporosis, AUSL 04 Teramo, 64100 Teramo, Italy
4. Pathological Anatomy Unit, Mazzini Hospital, AUSL04 Teramo, 64100 Teramo, Italy; gina.quaglione@aslteramo.it
5. Radiotherapy Unit, Department of Oncology, AUSL 04, 64100 Teramo, Italy; carlo.dugo@aslteramo.it
* Correspondence: demartinis@cc.univaq.it; Tel.: +39-0861-429862

Citation: Irelli, A.; Sirufo, M.M.; Quaglione, G.R.; De Pietro, F.; Bassino, E.M.; D'Ugo, C.; Ginaldi, L.; De Martinis, M. Invasive Ductal Breast Cancer with Osteoclast-Like Giant Cells: A Case Report Based on the Gene Expression Profile for Changes in Management. *J. Pers. Med.* 2021, 11, 156. https://doi.org/10.3390/jpm11020156

Academic Editor: Gianluca Franceschini

Received: 11 January 2021
Accepted: 16 February 2021
Published: 23 February 2021

Publisher's Note: MDPI stays neutral with regard to jurisdictional claims in published maps and institutional affiliations.

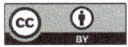

Copyright: © 2021 by the authors. Licensee MDPI, Basel, Switzerland. This article is an open access article distributed under the terms and conditions of the Creative Commons Attribution (CC BY) license (https://creativecommons.org/licenses/by/4.0/).

Abstract: We report the case of a 49-year-old woman diagnosed with a rare histotype of early breast cancer (BC), invasive ductal carcinoma with osteoclast-like giant cells (OGCs), from the perspective of gene profile analysis tests. The patient underwent a quadrantectomy of the right breast with removal of 2 cm neoplastic nodule and three ipsilateral sentinel lymph nodes. The Oncotype Dx gave a recurrence score (RS) of 23, and taking into account the patient's age, an RS of 23 corresponds to a chemotherapy benefit of 6.5%. After a multidisciplinary collegial discussion, and in consideration of the patient's age, the absence of comorbidity, the premenopausal state, the rare histotype and the Oncotype Dx report, the patient was offered adjuvant chemotherapy treatment followed by hormone therapy. This case may be an example of the utility of integrating gene expression profiling tests into clinical practice in the adjuvant treatment decision of a rare histotype BC. The Oncotype Dx test required to supplement the histological examination made us opt for the proposal of a combined treatment of adjuvant chemotherapy followed by adjuvant hormone therapy. It demonstrates the importance of considering molecular tests and, in particular, the Oncotype Dx, in estimating the risk of disease recovery at 10 years in order to identify patients who benefit from hormone therapy alone versus those who benefit from the addition of chemotherapy, all with a view toward patient-centered oncology. Here, we discuss the possible validity and limitations of the Oncotype Dx in a rare luminal A-like histotype with high infiltrate of stromal/inflammatory cells.

Keywords: rare breast cancer; osteoclast-like giant cells; gene profiling; Oncotype Dx; adjuvant treatment

1. Introduction

Breast cancer (BC) represents the most frequently diagnosed cancer among women regardless of age. Male BC is rare and affects about 1% of cases [1–4].

In Italy, about 55,000 new cases of BC have been reported among women in 2020, and there are 834,200 women who survive BC after a diagnosis. To date, BC represents the leading cause of death from cancer among women, with over 12,300 deaths in all age groups, although mortality is declining in all age groups, especially in women under the age of 50, probably due to the spread of screening programs and to therapeutic progress.

The 5-year survival of women with breast cancer BC patients is 87%, while survival 10 years after diagnosis is 89% [5].

Overall, BC accounts for 30% of female cancers among women and is the leading cause of cancer death among women between the ages of 20 and 59. Cancer screening programs and advances have resulted in a steep drop in BC mortality, so much so that, as of 2017, the death rate has dropped from its peak in 1989 by 40% [6]. BC diagnosis is based on clinical examination, radiological imaging and histological type.

The two most frequent subtypes of invasive BC are carcinoma not otherwise specified (70–75% of cases) and lobular carcinoma (12–15%). The other 18 subtypes exhibit specific morphological traits and are rare (0.5–5%) [7].

Invasive carcinomas have been classified by histological subtype as "favorable" (mucinous, tubular, cribriform, tubulo-lobular and lobular) and "unfavorable" (ductal, mixed ductal and lobular and micropapillary carcinoma). The histological subtypes with the highest percentage of high recurrence score (RS) were invasive micropapillary, pleomorphic lobular and ductal carcinoma [8].

The indication for systemic adjuvant therapy is decided on the basis of the biological characteristics of the tumor (the histological type, presence or absence of ductal carcinoma in situ, grade, Ki67, presence of peritumor vascular invasion, receptors for estrogen (ER), receptors for progesterone (PR), human epidermal growth factor receptor 2 (HER2) status, the number of regional lymph nodes involved, dimensions) and the patient's clinical characteristics (age, performance status, comorbidity), with the help of scales such as Activities of Daily Living (ADL), Instrumental Activities of Daily Living (IADL), Cumulative Illness Rating Scale (CIRS) and, considering the toxicities of the proposed therapy, the patient's life expectancy, as well as her preferences [9–13].

Multigenic prognostic tests help to identify hormone receptors (HR)-positive, luminal-like and HER2-negative early BC patients who could benefit from chemotherapy, providing an estimate of the risk of recurrence after 10 years [1].

Among different kind of tests, the Oncotype Dx, a molecular test that uses quantitative reverse transcription polymerase chain reaction (qRT-PCR) technology, has both a prognostic value for 10-year risk of recurrence and a predictive value in terms of survival advantage from adjuvant chemotherapy. This test was built as a mathematical model based on the analysis of 21 genes (16 genes that inform about the proliferative state of the tumor and 5 control genes) and allows for division of the operated items for early breast cancer into risk categories. By assessing the differential expression of these genes, it is possible to associate gives each tumor with a score from 0 to 100. The score is called the recurrence score (RS) and predicts the risk of distant relapse within 10 years in patients with luminal/HER2-negative tumor. A higher RS is associated with a greater risk of distant cancer relapse in the 10 years following the diagnosis of early BC [9,14,15].

A higher RS was observed in invasive ductal carcinoma with micropapillary features, followed by invasive ductal carcinoma not otherwise specified, invasive mucinous carcinoma, invasive lobular carcinoma, mixed ductal and lobular carcinoma, tubular carcinoma, mixed and mucinous ductal carcinoma and pleomorphic lobular carcinoma. For special histological types of BC, it is unclear whether RS is as significant as in nonspecial type carcinomas [16].

In particular, the prevalence of high RS has been observed to be lower in BC patients with lobular than in those with non-lobular histotype [17,18].

The combination of genomic and clinical information provides the clinician with a more accurate estimate of the BC patient's prognosis than considering genomic or clinical information, alone [19].

BC with osteoclast-like giant cells (OGCs) was first described by Leroux in 1931; then by Duboucher in 1933 and Factor in 1977 [20] and subsequently by Agnatis in 1979 [21], Holland in 1984 [22] and Pettinato in 1989 [23].

The origin and nature of multinucleated OGCs in extra-skeletal tumors are not defined. OGCs are a specific type of macrophage different from osteoclasts. Bone resorption by

OGCs isolated from breast tissue and the breast indicates that this transplanted cell into new tissue performs the bone resorption function of the osteoclast [24].

BC with OGCs is a rare histotype found in 0.5–1.2% of BC cases, with an unknown OGC mechanism of formation.

This histotype is characterized by the presence of OGCs, or giant cells similar to multinucleated osteoclasts, in association with ductal, lobular, papillary, cribriform, tubular, mucinous, scaly or other BC [25–27].

Among the histological types of breast cancer with OGCs reported, invasive ductal carcinoma is the most frequent histotype reported in association with OGCs [28], particularly, the luminal-like A subtype [29].

OGCs have similar characteristics to bone osteoclasts but have lost antigen presentation capabilities, such as an anticancer defense. The appearance of OGCs could result from a protumor differentiation of macrophages that respond to hypervascular microenvironments induced by BC. OGCs correspond to cells that strongly express the pan-macrophage marker CD68 and variably express CD163, a marker of the M2-macrophage with protumor function.

The high content of tumor-associated macrophages (TAMs) in the BC microenvironment is associated with a worse prognosis [30–32].

Genomic tests investigate genes associated with the proliferation and estrogen receptors of cancer cells for risk stratification but do not consider the tumor microenvironment, hence the perplexity of using these tests for tumors with special histology, particularly if they are rich in macrophages [33].

2. Case Report

We reported the case of an early BC, invasive ductal carcinoma with OGCs, from the perspective of gene profile analysis tests.

At the end of February 2020, a 49-year-old nonsmoking female patient with no comorbidity and unfamiliar with oncological diseases, underwent a screening mammography x-ray that showed the presence of a nodule of about 2 cm against the external quadrant of the right breast, which was suspected for heteroplasia in the absence of further suspect nodules and/or lymph nodes. The patient was then subjected to an ultrasound examination, which confirmed the presence of a lump with malignant characteristics, and was therefore subjected to true-cut of the breast lump with histological examination positive for invasive ductal carcinoma of the breast.

In March 2020, the patient underwent a quadrantectomy of the right breast with removal of 2 cm neoplastic nodule and three ipsilateral sentinel lymph nodes. The microscopic examination was positive for moderately differentiated invasive ductal carcinoma containing osteoclast-like giant cells (OGCs). According to immunohistochemical analysis, the tumor had the following characteristics: ER: + 100%, PR: + 85%, E-cadherin: positive, Ki67: +10% and HER2: negative, with a staging category corresponding to pT1c pN0, according to the TNM staging system.

Immunohistochemically, OGCs are positive for the histiocytic marker CD68 and negative for E-cadherin, an epithelial marker, and for ER, PR and HER2. In addition, they are CD163 positive (Figures 1–8).

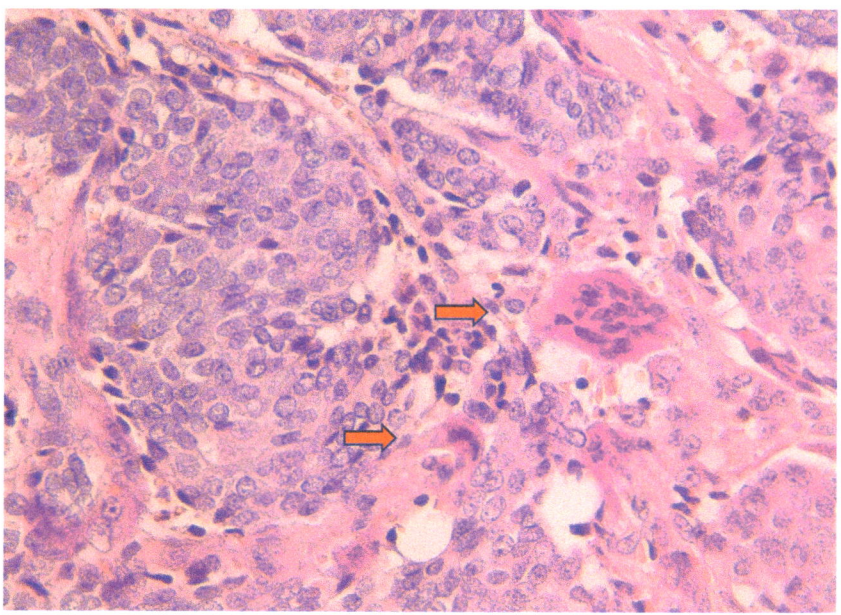

Figure 1. Hematoxylin and eosin stain 40× showing invasive ductal carcinoma with at least 2 osteoclast-like giant cells (↑).

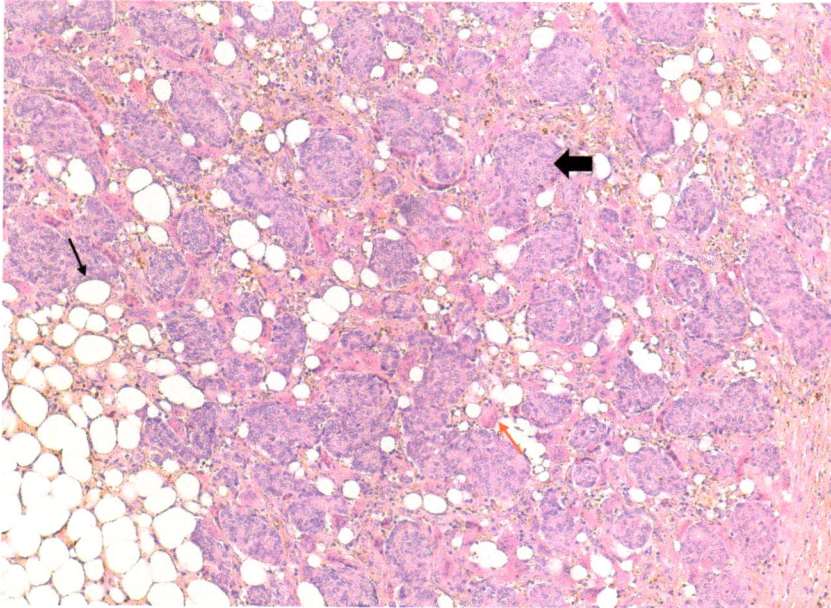

Figure 2. Hematoxylin and eosin stain 20× showing invasive ductal carcinoma with at least 30 osteoclast-like giant cells (↑), which are multinucleated cells and vary in shape and size with eosinophilic cytoplasm; grouped neoplastic cells (↑) are present immersed in the stroma containing adipocytes (↑).

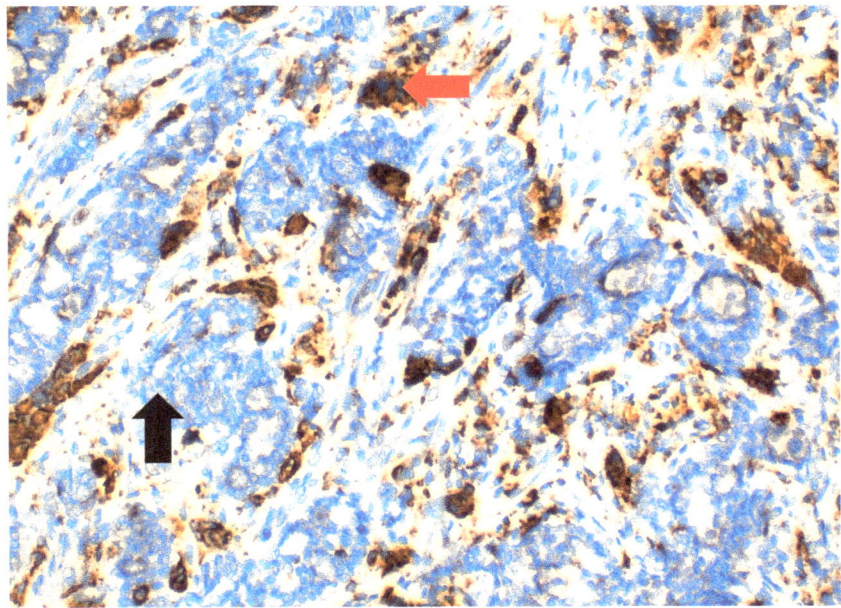

Figure 3. At 40× magnification. Immunohistochemical-positive reaction of macrophages included osteoclast-like giant cells (OGCs) for CD68 (🡅), unlike neoplastic cells, which are CD68-negative (🡅).

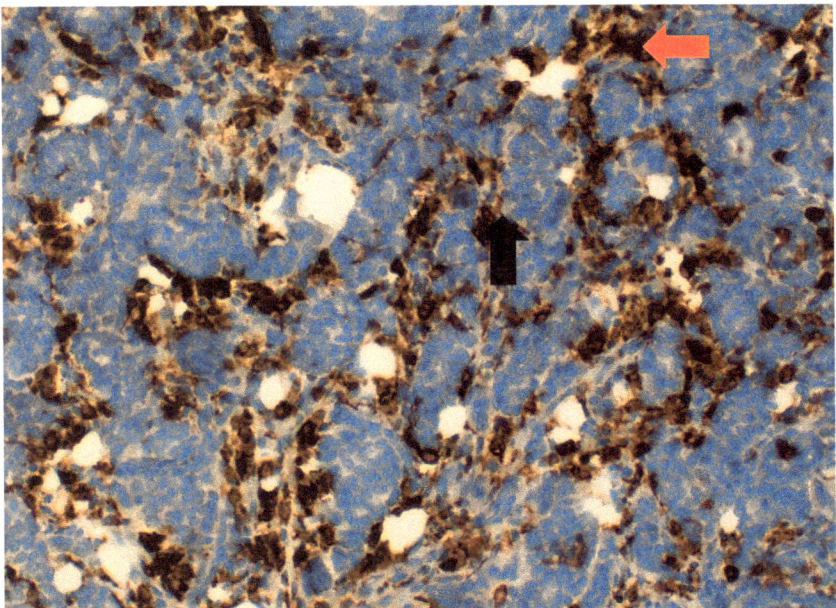

Figure 4. At 40× magnification. Immunohistochemical-positive reaction of OGCs and macrophages for CD163 (🡅), unlike neoplastic cells, which are CD163-negative (🡅).

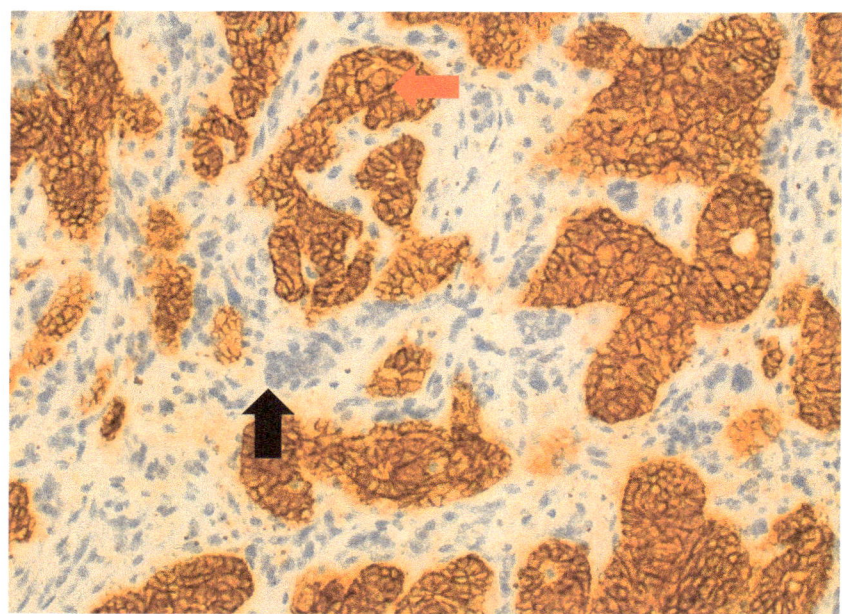

Figure 5. At 40× magnification. Immunohistochemical-positive reaction of neoplastic cells for E-cadherin (⬆), unlike OGCs, which are E-cadherin-negative (⬆).

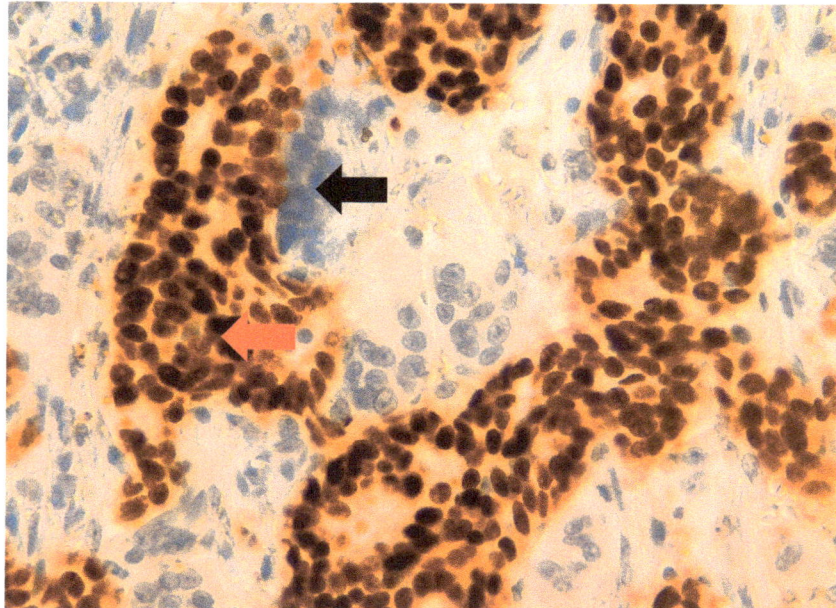

Figure 6. At 40× magnification. Immunohistochemical-positive reaction of neoplastic cells for estrogen receptor (⬆), unlike OGCs, which are estrogen receptor-negative (⬆).

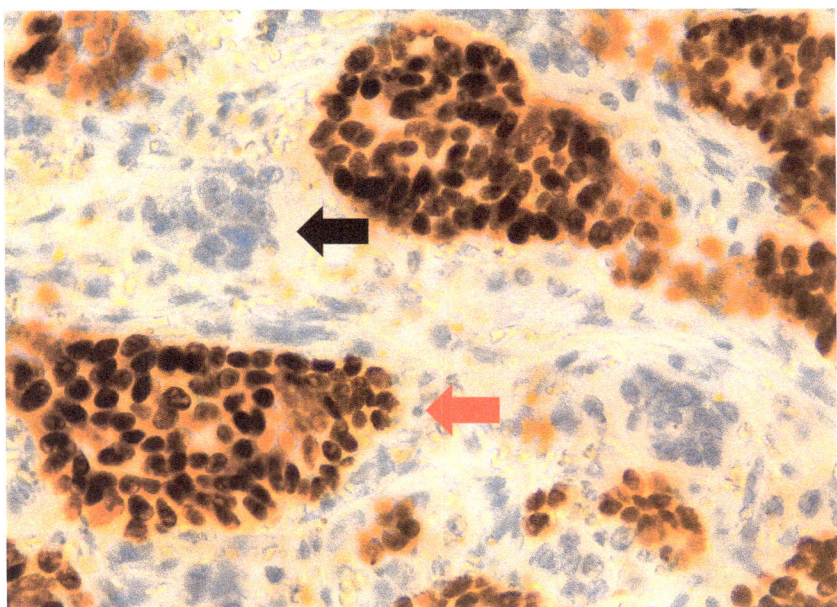

Figure 7. At 40× magnification. Immunohistochemical-positive reaction of neoplastic cells for progesterone receptor (🔴), unlike OGCs which are progesterone receptor-negative (⬆).

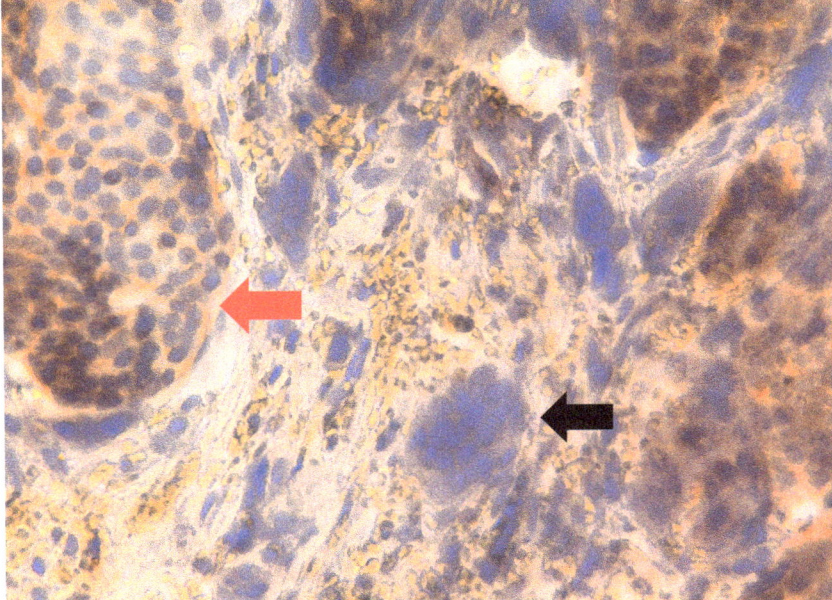

Figure 8. At 40× magnification. Immunohistochemical-negative reaction of neoplastic cells for human epidermal growth factor receptor 2 (🔴) and OGCs (⬆).

On the other hand, cancer cells are negative for CD68 and CD163 for the HER2 but are positive for cadherin E, estrogen receptor (ER: 100%) and progesterone receptor (PR: 85%) (Table 1).

Table 1. Immunohistochemical findings in invasive ductal carcinoma of the breast with osteoclast-like giant cells.

	Cancer Cells	Osteoclast-Like Giant Cells
Estrogen Receptor	+	-
Progesterone Receptor	+	-
Human Epidermal Growth Factor Receptor 2	-	-
E-cadherin	+	-
CD68	-	+
CD163	-	+

+: positive; -: negative.

Clinical–instrumental staging tests (blood chemistry tests with tumor markers, abdomen ultrasound, chest CT without bone and bone scan) were negative for distant neoplastic disease.

For the negative HER2 hormone-responsive disease, various analysis tests of gene profiles are available and are useful in determining the risk of relapse of disease in early breast cancer, in order to assess the need for chemotherapy in addition to hormone therapy.

In this clinical case, the Oncotype Dx test provided was used in our institute, with a recurrence score of 23. Considering the age of the patient, ≤ 50 years, the use of chemotherapy was found to correspond to a benefit of approximately 6.5%.

After a multidisciplinary collegial discussion, and considering the age, the absence of comorbidity, the premenopausal state, the rare histotype and the Oncotype Dx report, the patient underwent adjuvant chemotherapy treatment, according to the Docetaxel-Cyclophosphamide q21 scheme, for 4 cycles, followed by hormone therapy with luteinizing hormone-releasing hormone (LHRH) analogue and exemestane.

The patient, aware of the benefits and risks related to the aforementioned therapeutic proposal, decided to accept it. After chemotherapy, the patient will also undergo radiotherapy treatment on the residual breast.

3. Discussion

In several other diseases, such as tuberculosis, sarcoidosis and granulomatous mastitis, we can found the presence of OGCs. However, breast cancer does not have histological features consistent with granulomatous disease. The origin and mechanism for developing osteoclast-like giant cells is unknown. However, one hypothesis suggests that cancer cells secrete the vaso-endothelial growth factor, which promotes angiogenesis and migration of macrophages into the tumor; this eventually induces monocytic stromal cells to merge with each other to become OGCs [34].

Immunohistochemical studies suggest that OGCs originate from mesenchymal cells, particularly macrophages, in response to cytokines produced by cancer cells [28].

The secretion of cytokines, such as VEGF and MMP12, indeed determines an inflammatory and hypervascular stroma and improves macrophage migration. Therefore, the appearance of OGCs could be not an antitumor immunological reaction but a differentiation of macrophages that respond to the hypervascular tumor microenvironment induced by breast cancer. OGCs have a phenotypic similarity to osteoclasts in the bone and lack antigen presentation capabilities [30].

It has also been shown that when OGCs are isolated from breast carcinomas BC and placed in cell cultures on bone slices, they perform an osteoclast function with consequent formation of bone resorption pits [20].

While osteoclasts are activated by osteoblasts, OGCs are activated directly by the presence of the parathyroid hormone. Furthermore, OGCs are not inhibited by calcitonin, demonstrating another key distinction between OGCs and osteoclasts [35].

The histopathological diagnosis of BC with OGCs passes through the immunohistochemical determination of markers such as E-cadherin, CD68 and CD163. E-cadherin stains tumor cells but not OGCs; CD68 stains OGCs but not tumor cells; CD163 is expressed inconsistently by OGCs, i.e., with moderate- to high intensity [31], or is not expressed [32,36]. In the clinical case we present here, CD163 stains both macrophages and OGCs.

Due to the limited number of cases of this rare histological subtype in clinical practice, it is difficult to establish the prognosis in these patients [20].

The prognostic significance of the presence of OGCs in breast cancer remains controversial, as some authors have suggested a less favorable prognosis for invasive breast cancer with OGCs among BC [14], while others have reported a similar or better prognosis than infiltrative carcinomas without OGCs.

Given this discrepancy, the prognosis in these patients is much more likely associated with the BC histology than with the presence or absence of OGCs [26,28,35].

With the above doubts regarding the prognosis of this tumor, we decided to use the Oncotype Dx test for the patient under consideration.

The Oncotype Dx is used in early luminal-like and HER2-negative BC patients [37].

In the TAILORx study. Sparano et al. have enrolled 6711 early BC patients with hormonal-positive receptors, HER2 negative and without locoregional lymph node metastases. The Oncotype Dx allowed patients to be stratified into three groups based on the RS value: patients with RS ≤ 10 underwent exclusive hormone therapy; patients with RS > 25 underwent chemotherapy followed by hormone therapy and patients with RS = 11–25 were randomized to receive hormone therapy versus chemotherapy followed by hormone therapy. It was observed that, for patients with RS 16–25, the combination of RS and age <50 years identifies patients who benefit from the addition of chemotherapy to hormone therapy: for RS 16–20, approximately 1.6% benefit from chemotherapy; for RS 21–25, approximately 6.5% benefit from chemotherapy [38,39].

The Italian prospective study ROXANE assessed the impact of the Oncotype Dx in clinical practice in nine Italian cancer centers. This test was used when the recommendation of adjuvant treatment with chemotherapy was uncertain for 251 patients with early luminal-like/HER2 negative BC, T1-T3, N0-N1. The rate of change in the treatment decision was 30% (n = 75), mainly from chemotherapy plus hormone therapy to hormone therapy (76%, n = 57/75). The proportion of patients recommended to chemotherapy plus hormone therapy (n = 130) was significantly reduced from pre-RS to post-RS (from 52% to 36%, $p < 0.0001$). Among the 121 BC patients, candidates for exclusive hormone therapy without the Oncotype Dx, 18 (15%) patients obtained an RS that referred to chemotherapy treatment followed by hormone therapy. The percentage of patients initially recommended for hormone therapy alone for whom the recommendation changed to chemotherapy plus hormone therapy was low (7%) [40].

We reported the case of a patient with rare and grade 2 luminal A-like BC. Given the rarity of the histotype, the case was subjected to a second anatomopathological review at another hospital, which confirmed the histopathological characteristics reported. Given that luminal A-like tumors are more likely low-grade and with low RS than luminal B-like tumors [41], by subjecting this case to Oncotype Dx, we expected to obtain a low RS. We obtained an intermediate RS of 23, which, combined with the patient's age of 49, suggested a chemotherapy benefit of approximately 6.5%. The reliability of this result is questioned by the studies of Acs G. et al. [42,43], who recognized the inflammatory cells of the tumor microenvironment as factors influencing the RS by increasing it. For example, Mammostrat, an immunohistochemistry-based assay that analyzes only tumor cells, could represent a valid alternative to the Oncotype Dx that analyzes RNA extracted from both tumor cells and stromal/inflammatory cells in cases of BC with inflammatory infiltrate. In fact, tumors with intermediate/high risk in the Oncotype Dx but not with Mammostrat showed a tumor microenvironment rich in inflammatory cells. We can deduce that, in the case of inflammatory tumors, the Oncotype Dx could have less informative value, but further studies are needed to validate this hypothesis. However, it should be remembered that Mammostrat is not currently available on the market in Italy [15].

4. Conclusions

We presented a clinical case of early breast cancer with a rare histotype for which we used one of the gene expression profiling tests available, i.e., Oncotype Dx, in order to identify the best therapeutic procedure for the patient. Based exclusively on histopathological parameters, except histology, we would have offered the patient exclusive hormonal treatment. The Oncotype Dx together with the age of the patient and her premenopausal state, as well as the rare histology, made us opt for adjuvant chemotherapy followed by adjuvant hormone therapy. It follows the importance of considering molecular tests and, in particular, prospectively validated genomic tests such as Oncotype Dx, with the limits related to the literature data available on special histologies, in estimating the risk of disease recovery at 10 years, in order to identify the best treatment with a view to personalized, patient-centered oncology.

Author Contributions: Conceptualization, A.I., M.M.S., L.G. and M.D.M.; methodology, A.I., M.M.S., G.R.Q., C.D., E.M.B., F.D.P., L.G. and M.D.M.; validation, A.I., M.M.S., L.G. and M.D.M.; investigation, A.I., M.M.S., G.R.Q., L.G. and M.D.M.; resources, A.I., M.M.S., G.R.Q., C.D., E.M.B., F.D.P., L.G. and M.D.M.; data curation, A.I., M.M.S., G.R.Q., C.D., E.M.B., F.D.P., L.G. and M.D.M.; writing—original draft preparation, A.I., M.M.S., G.R.Q., C.D., E.M.B., F.D.P., L.G. and M.D.M.; writing—review and editing, A.I., M.M.S., G.R.Q., C.D., E.M.B., F.D.P., L.G. and M.D.M.; supervision, A.I., M.M.S., G.R.Q., C.D., E.M.B., F.D.P., L.G. and M.D.M. All authors have read and agreed to the published version of the manuscript.

Funding: This research received no external funding.

Informed Consent Statement: Informed consent was obtained from all subjects involved in the study.

Data Availability Statement: Data is contained within the article.

Conflicts of Interest: The authors declare no conflict of interest.

References

1. Cardoso, F.; Kyriakides, S.; Ohno, S.; Penault-Llorca, F.; Poortmans, P.; Rubio, I.; Zackrisson, S.; Senkus, E. Early breast cancer: ESMO Clinical Practice Guidelines for diagnosis, treatment and follow-up. *Ann. Oncol.* **2019**, *30*, 1194–1220. [CrossRef]
2. Irelli, A.; Sirufo, M.M.; Scipioni, T.; De Pietro, F.; Pancotti, A.; Ginaldi, L.; De Martinis, M. Denosumab in breast cancer patients receiving aromatase inhibitors: A single-center observational study of effectiveness in adjuvant setting. *Indian J. Cancer* **2020**. [CrossRef]
3. Irelli, A.; Sirufo, M.M.; D'Ugo, C.; Ginaldi, L.; De Martinis, M. Real-life use of denosumab 120 mg every 12 weeks in prolonged treatment over 2 years of patients with breast cancer bone metastases. *J. BUON* **2020**, *25*, 1799–1804.
4. Irelli, A.; Sirufo, M.M.; Scipioni, T.; De Pietro, F.; Pancotti, A.; Ginaldi, L.; De Martinis, M. Breast cancer patients receiving denosumab during adjuvant aromatase inhibitors treatment: Who are the "inadequate responders" patients to denosumab? *J. BUON* **2020**, *25*, 648–654.
5. Gori, S.; Dieci, M.V.; Modena, A.; AIRTUM Working Group. Neoplasie per single sedi. Mammella. I numeri del cancro in Italia 2020. Intermedia Editore 2020. Available online: https://www.registri-tumori.it/cms/sites/default/files/pubblicazioni/new_NDC2020-operatori-web.pdf (accessed on 11 January 2021).
6. Siegel, R.L.; Miller, K.D.; Jemal, A. Cancer statistics, 2020. *CA Cancer J. Clin.* **2020**, *70*, 7–30. [CrossRef] [PubMed]
7. Irelli, A.; Sirufo, M.M.; Morelli, L.; D'Ugo, C.; Ginaldi, L.; De Martinis, M. Neuroendocrine Cancer of the Breast: A Rare Entity. *J. Clin. Med.* **2020**, *9*, 1452. [CrossRef]
8. Wilson, P.C.; Chagpar, A.B.; Cicek, A.F.; Bossuyt, V.; Buza, N.; Mougalian, S.; Killelea, B.K.; Patel, N.; Harigopal, M. Breast cancer histopathology is predictive of low-risk Oncotype Dx recurrence score. *Breast J.* **2018**, *24*, 976–980. [CrossRef]
9. Parmelee, P.A.; Thuras, P.D.; Katz, I.R.; Lawton, M.P. Validation of the Cumulative Illness Rating Scale in a Geriatric Residential Population. *J. Am. Geriatr. Soc.* **1995**, *43*, 130–137. [CrossRef] [PubMed]
10. Katz, S.; Downs, T.D.; Cash, H.R.; Grotz, R.C. Progress in Development of the Index of ADL. *Gerontologist* **1970**, *10*, 20–30. [CrossRef]

11. Lawton, M.P.; Brody, E.M. Assessment of Older People: Self-Maintaining and Instrumental Activities of Daily Living. *Gerontol.* **1969**, *9*, 179–186. [CrossRef]
12. Irelli, A.; Sirufo, M.M.; Scipioni, T.; Aielli, F.; Martella, F.; Ginaldi, L.; Pancotti, A.; De Martinis, M. The VES-13 test as a predictor of toxicity associated with aromatase inhibitors in the adjuvant treatment of breast cancer in elderly patients: A single-center study. *Indian J. Cancer* **2020**. (In press)
13. Irelli, A.; Sirufo, M.M.; D'Ugo, C.; Ginaldi, L.; De Martinis, M. Sex and Gender Influences on Cancer Immunotherapy Response. *Biomedicines* **2020**, *8*, 232. [CrossRef]
14. Zhang, L.; Hsieh, M.-C.; Petkov, V.; Yu, Q.; Chiu, Y.-W.; Wu, X.-C. Trend and survival benefit of Oncotype DX use among female hormone receptor-positive breast cancer patients in 17 SEER registries, 2004–2015. *Breast Cancer Res. Treat.* **2020**, *180*, 491–501. [CrossRef]
15. Gori, S.; Dieci, M.V.; Biganzoli, L.; Calabrese, M.; Cortesi, L.; Criscitiello, C.; Del Mastro, L.; Dellepiane, C.; Fortunato, L.; Franco, P.; et al. Breast Neoplasms Guidelines, 2020 ed. Available online: https://www.aiom.it/wp-content/uploads/2020/10/20201218_LG_AIOM_NeoplasieMammella.pdf (accessed on 11 January 2021).
16. Bomeisl, P.E.; Thompson, C.L.; Harris, L.N.; Gilmore, H.L. Comparison of Oncotype DX Recurrence Score by Histologic Types of Breast Carcinoma. *Arch. Pathol. Lab. Med.* **2015**, *139*, 1546–1549. [CrossRef] [PubMed]
17. Christgen, M.; Gluz, O.; Harbeck, N.; Kates, R.E.; Raap, M.; Christgen, H.; Clemens, M.; Malter, W.; Nuding, B.; Aktas, B.; et al. West German Study Group PlanB Investigators. Differential impact of prognostic parameters in hor-mone receptor-positive lobular breast cancer. *Cancer* **2020**, *126*, 4847–4858. [CrossRef] [PubMed]
18. Singh, K.; He, X.; Kalife, E.T.; Ehdaivand, S.; Wang, Y.; Sung, C.J. Relationship of histologic grade and histologic sub-type with oncotype Dx recurrence score; retrospective review of 863 breast cancer oncotype Dx results. *Breast Cancer Res. Treat.* **2018**, *168*, 29–34. [CrossRef] [PubMed]
19. Sparano, J.A.; Gray, R.J.; Ravdin, P.M.; Makower, D.F.; Pritchard, K.I.; Albain, K.S.; Hayes, D.F.; Geyer, C.E.; Dees, E.C.; Goetz, M.P.; et al. Clinical and Genomic Risk to Guide the Use of Adjuvant Therapy for Breast Cancer. *N. Engl. J. Med.* **2019**, *380*, 2395–2405. [CrossRef]
20. Albawardi, A.S.; Awwad, A.A.; Almarzooqi, S.S. Mammary carcinoma with osteoclast-like giant cells: A case report. *Int. J. Clin. Exp. Pathol.* **2014**, *7*, 9038–9043. [PubMed]
21. Agnantis, N.T.; Rosen, P.P. Mammary carcinoma with osteoclast-like giant cells. A study of eight cases with fol-low-up data. *Am. J. Clin. Pathol.* **1979**, *72*, 383–389. [CrossRef] [PubMed]
22. Holland, R.; van Haelst, U.J. Mammary carcinoma with osteoclast-like giant cells. Additional observations on six cases. *Cancer* **1984**, *53*, 1963–1973. [CrossRef]
23. Pettinato, G.; Manivel, J.; Picone, A.; Petrella, G.; Insabato, L. Alveolar variant of infiltrating lobular carcinoma of the breast with stromal osteoclast-like giant cells. *Pathol. Res. Pr.* **1989**, *185*, 388–394. [CrossRef]
24. Athanasou, N.A.; Wells, C.A.; Quinn, J.; Ferguson, D.P.; Heryet, A.; McGee, J.O. The origin and nature of stromal osteo-clast-like multinucleated giant cells in breast carcinoma: Implications for tumour osteolysis and macrophage biology. *Br. J. Cancer.* **1989**, *59*, 491–498. [CrossRef]
25. Takahashi, T.; Moriki, T.; Hiroi, M.; Nakayama, H. Invasive Lobular Carcinoma of the Breast with Osteoclastlike Giant Cells. *Acta Cytol.* **1998**, *42*, 734–741. [CrossRef] [PubMed]
26. Niu, Y.; Liao, X.; Li, X.; Zhao, L. Breast carcinoma with osteoclastic giant cells: Case report and review of the litera-ture. *Int. J. Clin. Exp. Pathol.* **2014**, *7*, 1788–1791.
27. Khong, K.; Zhang, Y.; Tomic, M.; Lindfors, K.K.; Aminololama-Shakeri, S. Aggressive Metaplastic Carcinoma of the Breast with Osteoclastic Giant Cells. *J. Radiol. Case Rep.* **2015**, *9*, 11–19. [CrossRef] [PubMed]
28. Peña-Jaimes, L.; González-García, I.; Reguero-Callejas, M.E.; Pinilla-Pagnon, I.; Pérez-Mies, B.; Albarrán-Artahona, V.; Martínez-Jañez, N.; Rosa-Rosa, J.M.; Palacios, J. Pleomorphic lobular carcinoma of the breast with osteoclast-like giant cells: A case report and review of the literature. *Diagn. Pathol.* **2018**, *13*, 62. [CrossRef]
29. Zhou, S.; Yu, L.; Zhou, R.; Li, X.; Yang, W. Invasive breast carcinomas of no special type with osteoclast-like giant cells frequently have a luminal phenotype. *Virchows Arch.* **2014**, *464*, 681–688. [CrossRef] [PubMed]
30. Shishido-Hara, Y.; Kurata, A.; Fujiwara, M.; Itoh, H.; Imoto, S.; Kamma, H. Two cases of breast carcinoma with osteo-clastic giant cells: Are the osteoclastic giant cells pro-tumoural differentiation of macrophages? *Diagn Pathol.* **2010**, *23*, 55. [CrossRef] [PubMed]
31. Ohashi, R.; Yanagihara, K.; Namimatsu, S.; Sakatani, T.; Takei, H.; Naito, Z.; Shimizu, A. Osteoclast-like giant cells in invasive breast cancer predominantly possess M2-macrophage phenotype. *Pathol. Res. Pr.* **2018**, *214*, 253–258. [CrossRef]
32. Ohashi, R.; Hayama, A.; Matsubara, M.; Watarai, Y.; Sakatani, T.; Naito, Z.; Shimizu, A. Breast carcinoma with osteo-clast-like giant cells: A cytological-pathological correlation with a literature review. *Ann. Diagn Pathol.* **2018**, *33*, 1–5. [CrossRef]
33. Güth, U.; Borovecki, A.; Amann, E.; Rechsteiner, M.; Tinguely, M. Pleomorphic lobular breast carcinoma with osteo-clast like giant cells in the era of genomic testing. *Curr. Probl. Cancer Case Rep.* **2020**, *1*, 100008. [CrossRef]
34. Stratton, A.; Plackett, T.P.; Belnap, C.M.; Lin-Hurtubise, K.M. Infiltrating Mammary Carcinoma with Osteoclast-like Giant Cells. *Hawaii Med. J.* **2010**, *69*, 284–285.
35. Zagelbaum, N.K.; Ward, M.F.; Okby, N.; Karpoff, H. Invasive ductal carcinoma of the breast with osteoclast-like giant cells and clear cell features: A case report of a novel finding and review of the literature. *World J. Surg. Oncol.* **2016**, *14*, 227. [CrossRef]

36. Jamiyan, T.; Kuroda, H.; Hayashi, M.; Abe, A.; Shimizu, K.; Imai, Y. Ductal carcinoma in situ of the breast with osteoclast-like giant cells: A case report with immunohistochemical analysis. *Hum. Pathol. Case Rep.* **2020**, *20*, 200383. [CrossRef]
37. Andre, F.; Ismaila, N.; Henry, N.L.; Somerfield, M.R.; Bast, R.C.; Barlow, W.; Collyar, D.E.; Hammond, M.E.; Kuderer, N.M.; Liu, M.C.; et al. Use of Biomarkers to Guide Decisions on Adjuvant Systemic Therapy for Women With Early-Stage Invasive Breast Cancer: ASCO Clinical Practice Guideline Up-date-Integration of Results From TAILORx. *J. Clin. Oncol.* **2019**, *37*, 1956–1964. [CrossRef] [PubMed]
38. Sparano, J.A.; Gray, R.J.; Makower, D.F.; Pritchard, K.I.; Albain, K.S.; Hayes, D.F.; Geyer, C.E.; Dees, E.C.; Perez, E.A.; Olson, J.A.; et al. Prospective Validation of a 21-Gene Expression Assay in Breast Cancer. *N. Engl. J. Med.* **2015**, *373*, 2005–2014. [CrossRef]
39. Sparano, J.A.; Gray, R.J.; Makower, D.F.; Pritchard, K.I.; Albain, K.S.; Hayes, D.F.; Geyer, C.E., Jr.; Dees, E.C.; Goetz, M.P.; Olson, J.A., Jr.; et al. Adjuvant Chemotherapy Guided by a 21-Gene Expression Assay in Breast Cancer. *N. Engl. J. Med.* **2018**, *379*, 111–121. [CrossRef]
40. Dieci, M.V.; Guarneri, V.; Zustovich, F.; Mion, M.; Morandi, P.; Bria, E.; Merlini, L.; Bullian, P.; Oliani, C.; Gori, S.; et al. Impact of 21-Gene Breast Cancer Assay on Treatment Decision for Patients with T1–T3, N0–N1, Estrogen Receptor-Positive/Human Epidermal Growth Factor Receptor 2-Negative Breast Cancer: Final Results of the Prospective Multicenter ROXANE Study. *Oncologist* **2019**, *24*, 1424–1431. [CrossRef] [PubMed]
41. Mizuno, Y.; Fuchikami, H.; Takeda, N.; Yamada, J.; Inoue, Y.; Seto, H.; Sato, K. Comparing Oncotype DX Recurrence Score Categories with Immunohistochemically Defined Luminal Subtypes. *J. Cancer Ther.* **2016**, *7*, 223–231. [CrossRef]
42. Acs, G.; Esposito, N.N.; Kiluk, J.; Loftus, L.; Laronga, C. A mitotically active, cellular tumor stroma and/or inflammatory cells associated with tumor cells may contribute to intermediate or high Oncotype DX Recurrence Scores in low-grade invasive breast carcinomas. *Mod. Pathol.* **2011**, *25*, 556–566. [CrossRef] [PubMed]
43. Acs, G.; Kiluk, J.; Loftus, L.; Laronga, C. Comparison of Oncotype DX and Mammostrat risk estimations and corre-lations with histologic tumor features in low-grade, estrogen receptor-positive invasive breast carcinomas. *Mod. Pathol.* **2013**, *26*, 1451–1460. [CrossRef] [PubMed]

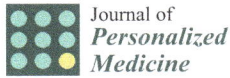 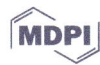

Article

Immediate Prosthetic Breast Reconstruction after Nipple-Sparing Mastectomy: Traditional Subpectoral Technique versus Direct-to-Implant Prepectoral Reconstruction without Acellular Dermal Matrix

Gianluca Franceschini [1,*,†], Lorenzo Scardina [1,†], Alba Di Leone [1], Daniela Andreina Terribile [1], Alejandro Martin Sanchez [1], Stefano Magno [1], Sabatino D'Archi [1], Antonio Franco [1], Elena Jane Mason [1], Beatrice Carnassale [1], Federica Murando [1], Armando Orlandi [2], Liliana Barone Adesi [3], Giuseppe Visconti [3], Marzia Salgarello [3] and Riccardo Masetti [1]

1. Department of Woman and Child Health and Public Health, Division of Breast Surgery, Fondazione Policlinico Universitario Agostino Gemelli IRCCS, Università Cattolica del Sacro Cuore, Largo Agostino Gemelli, 8, 00168 Rome, Italy; lorenzoscardina@libero.it (L.S.); alba.dileone@policlinicogemelli.it (A.D.L.); daniela.terribile@policlinicogemelli.it (D.A.T.); martin.sanchez@hotmail.it (A.M.S.); stefano.magno@policlinicogemelli.it (S.M.); sabatinodarchi@gmail.com (S.D.); antonio.franco89@icloud.com (A.F.); elenajanemason@gmail.com (E.J.M.); carnassale.beatrice@gmail.com (B.C.); murandofederica@gmail.com (F.M.); riccardo.masetti@policlinicogemelli.it (R.M.)
2. Comprehensive Cancer Center, Multidisciplinary Breast Unit, Fondazione Policlinico Universitario Agostino Gemelli IRCCS, Università Cattolica del Sacro Cuore, Largo Agostino Gemelli, 8, 00168 Rome, Italy; armando.orlandi@policlinicogemelli.it
3. Department of Woman and Child Health and Public Health, Division of Plastic Surgery, Fondazione Policlinico Universitario Agostino Gemelli IRCCS, Università Cattolica del Sacro Cuore, Largo Agostino Gemelli, 8, 00168 Rome, Italy; liliana.baroneadesi@policlinicogemelli.it (L.B.A.); joevisconti@hotmail.com (G.V.); marzia.salgarello@policlinicogemelli.it (M.S.)
* Correspondence: gianlucafranceschini70@gmail.com; Tel.: +39-3201803270
† Gianluca Franceschini and Lorenzo Scardina contributed equally to this work.

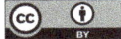

Abstract: Background: The aim of this study was to compare outcomes of immediate prosthetic breast reconstruction (IPBR) using traditional submuscular (SM) positioning of implants versus prepectoral (PP) positioning of micropolyurethane-foam-coated implants (microthane) without further coverage. Methods: We retrospectively reviewed the medical records of breast cancer patients treated by nipple-sparing mastectomy (NSM) and IPBR in our institution during the two-year period from January 2018 to December 2019. Patients were divided into two groups based on the plane of implant placement: SM versus PP. Results: 177 patients who received IPBR after NSM were included in the study; implants were positioned in a SM plane in 95 patients and in a PP plane in 82 patients. The two cohorts were similar for mean age (44 years and 47 years in the SM and PP groups, respectively) and follow-up (20 months and 16 months, respectively). The mean operative time was 70 min shorter in the PP group. No significant differences were observed in length of hospital stay or overall major complication rates. Statistically significant advantages were observed in the PP group in terms of aesthetic results, chronic pain, shoulder dysfunction, and skin sensibility ($p < 0.05$), as well as a trend of better outcomes for sports activity and sexual/relationship life. Cost analysis revealed that PP-IPBR was also economically advantageous over SM-IPBR. Conclusions: Our preliminary experience seems to confirm that PP positioning of a polyurethane-coated implant is a safe, reliable and effective method to perform IPBR after NSM.

Keywords: breast cancer; nipple-sparing mastectomy; immediate breast reconstruction; acellular dermal matrix (ADM); aesthetic and oncological outcomes; quality of life

1. Introduction

Immediate prosthetic breast reconstruction (IPBR) is considered as an integral part of the surgical treatment of patients undergoing nipple-sparing mastectomy (NSM) for breast cancer, as it positively affects psychological health, sexuality, body image, and self-esteem.

Traditionally, IPBR has been performed by placement of the prosthetic implant in a submuscular (SM) pocket created beneath the pectoralis major muscle, in order to protect the integrity of the implant and reduce its visibility and palpability [1,2]. Although this technique has shown increasingly good results, it still yields a higher risk of undesirable outcomes such as significant postoperative pain, injury-induced muscular deficit, breast animation deformity, lateral deviation of the breast mound with poor inframammary fold definition, and insufficient lower pole fullness [3,4].

In recent years, placement of the implant in a prepectoral (PP) plane has been increasingly employed. When this technique is performed, the implant is usually covered with an acellular dermal matrix (ADM) to shield it in the subcutaneous space underneath the skin flaps; however, the use of ADM has been reported to increase risks of seroma, infection, and skin/nipple-areola complex (NAC) necrosis, and associated with higher medical costs [1]. To limit these inconveniences, the use of implants with a special micropolyurethane-foam-coated shell surface (microthane) that does not require ADM coverage has recently been proposed [2,5].

The aim of this study was to compare outcomes between traditional SM-IPBR and a PP technique using microthane implants without ADMs in patients undergoing NSM.

2. Materials and Methods

After approval from the Institutional Review Board of our hospital, a retrospective review of the medical records of breast cancer patients who underwent NSM followed by IPBR over the two-year period of January 2018–December 2019 was performed. Patients treated before January 2018 were not enrolled because before that date, PP-IPBR in our institution was routinely performed with ADMs, which would have added heterogeneity to our population.

Patients were divided into two cohorts based on the site of implant placement: in SM-IPBR, anatomical textured implants were positioned in the subpectoral pocket according to a previously described standardized technique, while in PP-IPBR, a definitive Polytech implant with a micropolyurethane-foam-coated shell surface was placed in the subcutaneous plane [5,6].

2.1. Operative Protocol and Surgical Technique

A complete preoperative workup including clinical assessment, ultrasonography, mammography, breast MRI, and disease staging was performed in all patients; surgical planning was always discussed in a multidisciplinary dedicated surgery board. Common indications to NSM included large tumor-to-breast size, inability to obtain clear surgical margins with breast-conserving surgery, extensive or multicentric disease, contraindications to adjuvant radiotherapy, and patient preference; absolute contraindications to NSM with both types of reconstruction were inflammatory carcinoma, a locally advanced tumor infiltrating the skin or NAC, and previous radiotherapy. Obesity (BMI > 30 kg/m^2), large breasts with severe ptosis, and active smoking were considered as relative contraindications due to the increased risk of skin or NAC necrosis, breast asymmetry, and nipple displacement [2–6]. Bilateral NSM was performed in patients with a bilateral breast tumor or in women with unilateral disease and a high risk of contralateral breast cancer, such as BRCA mutation carriers.

A specific algorithm shared with the plastic surgeons, based on anamnestic, morphological, functional, and oncological criteria, was used to define the most appropriate reconstruction technique [7,8]. The Rancati classification, based on digital mammographic imaging, was used to predict thickness of post-mastectomy skin flaps [9].

In the vast majority of cases, NSM was carried out through a radial incision on the external quadrants; axillary or inframammary crease incisions were used only in selected cases. Skin flaps and NAC were progressively elevated from glandular tissue. The entire gland was then separated from the muscular plane and removed, preserving the superficial pectoralis fascia. An accurate circumferential palpation of the surgical cavity after removal of the gland was always performed to rule out the possibility of residual breast tissue. Intraoperative pathology evaluation of retroareolar tissue was performed in all cases to confirm secure margins. The removed gland was always weighed to better determine the subsequent reconstruction volume.

The final decision on the type of reconstructive technique (SM versus PP) was made in the operating room based on flap thickness and perfusion assessment [2,10]. Skin-flap thickness was measured using pliers, and perfusion was assessed using indocyanine green dye fluoroangiography and a photodynamic eye (PDE) imaging system (Figures 1 and 2).

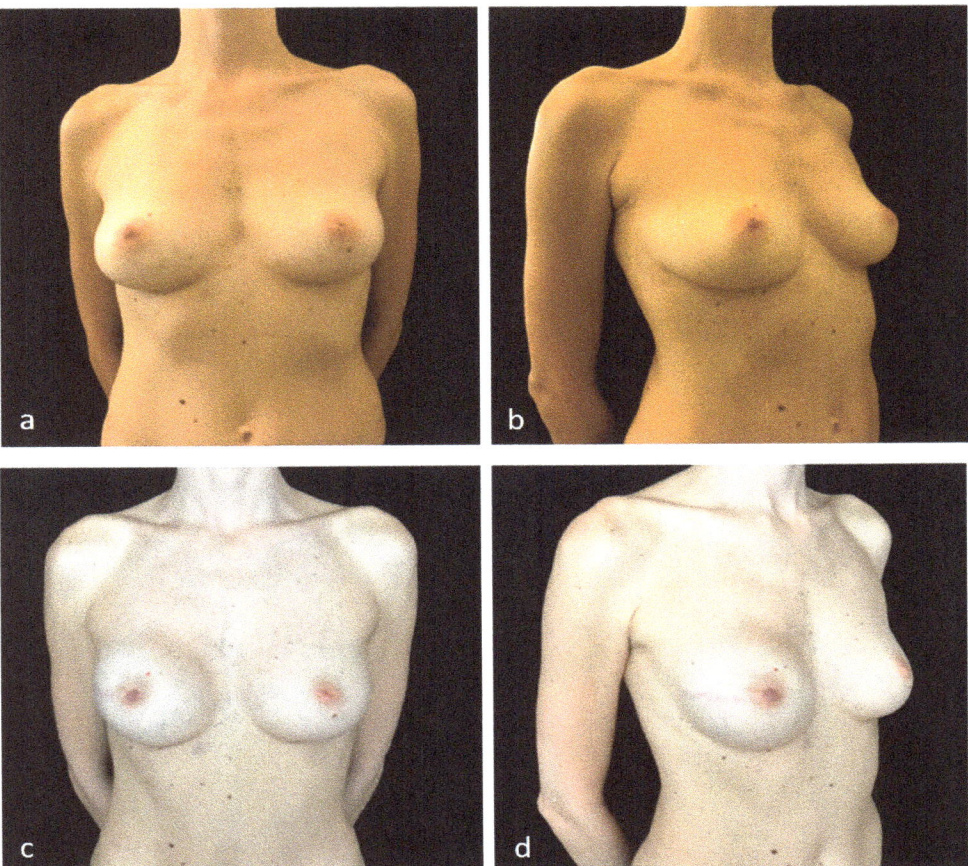

Figure 1. A case of nipple-sparing mastectomy and direct-to-implant prepectoral reconstruction without acellular dermal matrix. (**a**,**b**) Preoperative pictures of a 43-year-old right-breast cancer patient for whom right nipple-sparing mastectomy and direct-to-implant prepectoral reconstruction without acellular dermal matrix were planned. (**c**,**d**) Six-month postoperative pictures after right nipple-sparing mastectomy through a radial lateral incision (mastectomy specimen 190 g) and prepectoral reconstruction using a definitive anatomical implant (Polytech 30746, 295cc) with a micropolyurethane-foam-coated shell surface, placed in the subcutaneous plane.

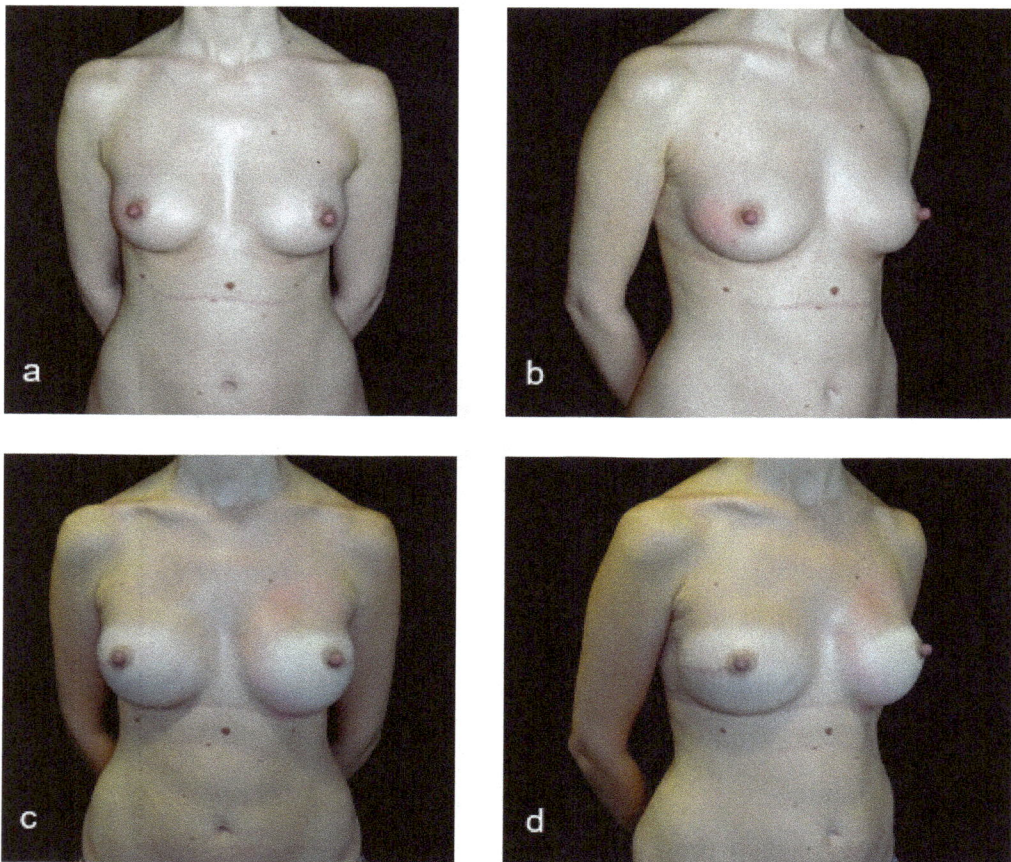

Figure 2. A case of nipple-sparing mastectomy and direct-to-implant submuscular reconstruction. (**a,b**) Preoperative pictures of a 47-year-old bilateral-breast cancer patient for whom bilateral nipple-sparing mastectomy and direct-to-implant submuscular reconstruction without acellular dermal matrix were planned. (**c,d**) Six-month postoperative pictures after bilateral nipple-sparing mastectomy through a radial lateral incision.

A single-stage SM reconstruction was performed using total coverage of the implant beneath the pectoralis major and serratus anterior [7]; PP-IPBR was realized with the placement of the prosthesis into the same anatomical space of the excised mammary gland [2,5]; textured implants were used for SM-IPBR and Polytech implants with a micropolyurethane-foam-coated shell surface for PP-IBPR [2,5]; and a contralateral procedure to achieve better symmetry was performed when deemed necessary [10,11].

We chose to position a prepectoral implant every time we had good soft-tissue coverage after mastectomy (defined as flap thickness of at least 1 cm and good perfusion with indocyanine green dye fluoroangiography and the photodynamic eye imaging system). In SM-IBPR, we performed a submuscular–subfascial pocket dissection, which allows, with time, a good ptosis. In these cases, any exceeding skin can usually be nicely managed by intraoperative redraping with taping. In SM-IBPR, reduction–augmentation procedures were performed as previously reported.

Two Jackson Pratt drains were always placed in the reconstructive space, usually left in place at the time of hospital discharge and later removed when the amount of fluid collected over 24 h was <30 mL. Patients received levofloxacin at a dosage of 500 mg every 12 h until drain removal and were advised to continue wearing a sports bra for 1 month.

The operative time (from incision to the end of skin suture) and length of hospitalization were recorded.

2.2. Clinical Assessment and Statistical Analysis

Patients were assessed at weekly intervals during the first month and then every 6 months by breast surgeons, plastic surgeons, and oncologists.

Major complications (requiring surgical revision), loco-regional recurrences (defined as local recurrence if involving the ipsilateral skin flap, chest wall, or NAC; or as regional recurrence if involving ipsilateral axillary, internal mammary, or supraclavicular nodes), cosmetic outcomes, quality of life, and economic costs were assessed in all patients.

An automated breast volume scanner (ABVS), a dedicated imaging system that can obtain full-field high-resolution views of skin flaps, was used to better evaluate possible local recurrence in the usually thicker skin flaps of patients with PP-IPBR [10].

The "QOL assessment PRO" is a questionnaire created through a multidisciplinary effort by all specialists working in the Breast Unit of Fondazione Policlinico Universitario Agostino Gemelli IRCCS. It was developed based on the experiences reported in the literature, and has been proficiently employed in our center for several years [12–17]. The questionnaire condenses in seven simple questions the essential patient-reported outcomes (PROs) involving pain, arm motility, aesthetic satisfaction, and general quality of life (QOL), and is therefore a practical tool that in our experience gives results more agreeable to patients than BREAST-Q, and increases their compliance to participate in the study [18]. The QOL assessment PRO was administered six months after surgery via a telephone call by a member of hospital staff, and consisted of five close-ended questions (requiring a yes/no answer) and two scoring questions (requiring a score between 0 and 5 as an answer) (Table 1).

Table 1. QOL assessment PRO survey.

Smart QoL Assessment
Quality of life
• What score would you give to your pain, from 0 (no pain) to 5 (very intense)?
• Is arm motility impaired after surgery? (YES/NO)
• Did you do sports before surgery? (YES/NO) • Have you practiced sports since surgery? (YES/NO)
• Was the sensitivity of the skin and the areola-nipple complex maintained after surgery? (YES/NO)
Satisfaction
• How would you evaluate, from 1 (poor) to 5 (excellent), the aesthetic result of your operation?
Psychological and relational field
• Did the operation compromise your womanhood, sexuality, or relationship life? (YES/NO)

Abbreviations: QOL = quality of life; PRO = patient-reported outcomes.

Results were expressed as means with associated median and range. Statistical analysis was performed using SPSS (version 24.0 for Windows). A Fisher exact test was used for comparison of categorical variables. A p-value equal to or less than 0.05 was considered statistically significant. A cost analysis was performed according to a standardized method [19].

3. Results

Over the two-year study period from January 2018 to December 2019, 177 breast cancer patients with IPBR after NSM were included. SM-IPBR was performed in 95 cases, while PP-IPBR was performed in 82 cases. Patient characteristics are reported in Table 2. Ptosis degree, Rancati score, and intraoperative flap thickness assessment were decisive in determining the kind of reconstruction performed, and therefore differed significantly between the PP and SM group. The remaining aspects were similar in both populations. Adjuvant radiotherapy did not affect aesthetic and oncological outcomes.

Table 2. Patient characteristics.

Characteristics	PP-IPBR	SM-IPBR	p
Patients, n (%)	82 (46.3%)	95 (53.6%)	
Age (years)	47 (27–73)	44 (28–73)	0.113
FUP (months)	15.9 (5–28)	20 (6–28)	0.254
Radiotherapy adjuvant, n (%)	23/82 (28.0%)	22/95 (23.2%)	0.355
Body Mass Index (BMI)	23.95 (17.5–29.4)	24.77 (18.2–28.9)	0.135
Neoadjuvant chemotherapy, n (%)	35/82 (42.7%)	38/95 (40.0%)	0.938
BRCA 1/2 mutation, n (%)	13/82 (15.8%)	12/95 (12.6%)	0.539
Ptosis degree			**<0.001**
➢ 0	19 (23.2%)	41 (43.2%)	
➢ 1	31 (37.8%)	48 (50.5%)	
➢ 2	32 (39%)	6 (6.3%)	
Rancati score			**<0.001**
➢ 1	0	36 (37.9%)	
➢ 2	44 (53.7%)	38 (40%)	
➢ 3	38 (46.3%)	21 (22.1%)	
Intraoperative flap thickness assessment (Indocyanine green visualization < 60 s)	82 (100%)	12 (12.6%)	**<0.001**

Abbreviations: FUP = follow-up; BRCA = breast cancer gene. Statistically significant p values (<0.05) are marked in bold.

The mean ages were 44 (28–73) and 47 (27–73) years respectively. After unilateral NSM, a simultaneous contralateral symmetrization procedure was deemed necessary and carried out in 44/44 (100%) patients of the SM group and in 2/55 (3.6%) patients of the PP group. The type of surgical treatment is summarized in Table 3.

Table 3. Type of surgical treatment.

Surgical Procedures	PP-IPBR	SM-IPBR	p
Bilateral NSM with IPBR, n (%)	27/82 (32.9%)	51/95 (53.7%)	**0.006**
Unilateral NSM with IPBR, n (%)	55/82 (67.1%)	44/95 (46.3%)	**0.008**
Contralateral implant-based symmetrisation mammoplasty after unilateral NSM with IPBR, n (%)	2/55 (3.6%)	44/44 (100%)	**<0.001**

Abbreviations: NSM = nipple-sparing mastectomy; IPBR = immediate prosthetic breast reconstruction. Statistically significant p values (<0.05) are marked in bold.

3.1. Duration of Surgery and of Hospitalization

For patients undergoing unilateral NSM and IPBR, the mean total operative time was 319 min in the SM group and 247 min in the PP group; for patients undergoing bilateral NSM, it was 368 min and 306 min, respectively.

The longest surgery (510 min) was for a patient who underwent a transaxillary bilateral mastectomy with sentinel node biopsy, axillary dissection, and bilateral SM reconstruction. Operative times are summarized in Table 4. Length of hospitalization did not significantly differ between the two populations.

Table 4. Operative time (minutes).

	PP-IPBR	SM-IPBR	p
Bilateral NSM + IPBR	306 (202–381)	368 (276–478)	**0.041**
Unilateral NSM + IPBR + contralateral symmetrization	247 (182–305)	319 (254–393)	**<0.001**

Statistically significant p values (<0.05) are marked in bold.

3.2. Perioperative and Oncological Outcomes

Median follow-up was similar: 20 (6–28) months in the SM group and 16 (5–28) months in the PP group. There was no significant difference in length of stay, overall major complication rates, and oncological outcomes between the two reconstructive cohorts.

Implant loss caused by infection was observed in one patient in the SM group (1.05%) and one patient in the PP group (1.2%). One patient in the PP group (1.2%) developed a full-thickness NAC necrosis that required secondary excision.

During follow-up, NAC recurrence occurred in one patient of the SM group (1.05%), while in the PP group, no local relapse was observed. Regional recurrences occurred in 2/95 (2.1%) patients in the SM group and in 1/82 patients (1.2%) in the PP cohort.

Regarding disease-free survival, one patient in the SM group with triple negative breast cancer developed brain metastases six months after surgery.

3.3. Cosmetic Outcomes and Health-Related Quality of Life

A total of 126/177 patients completed our survey assessing their postoperative quality of life (64.2% and 78%, respectively, for the SM and PP groups).

Statistically significant ($p < 0.05$) advantages in terms of cosmetic results, chronic pain, shoulder dysfunction, and skin sensibility were observed in the PP group.

A not statistically significant difference in favor of the PP group was shown for sports activity and sexual/relationship life (Table 5).

Table 5. QOL assessment PRO survey replies.

	N° Total Patients	PP-IPBR	SM-IPBR	p
Patients who completed our survey	126/177 (71.2%)	64/82 (78%)	62/95 (64.2%)	
Aesthetic satisfaction				**<0.001**
VOTE 1 (poor)	5	0 (0%)	5 (8.1%)	
VOTE 2 (insufficient)	9	1 (1.6%)	8 (12.9%)	
VOTE 3 (satisfactory)	33	4 (6.3%)	29 (46.8%)	
VOTE 4 (good)	30	17 (26.6%)	13 (21.0%)	
VOTE 5 (excellent)	49	42 (65.6%)	7 (11.3%)	
Skin sensibility				**0.025**
YES	49	31 (48.4%)	18 (29.0%)	
NO	77	33 (51.6%)	44 (71.0%)	
Compromised relationship life				0.208
YES	42	18 (28,1%)	24 (38,7%)	
NO	84	46 (71,9%)	38 (61,3%)	
Sports before surgery				0.472
YES	65	31 (48.4%)	34 (54.8%)	
NO	61	33 (51.6%)	28 (45.2%)	
Sports after surgery				0.881
YES	52	26 (40.6%)	26 (41.9%)	
NO	74	38 (59.4%)	36 (58.1%)	
Chronic pain in pectoral region				**<0.001**
0 (no pain)	40	32 (50.0%)	8 (12.9%)	
1 (very mild)	24	19 (29.7%)	5 (8.1%)	
2 (mild)	16	8 (12.5%)	8 (12.9%)	
3 (tolerable)	31	4 (6.3%)	27 (43.5%)	
4 (distressing)	12	1 (1.6%)	11 (17.7%)	
5 (very intense)	3	0 (0%)	3 (4.8%)	
Impaired arm motility				**<0.001**
YES	28	3 (4.7%)	25 (40.3%)	
NO	98	61 (95.3%)	37 (59.7%)	

Statistically significant p values (<0.05) are marked in bold.

3.4. Economic Performance

Whenever a surgical procedure is performed, different resources (including personnel, equipment, facilities, time, and materials) are utilized. A cost analysis was performed according to a standardized method and direct cost comparison [19]. The analysis showed better economic performances in the PP group due to shorter operative times, less-frequent need of contralateral breast symmetrization, and less-frequent use of contralateral implants. The average savings with PP-IPBR were EUR 1503 for unilateral NSMs and EUR 1568 for bilateral procedures (Table 6).

Table 6. Economic analysis.

	Costs		
	PP-IPBR	SM-IPBR	p
OR cost for unilateral NSMs (EUR 6.5/min)	EUR 1605.5	EUR 2073.5	**<0.001**
OR cost for bilateral NSMs (EUR 6.5/min)	EUR 1989	EUR 2392	**<0.001**
Implant (EUR 1100/implant)	EUR 1100	EUR 2200	**<0.001**
	Savings		
PP-IPBR without ADM vs. SM-IPBR	Unilateral NSM	Bilateral NSM	
	EUR 1503	EUR 1568	0.543

Abbreviations: PP-IPBR = prepectoral immediate prosthetic breast reconstruction; SM-IPBR = submuscular immediate prosthetic breast reconstruction; OR = operating room; NSM = nipple-sparing mastectomy; ADM = acellular dermal matrix. Statistically significant p values (<0.05) are marked in bold.

4. Discussion

In our institution, we offer IPBR to all patients undergoing NSM. For many years, we have used only SM placement of the implants, but since 2016, we also started to perform PP-IPBR in selected cases, initially with ADM coverage and only recently without the use of matrices [2,6,20].

PP placement of the prosthesis into the space of the excised mammary gland allows a more natural breast appearance with a more harmonious breast slope and ptosis [21–23]. It also allows, in most cases of unilateral NSM, the avoidance of symmetrization procedures on the contralateral breast [24,25]. In our experience, a symmetrization procedure was performed for 44/44 (100%) patients in the SM group, compared to only 2/55 (3.6%) cases in the PP group with polyurethane-covered implants.

Initially, when performing PP-IPBR, we used ADM coverage of the implant. ADMs are biologic scaffolds of human, bovine, or porcine origin that lack immunogenic epitopes and are therefore easily revascularized and integrated into host tissue without encapsulation or contracture [23–26].

The use of ADM, however, may be hampered by surgical and economic issues. Some authors reported higher medical costs, with a variable additional expense between USD 2100 and USD 3400, depending on the size of the dermal sheet utilized [17,27].

For these reasons, in January 2018 we started to perform PP-IPBR using a Polytech implant with a micropolyurethane-foam-coated shell surface (microthane) that does not require further ADM coverage [2,5]. The 1.4 mm micropolyurethane sponge coating is reabsorbed by the body and contributes to form an ideal capsule that protects the implant and reduces capsular contracture, resulting in softer and more natural-appearing breasts. Furthermore, the extremely adherent texture of this implant reduces the risks of rotation and displacement, and consequently the possible need for revision surgery [5].

Careful patient selection and surgical conduct are mandatory to perform PP-IPBR successfully. This technique should be considered only for patients in which adequate thickness and perfusion of skin flaps can be ensured during mastectomy [2,24,28].

To minimize the risk of learning-curve-related complications and technical problems, we considered exclusion criteria of BMI > 30kg/m^2, oversized breasts, ptosis of grade >2, obese patients, heavy smokers, and previous radiation therapy [24,29].

Regarding the surgical conduct, lateral–radial incisions or axillary or inframammary crease incisions are preferable in order to better preserve vascular integrity of the NAC [20,29,30]; skin flaps of adequate thickness should be separated from the mammary gland using blunt dissection and preserving medial perforators, and real-time skin-perfusion testing with a fluorescence imaging system should be performed intraoperatively to assess skin-flap viability with immediate resection of potential ischemic tissues. Choice of implant size and shape should be based on evaluation of the breast and chest-wall conformation and accurate weight of the surgical specimen (in this regard, we recommend using fill volumes similar to those of the removed gland).

With proper patient and implant selection and careful surgical conduct, PP-IPBR can be performed with results similar to SM-IPBR in terms of postoperative complication rates and oncologic safety [1,27,30,31]. In our series, there were no statistically significant differences in terms of implant failure and local, regional, or systemic recurrence between the two groups. We observed only two cases of major complications that led to implant loss: one case of infection in the PP group, and one in the SM group. One patient in the PP group developed NAC necrosis. We classified this complication as minor because it required no surgical revision and was treated successfully in outpatient regime, as the necrosis involved only a small portion of the NAC and was not full thickness.

Regarding patient quality of life, we observed statistically significant improvements in aesthetic results, chronic pain, shoulder dysfunction, and skin sensibility ($p < 0.05$) in the PP group, and a trend of better outcomes (even if statistically not significant) regarding sports activity and sexual/relationship life in this group.

These better results are probably explained by the avoidance of chest-wall musculature manipulation in PP-IPBR [1,2,5].

PP-IPBR significantly reduces operative time as there is no need for submuscular pocket creation, and, in most cases, for contralateral breast symmetrization. When using microthane-coated implants, operative time is further reduced by the avoidance of ADM coverage [2,5,27].

In our series, this shorter operative time, coupled with the reduced need for contralateral implants, generated an average saving of EUR 1500 for unilateral procedures; this saving significantly increased when using a Polytech implant, as the costs of ADM coverage are also avoided (the cost of a 30 × 20 cm sheet of ADM in our hospital is EUR 4056). Furthermore, because PP reconstruction averts the issues related to pectoralis major muscle manipulation, it also minimizes postoperative costs of painkillers and postoperative physiotherapy, with additional benefit for the healthcare system [32–35].

5. Conclusions

Our study presents several limitations, as it is a retrospective unicentric analysis with a relatively limited duration of follow-up, and may include a small selection bias, as PP-IPBR without ADM has been adopted in our institution only recently, and therefore grants less expertise and more potential for technical mistakes than SM-IPBR. However, this work provides encouraging preliminary data on the safety and efficacy of PP positioning of microthane-coated implants without ADM in patients undergoing NSM with IPBR.

PP-IPBR can represent a valid alternative to traditional IPBR, improving outcomes and patient quality of life; it is easier to perform, reduces operative time, and minimizes complications related to manipulation of the pectoralis major muscle, while also contributing to the containment of costs.

Careful patient selection, adequate surgical experience, and repetitive practice of specific tasks are mandatory to optimize the outcomes and reduce the risk of minor and major complications. Further prospective trials with a larger number of patients and a longer follow-up are necessary to draw more validated conclusions.

Author Contributions: Conceptualization, G.F. and L.S.; methodology, G.F., A.D.L., L.S. and A.O.; software, A.F. and S.M.; validation, G.F., R.M., D.A.T.; formal analysis, E.J.M. and B.C.; investigation, A.M.S.; resources, L.B.A. and G.V.; data curation, S.D. and F.M.; G.F. and L.S.; writing—review and editing, G.F. and R.M.; visualization, G.F. and G.V.; supervision, G.F., R.M. and M.S., G.F. and L.S. contributed equally to this work. All authors have read and agreed to the published version of the manuscript.

Funding: This research received no external funding.

Institutional Review Board Statement: The study was conducted according to the guidelines of the Declaration of Helsinki, and approved by the Institutional Review Board and Ethics Committee of Fondazione Policlinico Universitario Agostino Gemelli IRCCS; Università Cattolica del Sacro Cuore, Rome, Italy.

Informed Consent Statement: Informed consent was obtained from all subjects involved in the study.

Data Availability Statement: The data presented in this study are available on request from the corresponding author.

Conflicts of Interest: The authors declare no conflict of interest.

References

1. Manrique, O.J.; Huang, T.C.; Martinez-Jorge, J.; Ciudad, P.; Forte, A.J.; Bustos, S.S.; Boughey, J.C.; Jakub, J.W.; Degnim, A.C.; Galan, R. Prepectoral Two-Stage Implant-Based Breast Reconstruction with and without Acellular Dermal Matrix: Do We See a Difference? *Plast Reconstr. Surg.* **2020**, *145*, 263e–272e. [CrossRef] [PubMed]
2. Franceschini, G.; Masetti, R. Immediate implant-based breast reconstruction with acellular dermal matrix after conservative mastectomy: Can a more effective alternative be used in the near future? *Eur. J. Surg. Oncol. (EJSO)* **2020**. [CrossRef]
3. Sbitany, H.; Piper, M.; Lentz, R. Prepectoral Breast Reconstruction: A Safe Alternative to Submuscular Prosthetic Reconstruction following Nipple-Sparing Mastectomy. *Plast. Reconstr. Surg.* **2017**, *140*, 432–443. [CrossRef]
4. Mirhaidari, S.J.; Azouz, V.; Wagner, D.S. Prepectoral Versus Subpectoral Direct to Implant Immediate Breast Reconstruction. *Ann. Plast. Surg.* **2020**, *84*, 263–270. [CrossRef] [PubMed]
5. De Vita, R.; Buccheri, E.M.; Villanucci, A.; Pozzi, M. Breast Reconstruction Actualized in Nipple-sparing Mastectomy and Direct-to-implant, Prepectoral Polyurethane Positioning: Early Experience and Preliminary Results. *Clin. Breast Cancer* **2019**, *19*, e358–e363. [CrossRef]
6. Salgarello, M.; Barone-Adesi, L.; Terribile, D.; Masetti, R. Update on one-stage immediate breast reconstruction with definitive prosthesis after sparing mastectomies. *Breast* **2011**, *20*, 7–14. [CrossRef] [PubMed]
7. Rancati, A.O.; Angrigiani, C.H.; Hammond, D.C.; Nava, M.B.; Gonzalez, E.G.; Dorr, J.C.; Gercovich, G.F.; Rocco, N.; Rostagno, R.L. Direct to Implant Reconstruction in Nipple Sparing Mastectomy: Patient Selection by Preoperative Digital Mammogram. *Plast. Reconstr. Surg. Glob. Open* **2017**, *5*, e1369. [CrossRef]
8. Robertson, S.A.; Rusby, J.E.; Cutress, R.I. Determinants of optimal mastectomy skin flap thickness. *BJS* **2014**, *101*, 899–911. [CrossRef]
9. Salgarello, M.; Visconti, G.; Barone-Adesi, L.; Franceschini, G.; Masetti, R. Contralateral Breast Symmetrisation in Immediate Prosthetic Breast Reconstruction after Unilateral Nipple-Sparing Mastectomy: The Tailored Reduction/Augmentation Mammaplasty. *Arch. Plast. Surg.* **2015**, *42*, 302–308. [CrossRef]
10. Rella, R.; Belli, P.; Giuliani, M.; Bufi, E.; Carlino, G.; Rinaldi, P.; Manfredi, R. Automated breast ultrasonography (ABUS) in the screening and diagnostic setting: Indications and practical use. *Acad. Radiol.* **2018**, *25*, 1457–1470. [CrossRef] [PubMed]
11. Salgarello, M.; Visconti, G.; Barone-Adesi, L. Nipple-Sparing Mastectomy with Immediate Implant Reconstruction: Cosmetic Outcomes and Technical Refinements. *Plast. Reconstr. Surg.* **2010**, *126*, 1460–1471. [CrossRef] [PubMed]
12. Porter, M.E.; Larsson, S.; Lee, T.H. Standardizing Patient Outcomes Measurement. *N. Engl. J. Med.* **2016**, *374*, 504–506. [CrossRef]
13. Franceschini, G.; Sanchez, A.M.; Di Leone, A.; Magno, S.; Moschella, F.; Accetta, C.; Natale, M.; Di Giorgio, D.; Scaldaferri, A.; D'Archi, S.; et al. Update on the surgical management of breast cancer. *Ann Ital Chir.* **2015**, *86*, 89–99. [PubMed]
14. Van Egdom, L.S.; Oemrawsingh, A.; Verweij, L.M.; Lingsma, H.F.; Koppert, L.B.; Verhoef, C.; Klazinga, N.S.; Hazelzet, J.A. Implementing Patient-Reported Outcome Measures in Clinical Breast Cancer Care: A Systematic Review. *Value Health* **2019**, *22*, 1197–1226. [CrossRef]
15. Franceschini, G.; Visconti, G.; Sanchez, A.M.; Di Leone, A.; Salgarello, M.; Masetti, R. Oxidized regenerated cellulose in breast surgery: Experimental model. *J. Surg. Res.* **2015**, *198*, 237–244. [CrossRef]
16. Dean, N.R.; Crittenden, T. A five year experience of measuring clinical effectiveness in a breast reconstruction service using the BREAST-Q patient reported outcomes measure: A cohort study. *J. Plast. Reconstr. Aesthetic Surg.* **2016**, *69*, 1469–1477. [CrossRef]
17. Chen, C.M.; Cano, S.J.; Klassen, A.F.; King, T.; McCarthy, C.; Cordeiro, P.G.; Morrow, M.; Pusic, A.L. Measuring Quality of Life in Oncologic Breast Surgery: A Systematic Review of Patient-Reported Outcome Measures. *Breast J.* **2010**, *16*, 587–597. [CrossRef] [PubMed]
18. Ghilli, M.; Mariniello, M.; Camilleri, V.; Murante, A.; Ferrè, F.; Colizzi, L.; Gennaro, M.; Caligo, M.; Scatena, C.; Del Re, M.; et al. PROMs in post-mastectomy care: Patient self-reports (BREAST-Q™) as a powerful instrument to personalize medical services. *Eur. J. Surg. Oncol. (EJSO)* **2020**, *46*, 1034–1040. [CrossRef]
19. Ziolkowski, N.I.; Voineskos, S.H.; Ignacy, T.A.; Thoma, A. Systematic Review of Economic Evaluations in Plastic Surgery. *Plast. Reconstr. Surg.* **2013**, *132*, 191–203. [CrossRef] [PubMed]
20. Franceschini, G.; Visconti, G.; Garganese, G.; Adesi, L.B.-; Di Leone, A.; Sanchez, A.M.; Terribile, D.; Salgarello, M.; Masetti, R. Nipple-sparing mastectomy combined with endoscopic immediate reconstruction via axillary incision for breast cancer: A preliminary experience of an innovative technique. *Breast J.* **2019**, *26*, 206–210. [CrossRef] [PubMed]

21. Nahabedian, M.Y.; Cocilovo, C. Two-stage prosthetic breast reconstruction: A comparison between prepectoral and partial subpectoral techniques. *Plast. Reconstr. Surg.* **2017**, *140*, 22S–30S. [CrossRef] [PubMed]
22. Bernini, M.; Calabrese, C.; Cecconi, L.; Santi, C.; Gjondedaj, U.; Roselli, J.; Nori, J.; Fausto, A.; Orzalesi, L.; Casella, D. Subcutaneous Direct-to-Implant Breast Reconstruction: Surgical, Functional, and Aesthetic Results after Long-Term Follow-Up. *Plast. Reconstr. Surg. Glob. Open* **2015**, *3*, e574. [CrossRef]
23. Zhu, L.; Mohan, A.T.; Abdelsattar, J.M.; Wang, Z.; Vijayasekaran, A.; Hwang, S.M.; Tran, N.V.; Saint-Cyr, M. Comparison of subcutaneous versus submuscular expander placement in the first stage of immediate breast reconstruction. *J. Plast. Reconstr. Aesthetic Surg.* **2016**, *69*, e77–e86. [CrossRef] [PubMed]
24. Yang, J.Y.; Kim, C.W.; Lee, J.W.; Kim, S.K.; Lee, S.A.; Hwang, E. Considerations for patient selection: Prepectoral versus subpectoral implant-based breast reconstruction. *Arch. Plast. Surg.* **2019**, *46*, 550–557. [CrossRef]
25. Tasoulis, M.-K.; Iqbal, F.M.; Cawthorn, S.; MacNeill, F.; Vidya, R. Subcutaneous implant breast reconstruction: Time to reconsider? *Eur. J. Surg. Oncol. (EJSO)* **2017**, *43*, 1636–1646. [CrossRef]
26. Sorkin, M.; Qi, J.; Kim, H.M.; Hamill, J.B.; Kozlow, J.H.; Pusic, A.L.; Wilkins, E.G. Acellular Dermal Matrix in Immediate Expander/Implant Breast Reconstruction: A Multicenter Assessment of Risks and Benefits. *Plast. Reconstr. Surg.* **2017**, *140*, 1091–1100. [CrossRef]
27. Cuomo, R. Submuscular and Pre-pectoral ADM Assisted Immediate Breast Reconstruction: A Literature Review. *Medicina* **2020**, *56*, 256. [CrossRef] [PubMed]
28. Li, L.; Su, Y.; Xiu, B.; Huang, X.; Chi, W.; Hou, J.; Zhang, Y.; Tian, J.; Wang, J.; Wu, J. Comparison of prepectoral and subpectoral breast reconstruction after mastectomies: A systematic review and meta analysis. *Eur. J. Surg. Oncol. (EJSO)* **2019**, *45*, 1542–1550. [CrossRef] [PubMed]
29. Franceschini, G.; Masetti, R. Evidence-based nipple-sparing mastectomy in patients with higher body mass index: Recommendations for a successful standardized surgery. *Am. J. Surg.* **2020**, *220*, 393–394. [CrossRef]
30. Braun, S.E.; Bs, M.D.; Butterworth, J.A.; Larson, K.E. Do Nipple Necrosis Rates Differ in Prepectoral Versus Submuscular Implant-Based Reconstruction After Nipple-Sparing Mastectomy? *Ann. Surg. Oncol.* **2020**, *27*, 4760–4766. [CrossRef]
31. Atisha, D.; Alderman, A.K.; Lowery, J.C.; Kuhn, L.E.; Davis, J.; Wilkins, E.G. Prospective analysis of long-term psychosocial outcomes in breast reconstruction: Two-year postoperative results from the Michigan Breast Reconstruction Outcomes Study. *Ann. Surg.* **2008**, *247*, 1019–1028. [CrossRef] [PubMed]
32. Glasberg, S.B. The Economics of Prepectoral Breast Reconstruction. *Plast Reconstr. Surg.* **2017**, *140*, 49S–52S. [CrossRef]
33. Bank, J.; Phillips, N.A.; Park, J.E.; Song, D.H. Economic Analysis and Review of the Literature on Implant-Based Breast Reconstruction With and Without the Use of the Acellular Dermal Matrix. *Aesthetic Plast. Surg.* **2013**, *37*, 1194–1201. [CrossRef] [PubMed]
34. Krishnan, N.M.; Chatterjee, A.; Van Vliet, M.M.; Powell, S.G.; Rosen, J.M.; Nigriny, J.F. A comparison of acellular dermal matrix to autologous dermal flaps in single-stage, implant-based immediate breast reconstruction: A cost-effectiveness analysis. *Plast. Reconstr. Surg.* **2013**, *131*, 953–961. [CrossRef] [PubMed]
35. Garreffa, E.; Agrawal, A. Cost-effectiveness of pre-pectoral implant-based breast reconstruction: A pilot comparative analysis. *J. Plast. Reconstr. Aesthetic Surg.* **2019**, *72*, 1700–1738. [CrossRef] [PubMed]

Article

The Assisi Think Tank Meeting Breast Large Database for Standardized Data Collection in Breast Cancer—ATTM.BLADE

Fabio Marazzi [1], Valeria Masiello [1,*], Carlotta Masciocchi [2], Mara Merluzzi [3], Simonetta Saldi [4], Paolo Belli [5], Luca Boldrini [1,6], Nikola Dino Capocchiano [6], Alba Di Leone [7], Stefano Magno [7], Elisa Meldolesi [1], Francesca Moschella [7], Antonino Mulé [8], Daniela Smaniotto [1,6], Daniela Andreina Terribile [8], Luca Tagliaferri [1], Gianluca Franceschini [6,7], Maria Antonietta Gambacorta [1,6], Riccardo Masetti [6,7], Vincenzo Valentini [1,6], Philip M. P. Poortmans [9,10] and Cynthia Aristei [11]

1. Fondazione Policlinico Universitario "A. Gemelli" IRCCS, UOC di Radioterapia Oncologica, Dipartimento di Diagnostica per Immagini, Radioterapia Oncologica ed Ematologia, 00168 Roma, Italy; fabio.marazzi@policlinicogemelli.it (F.M.); luca.boldrini@policlinicogemelli.it (L.B.); elisa.meldolesi@guest.policlinicogemelli.it (E.M.); daniela.smaniotto.rt@gmail.com (D.S.); luca.tagliaferri@policlinicogemelli.it (L.T.); mariaantonietta.gambacorta@policlinicogemelli.it (M.A.G.); vincenzo.valentini@policlinicogemelli.it (V.V.)
2. Fondazione Policlinico Universitario "A. Gemelli" IRCCS, 00168 Roma, Italy; carlotta.masciocchi@guest.policlinicogemelli.it
3. Radiation Oncology Section, Department of Medicine and Surgery, University of Perugia, 06123 Perugia, Italy; maramerluzzi@libero.it
4. Radiation Oncology Section, Perugia General Hospital, 06123 Perugia, Italy; saldisimonetta@gmail.com
5. Fondazione Policlinico Universitario "A. Gemelli" IRCCS, UOC di Diagnostica per Immagini, Dipartimento di Diagnostica per Immagini, Radioterapia Oncologica ed Ematologia, 00168 Roma, Italy; paolo.belli@policlinicogemelli.it
6. Istituto di Radiologia, Università Cattolica del Sacro Cuore, 00168 Roma, Italy; nikoladino.capocchiano@unicatt.it (N.D.C.); gianluca.franceschini@policlinicogemelli.it (G.F.); riccardo.masetti@policlinicogemelli.it (R.M.)
7. Fondazione Policlinico Universitario "A. Gemelli" IRCCS, UOC di Chirurgia Senologica, Dipartimento di Scienze della Salute della Donna e del Bambino e di Sanità Pubblica, 00168 Roma, Italy; alba.dileone@policlinicogemelli.it (A.D.L.); stefano.magno@policlinicogemelli.it (S.M.); francesca.moschella@policlinicogemelli.it (F.M.)
8. Fondazione Policlinico Universitario "A. Gemelli" IRCCS, UOC di Anatomia Patologica, Dipartimento di Scienze della Salute della Donna e del Bambino e di Sanità Pubblica, 00168 Roma, Italy; antonino.mule@policlinicogemelli.it (A.M.); danielaandreina.terribile@policlinicogemelli.it (D.A.T.)
9. Department of Radiation Oncology, Iridium Kankernetwerk, 2170 Wilrijk-Antwerp, Belgium; philip.poortmans@telenet.be
10. Faculty of Medicine and Health Sciences, University of Antwerp, 2170 Wilrijk-Antwerp, Belgium
11. Radiation Oncology Section, University of Perugia and Perugia General Hospital, 06123 Perugia, Italy; cynthia.aristei@unipg.it
* Correspondence: valeria.masiello@guest.policlinicogemelli.it

Abstract: Background: During the 2016 Assisi Think Tank Meeting (ATTM) on breast cancer, the panel of experts proposed developing a validated system, based on rapid learning health care (RLHC) principles, to standardize inter-center data collection and promote personalized treatments for breast cancer. **Material and Methods:** The seven-step *Breast LArge DatabasE (BLADE)* project included data collection, analysis, application, and evaluation on a data-sharing platform. The multidisciplinary team developed a consensus-based ontology of validated variables with over 80% agreement. This English-language ontology constituted a breast cancer library with seven knowledge domains: baseline, primary systemic therapy, surgery, adjuvant systemic therapies, radiation therapy, follow-up, and toxicity. The library was uploaded to the *BLADE* domain. The safety of data encryption and preservation was tested according to General Data Protection Regulation (GDPR) guidelines on data from 15 clinical charts. The system was validated on 64 patients who had undergone post-mastectomy radiation therapy. In October 2018, the *BLADE* system was approved by the Ethical Committee of Fondazione Policlinico Gemelli IRCCS, Rome, Italy (Protocol No. 0043996/18). **Results:** From June 2016 to July 2019, the multidisciplinary team completed the work plan. An ontology of 218 validated variables was uploaded to the *BLADE* domain. The GDPR safety test confirmed encryption and data preservation (on 5000 random cases). All validation benchmarks were met. **Conclusion:** *BLADE* is a support system for follow-up and assessment of breast cancer care. To successfully develop and validate it as the first standardized data collection system, multidisciplinary collaboration was crucial in selecting its ontology and knowledge domains. *BLADE* is suitable for multi-center uploading of retrospective and prospective clinical data, as it ensures anonymity and data privacy.

Keywords: breast cancer; large database; standardized data collection; networks

1. Introduction

Breast cancer, one of the main causes of women's mortality, is characterized by highly complex presentation patterns [1]. Even though population-based screening programs [1], new therapies [2], advanced technologies [3], and multidisciplinary approaches [4] have improved survival and quality of life [4] in the previous decades, cure remains a challenge in some sub-groups of patients. Consequently, hypothesis-based tailored treatments that are adapted to each individual patient's specific features are being explored in an approach termed personalized medicine. Due to complex information systems, personalized medicine overcomes uncertainties about particular conditions in small sub-groups of patients, which increase the complexity of decision-making [5,6]. Despite growing interest, a literature review revealed no consensus on how to define and apply personalized medicine [5]. Semantic approaches include patient stratification and treatment tailoring. In the former, individual patients are grouped into subpopulations according to the probability that a specific drug or treatment regimen will be of benefit, whereas in the latter, the individual patient's status is used as the rationale for treatment choice [6,7].

The application of personalized medicine may be limited in clinical practice by the results of randomized controlled trials (RCTs). Patient selection, as defined by inclusion and exclusion criteria, leads to adaptive randomization, so outcomes refer only to the RCT-eligible population [8]. Furthermore, since the selected patients are usually in good clinical condition, with few or no comorbidities, the results cannot be extrapolated to all cases that physicians may encounter in clinical practice [9]. Additionally, due to long recruitment and follow-up times, RCT evidence may be out-of-date when it is made available, and progress may have already been made in developing treatments beyond old standards. Lambin et al. [10,11] reported that high quantity, low quality data from clinical charts reflected reality better than RCT data, and therefore provided valuable information for applying personalized medicine in clinical practice [9,12]. However, new instruments are needed to include the data and address uncertainties in clinical decision-making.

Rapid learning health care fills this gap, since it extracts and applies knowledge from routine clinical care data rather than RCT evidence alone. Since data management of cross-linked information from diverse sources is complex, data analysis should be managed by machine learning to create decision support systems, i.e., software applications that apply knowledge-driven healthcare to clinical practice. Another rapid learning principle is that these systems need constant updating.

In February 2016, a group of expert radiation oncologists organised the Assisi Think Tank Meeting (ATTM) to discuss research, controversies, and grey areas in breast cancer [13], and proposed a validated system based on rapid learning health care for standardized data collection to generate evidence for personalized medicine. In one of the participating centers, the Fondazione Policlinico Gemelli IRCCS, an umbrella protocol [14,15] was already approved by the Ethical Committee. The Beyond Ontology Awareness (BOA) platform (Figure 1) had been developed and implemented in close collaboration with physicians and informatics technology researchers [8,13]. It safely stores, analyzes, and shares data on diverse cancer types in a standardized manner [9,16] as well as reproducing the ontology structure and managing data legacy and privacy. BOA software converts the center's legacy archives in accordance with a global data dictionary and anonymously replicates clinical data in a large cloud-based database.

In the present project, the BOA platform was expanded for specific use in breast cancer care. A multi-disciplinary panel of experts from the Fondazione Policlinico Gemelli IRCCS, Perugia University, and General Hospital designed a standardized data collection system and developed the *Breast LArge DatabasE (BLADE)*. Its primary objective was to offer radiation oncology centers worldwide treating breast cancer the opportunity to collect and share data in a standardized large database, and thus develop descriptive, predictive, and prognostic models for supportive care, survival, and toxicity. Its long-term aim is to build decision support systems to personalize treatments, use resources in terms of cost-effectiveness, and make therapies more effective and less toxic.

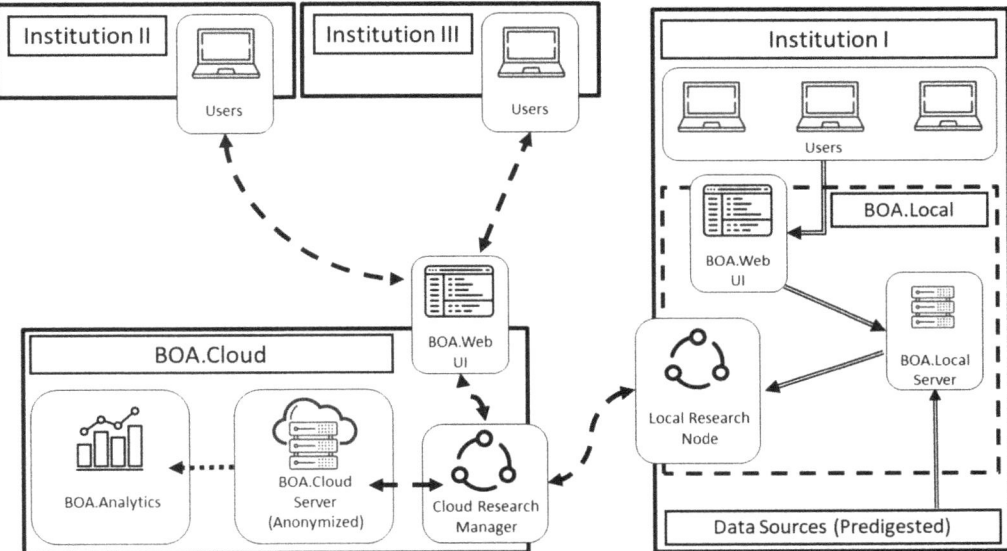

Figure 1. General beyond awareness ontology (BOA) architecture, with both the BOA.Local and BOA.Cloud servers. An infinite number of external institutions without a BOA.Local installation can be added at needed to this infrastructure. Double-line arrows represent non-anonymized patient data, dashed arrows represent anonymized patient data, and dotted arrows represent aggregate data.

2. Materials and Methods

After a review of breast cancer literature and current guidelines, a multi-step process was set up for data collection, analysis, application, and evaluation. Benchmarks were the rapid learning criteria by Lambin et al. [11]. The project was organized in a 7-step working plan as defined in a GANNT chart, and the time-frame for each step was established [17] (Figure 2). Data collection was structured to capture volume, variety, velocity, and veracity [11] and aimed to achieve a standardized ontology and overcome privacy issues. Approval was acquired from the Ethical Committee.

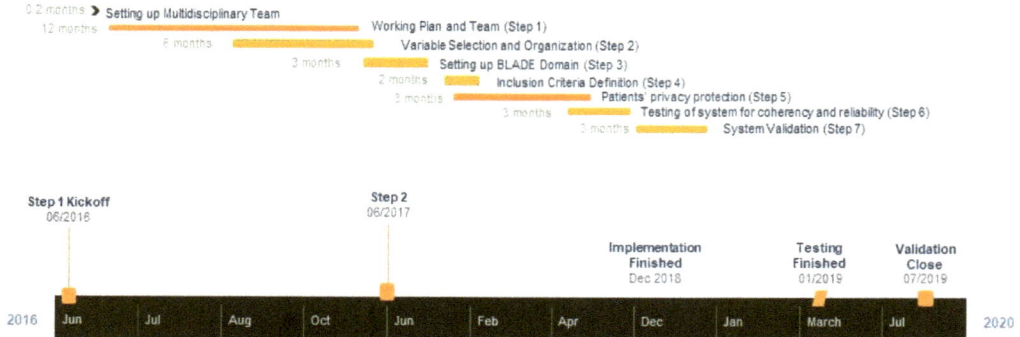

Figure 2. Timeline framework for ATTM.BLADE project.

2.1. Data Collection Methodology

Working Plan and Team (Step 1). Members of the working group from the Fondazione Policlinico Gemelli and Perugia University, and General Hospital included 6 radiation oncologists; 1 medical oncologist; 1 pathologist; 3 breast surgeons; 1 radiologist; 2 informatics experts; 1 data manager. The working group established a timeframe of 12 months for developing the *BLADE* system. Responsibilities and times to complete each step were defined. Progress was updated every 3 months via live meetings or conference calls.

Variable Selection and Organization (Step 2). Each team member reviewed the literature, focusing on RCTs and international guidelines, e.g., NCCN, ASTRO, ESTRO, and AIRO for radiation oncology [18–20] and established 7 domains of knowledge: baseline, primary systemic therapy, surgery, adjuvant systemic therapies, radiation therapy, follow-up, and toxicity. Major variables were chosen for each domain to create a shared-language ontology (terminology system). Variables were related to patients (e.g., age, sex, and gene profiling), clinical presentations (e.g., disease stage, markers, and pathology findings), treatments (e.g., surgery, systemic therapies, radiation therapy, and palliative care), and imaging (at diagnosis, treatment, and follow-up).

Variables were validated by a consensus panel that indicated the response type for each variable (yes/no, single, or multi-options), selected and voted on multi-options. Consensus was reached with 80% agreement.

Setting up the BLADE domain (Step 3). BOA was configured to include *BLADE* and process breast cancer data. It is equipped with local and cloud servers (Figure 1) depending on the desired configuration package. Users can access the BOA services through an intranet or internet connection and need only a standard web browser to connect, with no additional software. In the BOA.Local configuration, which only allows access through the local intranet, each institution has complete control over its data repository, and collected records are saved without any automated pseudo-anonymization procedures. The internet-facing server installation on the BOA.Cloud has the same features as the BOA.Local service, but it automatically and mandatorily pseudo-anonymizes all data. Before storage, each patient is assigned an ad hoc universally unique identifier (UUID), and all personal data or connections to existing records are severed. BOA.Cloud and BOA.Local store and process data in accordance with General Data Protection Regulation (GDPR). BOA.Local data can be dynamically cloned, automatically anonymized, and consolidated onto the BOA.Cloud server through a research manager—research node connection algorithm, and the data are then ready to be processed or analysed as needed. Figure 3 illustrates the underlying data model used in the databases of both BOA services.

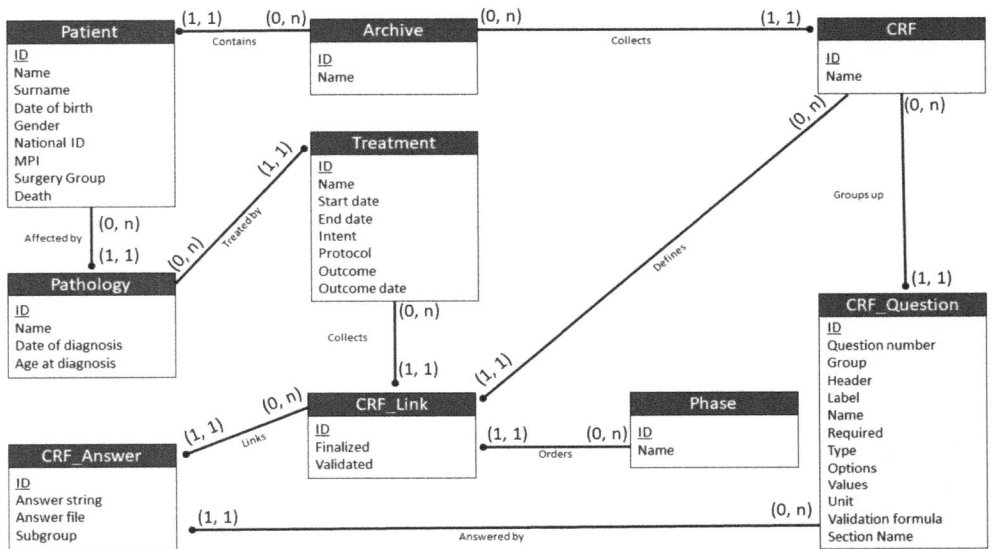

Figure 3. Underlying BOA data model visualized through an entity–relationship model that highlights all relationships between the different objects in the database. As an example (and using imaginary values), the archive named *BLADE* would contain a patient named John Doe, affected by a pathology of breast cancer, for which he was treated through a treatment of first treatment. This treatment would have a compiled version of the case report form (CRF) radiotherapy linked to the phase called neoadjuvant, and an answer of prone, to the question of radiotherapy treatment position present in the previously mentioned CRF.

To create the *BLADE* domain, Excel spreadsheet files with all ontology-related variables were uploaded on to the BOA platform. *BLADE*'s 7 specific case report forms (CRFs), which were devised according to OpenClinica system criteria [21], are compatible with the BOA ontology framework. CRFs are available in Supplementary Materials file 1, with explanations of CRF definitions in Supplementary Materials file 2.

Inclusion Criteria (Step 4). The working group defined patient selection criteria, agreeing that retrospective and prospective data from all selected breast cancer patients can be included in *BLADE*.

Retrospective data: When *BLADE* is installed on the BOA platform, patient data will be derived from existing retrospective electronic or paper databases in each participating center. The data will be anonymized and shared only for research purposes.

Prospective data: Patients whose data are eligible for enrolment in prospective *BLADE* studies will be informed about the opportunity to share their data for research purposes at their first medical examination, and invited to participate. The patients' written informed consent will be obtained and archived.

Patients' privacy protection (Step 5). Privacy needs to be guaranteed according to GDPR guidelines [22] for data protection. *BLADE* and BOA manage data using an AES-256 encryption system and an automatic data pseudo-anonymization algorithm. Each case is associated with a UUID code number with no reference to the individual's identity, and is only accessible to specifically authorized health operators through their personal access codes and accounts. All changes in *BLADE* are automatically tracked and logged, including past and present values for form fields and the account identifiers of operators that modified existing data or inserted new data into CRFs.

2.2. Testing the BLADE Domain for Coherency and Reliability (Step 6)

A data entry expert in the CRF system inserted data from 15 clinical charts of breast cancer patients that were randomly selected from Policlinico Gemelli records. According to GDPR principles, informatics verified accuracy, data conservation, limitations, and integrity during uploading. Criteria for coherency and reliability tests of the *BLADE* domain were the following (Article. 32 of GDPR):

- Data pseudo-anonymization and encryption;
- Permanent assurance of confidentiality, integrity, availability, and resiliency of treatment systems and services;
- Prompt restoration of availability and access to personal data in case of physical or technical accident;
- Regular tests, verifications, and assessments of technical and organizational effectiveness measures to ensure data safety.

2.3. System Validation (Step 7)

BLADE was validated after checking adhesion to the GDPR criteria, and uploading and extracting data for statistical analysis from the clinical records of 64 patients who had undergone post-mastectomy radiation therapy (RT). All patients gave permission for their data from local databases to be transferred to *BLADE*.

Physicians asked the informatics expert to extract the following data from *BLADE*:

- Clinical-, treatment-, and tumor-related data: age, date of diagnosis, primary systemic treatments, histological sub-type, receptor status, multi-focality, and clinical and pathological stages;
- Reconstruction data: type of reconstructive surgery, prosthesis material, time to prosthesis-related complication (TPC), time to prosthesis reoperation (TPR), and ratio of TPC/time from reconstructive surgery;
- Dosimetric data referring to the chest wall: prescribed dose, conformity index, homogeneity index, and V95% and V105%.

Records were automatically extracted and the output was structured according to the standard needs of a data science team (e.g., a .csv file with all selected records processed on a flat table with specific column names and without any identifying information).

Validation benchmarks were:

- Uploading at least 80% of chart data by the data manager without physician assistance;
- Physician correction of <20% of uploaded data;
- Extraction of at least 80% of data for statistical analyses;
- Joint physician and statistician correction of <20% of extracted data;
- Performance of at least 80% of planned statistical analyses on RStudio$^©$.

3. Results

3.1. Setting up BLADE (June 2016)

The 12-month timeline for completing *BLADE* overran by more than 1 year due to the quantity and complexity of the information. For example, Step 2 lasted 18 months, during which the working group met three times for variable selection and three times for variable validation. In July 2018, after reaching 80% consensus, a total of 218 variables were successfully uploaded to constitute the *BLADE* domain. Figure 4 reports as an example, the definition of the radiotherapy variable according to OpenClinica criteria.

	ID	CRF_NAME	QUESTION_NUMBER	SECTION_NAME	SECTION_LABEL	ITEM_NAME	DESCRIPTION_LABEL
0	6518	Radiotherapy	1	Radiotherapy	Radiotherapy	DateofRadiotherapyStarting	Date of Radiotherapy Starting
1	6519	Radiotherapy	2	Radiotherapy	Radiotherapy	DateofRadiotherapyEnding	Date of Radiotherapy Ending
2	6520	Radiotherapy	3	Radiotherapy	Radiotherapy	RadiotherapyTargetVolumes	Target Volumes prescribed
3	6521	Radiotherapy	4	Radiotherapy	Radiotherapy	VolumeCTVTumorBed	Volume (cc) CTV Tumor Bed
4	6522	Radiotherapy	5	Radiotherapy	Radiotherapy	VolumePTVTumorBed	Volume (cc) PTV Tumor Bed
5	6523	Radiotherapy	6	Radiotherapy	Radiotherapy	TimingTumorBed	Timing of Tumor Bed Administration
6	6524	Radiotherapy	7	Radiotherapy	Radiotherapy	TotalDoseTumorBed	Total Dose at Tumor Bed
7	6525	Radiotherapy	8	Radiotherapy	Radiotherapy	FractionDoseTumorBed	Dose for fraction at Tumor Bed
8	6526	Radiotherapy	9	Radiotherapy	Radiotherapy	FractionforDayTumorBed	Number of Daily Fraction at Tumor Bed
9	6527	Radiotherapy	10	Radiotherapy	Radiotherapy	RadiotherapyTeciniqueTumorBed	Radiotherapy Tecnique used for treat Tumor Bed
10	6528	Radiotherapy	11	Radiotherapy	Radiotherapy	VolumeCTVBreast/ChestWall	Volume (cc) CTV Breast/ChestWall
11	6529	Radiotherapy	12	Radiotherapy	Radiotherapy	VolumePTVBreast/ChestWall	Volume (cc) PTV Breast/ChestWall
12	6530	Radiotherapy	13	Radiotherapy	Radiotherapy	TotalDoseBreast/ChestWall	Total Dose at Breast/ChestWall
13	6531	Radiotherapy	14	Radiotherapy	Radiotherapy	FractionDoseBreast/ChestWall	Dose for fraction at Breast/ChestWall
14	6532	Radiotherapy	15	Radiotherapy	Radiotherapy	FractionforDayBreast/ChestWall	Number of Daily Fraction at Breast/ChestWall
15	6533	Radiotherapy	16	Radiotherapy	Radiotherapy	RadiotherapyTeciniqueBreast/ChestWall	Radiotherapy Tecnique used for treat Breast/ChestWall

Figure 4. Example of a CRF configuration file. The columns represent various mandatory configuration settings for BOA and are to be interpreted as follows: The ID column represents an internal identifier and is generated automatically when the CRF is first uploaded. CRF_NAME refers to the name by which the CRF is to be visualized in the UI. QUESTION_NUMBER can either be automatically assigned or manually set, and refers to the ordering of the various questions inside the CRF, with SECTION_NAME and SECTION_LABEL working as visual dividers when the questions are displayed in the interface, with the former being the name to be used in the UI code, and the latter being the name to be displayed. ITEM_NAME and DESCRIPTION_LABEL work in a similar manner, with the former being the identifier in the underlying code and the latter being the name of the text to be displayed with the question in the UI.

The variables were organized into seven main CRFs corresponding to the knowledge domains, which were the interfaces for uploading encrypted patient data. In parallel with the data entry expert's work, automatic testing tools in BOA tested specific characteristics in reference to the *BLADE* domain and generated synthetic patients. BOA tested both itself and the linked infrastructure by generating 5000 synthetic patients with a variable number of CRFs, and randomly created data in the space of nearly 20 min. To test performance, 30 fake user agents were connected to the interface and random pages from the web-service were requested for deletion or modification. Numbers for testing tool input were over a hypothetical maximum simultaneous workload for the *BLADE* project. Throughout these tests, no noticeable performance degradations were revealed, no abnormalities in the data structure or integrity were found, and no information leaked in the fake user sessions due to, for example, wrongly configured page-caching settings.

The privacy protection protocol was initially approved by the Ethical Committee of Fondazione Policlinico Gemelli IRCCS with protocol no. 0043996/18 in October 2018.

3.2. BLADE Data Safety Tests (January 2019)

To check that the *BLADE* domain was uploaded correctly, informatics analyzed accuracy, conservation limitation of data, data integrity, and data flows between application and data processing on 15 charts from randomly chosen patients. They completely adhered to EU GDPR criteria as reported in Article 32 Security of Processing [22,23]. Uploaded data were not linked to individual patients. Technical and organizational effectiveness measures did not break confidentiality, integrity, availability, and resiliency. Simulated physical and technical accidents showed no loss of data.

3.3. Validation (February–July 2019)

The physician's review increased 81.5% of uploaded data from 64 patients to 84% and corrected 10% of uploaded and missing data. The following were corrected: compile-time errors due to the data manager's lack of experience with *BLADE* (7.5%); missing data (8.5%).

For statistical analysis, 100% of clinical, treatment and tumor-related data, 80% of reconstruction data, and 98% of dosimetric data were available. Mean available data ranged from 92.6% to 94.5%, corresponding to <20% validation benchmarks. All the planned statistical analyses were performed.

4. Discussion

The *BLADE* project was set up to support ATTM research into breast cancer, with the aim of providing decision support systems to facilitate clinical decision-making and treatment tailoring. In the 2016 ATTM [13], attention focused on developing such a system from the potentially large database that was available from clinical records, not only in radiation oncology centers, but in many other specialty units (e.g., surgery, pathology, medical oncology, etc.) that are dedicated to the diagnosis and treatment of breast cancer.

The present results showed that *BLADE* is a valid system for collecting data anonymously, as its encryption system successfully passed the tests, satisfying GDPR criteria and benchmarks. Data managers were accountable for only 7.5% of errors, some of which were corrected during the physician's review. Regarding radiation therapy, *BLADE* uniquely focuses on clinical, technical and dosimetric parameters, which makes it particularly suitable for analyzing radiation-therapy-related outcomes and toxicity.

One of the strengths of *BLADE*'s ontology lies in its validated variables that were uploaded after a multi-step process involving the consensus of a multidisciplinary team. Unlike other large databases for breast cancer, *BLADE* provides health workers with the opportunity to focus on diverse fields in the diagnosis and treatment of breast cancer, as it is based on the acquisition of the pathways and the heterogeneity characterizing breast cancer [24–28]. Although several large national databases were set up, none were based on validated, published ontologies [25–28], and few could offer decision support systems [29–33]. Most were developed to investigate long-term survival outcomes such as, for example, the Surveillance, Epidemiology, and End Results (SEER) database, which was set up by the U.S. National Cancer Institute (NCI) and reports annually on the data it has collected on breast cancer from nine American oncological centers [29–31].

Another strength of the *BLADE* system is its capacity to incorporate new, validated variables or mathematical algorithms for assessing, for example, the success of treatment or a strategy for monitoring clinical outcomes and cost-effectiveness. In the future, it might include accreditation or valuation indicators for associated centers, update evidence or guidelines, and incorporate new sectors such as proteomics, complementary medicines, etc.

One limiting factor of the present study was linked to *BLADE*'s small homogeneous sample and its inability to upload digital imaging and communications in medicine (DICOM) data, which will be very relevant when *BLADE* is used to develop prediction models. DICOM data and RT planning information will be uploaded with the 2022 *BLADE* upgrade, which will create a unique data repository [34]. A lack of testing of *BLADE*'s ability to perform machine learning analysis, an upcoming modality in cancer care, especially for predicting response to treatment, is a current limitation that is expected to be eliminated in the future. Using algorithms that iteratively learn from data, machine learning allows computers to find hidden insights without being explicitly programmed where to look, while inferential statistics need different tools to achieve this purpose, such as Bayesian networks, support vector machines, neural networking, and Cox regression. Machine learning is now starting to flank inferential statistical models (e.g., linear models, generalized linear models, and survival models), and its success over inferential statistics has already been reported together with the first promising results of its use in building predictive models of cancer survival [10,15,19]. We are confident that when *BLADE* is expanded to systematic multi-center use, machine learning analysis will become a reality and systems for decision-making support will be developed and validated, as *BLADE* is projected for a huge number of patients who will provide millions of data for analyses.

In the near future, we will use *BLADE* in our clinical daily practice to collect retrospective and prospective data and analyze outcomes to assess the role of post-mastectomy radiation therapy in ductal in situ patients. This approach is derived from a 2019 survey by an ATTM research group [35], identifying this topic as a grey area in current practice.

5. Conclusions

BLADE, one of the projects emerging from the 2016 ATTM [13], is a support system for breast cancer care. In successfully developing and validating it as a standardized data collection system, multidisciplinary collaboration was crucial for selecting its ontology and knowledge domains. BLADE is suitable for multi-center uploading of retrospective and prospective clinical data, as it ensures anonymity and data privacy.

Finally, BLADE may constitute an international instrument for research purposes to be used by ATTM-like research groups [36].

Supplementary Materials: The following are available online at https://www.mdpi.com/2075-442 6/11/2/143/s1, Supplementary Materials file 1: CRFs, Supplementary Materials file 2: Explanations of CRF Definitions.

Author Contributions: Conceptualization, C.A., V.V. and P.M.P.P.; methodology C.A., N.D.C., F.M. (Fabio Marazzi), C.M., M.M. and V.M.; software, N.D.C.; validation, C.A., V.V. and P.M.P.P.; formal analysis C.A., F.M. (Fabio Marazzi), V.M., M.M. and N.D.C.; investigation C.A., F.M. (Fabio Marazzi), V.M., M.M. and N.D.C.; resources V.V.; data curation C.A, F.M. (Fabio Marazzi), V.M., M.M. and N.D.C.; writing—original draft preparation C.A., F.M. (Fabio Marazzi), M.M. and V.M.; writing—review and editing, F.M. (Fabio Marazzi), V.M., M.M., S.S., P.B., L.B., N.D.C., A.D.L., S.M., E.M., F.M. (Francesca Moschella), A.M., D.S., D.A.T., L.T., G.F., M.A.G., R.M., V.V., P.M.P.P. and C.A.; visualization F.M. (Fabio Marazzi), V.M., M.M., S.S., P.B., L.B., N.D.C., A.D.L., S.M., E.M., F.M. (Francesca Moschella), A.M., D.S., D.A.T., L.T., G.F., M.A.G., R.M., V.V., P.M.P.P. and C.A.; supervision C.A., P.M.P.P. and V.V.; project administration, C.A., V.V., P.M.P.P., F.M. (Fabio Marazzi) and V.M.; funding acquisition V.V. All authors have read and agreed to the published version of the manuscript.

Funding: This research received no external funding.

Institutional Review Board Statement: The study was conducted according to the guidelines of the Declaration of Helsinki, and approved by the Institutional Review Board (or Ethics Committee) of Fondazione Policlinico A. Gemelli IRCCS (protocol code N. 0043996/18—31.10.2018).

Informed Consent Statement: Not applicable.

Conflicts of Interest: The authors declare no conflict of interest.

Information to Join ATTM.BLADE Network and/or Propose Research Project: MD. Vincenzo Valentini—vincenzo.valentini@policlinicogemelli.it; Prof. MD. Cynthia Aristei—cynthia.aristei@unipg.it; MD. Fabio Marazzi—fabio.marazzi@policlinicogemelli.it; MD. Valeria Masiello—valeria.masiello@guest.policlinicogemelli.it.

References

1. Torre, L.A.; Islami, F.; Siegel, R.L.; Ward, E.M.; Jemal, A. Global Cancer in Women: Burden and Trends. *Cancer Epidemiol. Biomark. Prev.* **2017**, *26*, 444–457. [CrossRef]
2. Martin, E.; Pourtau, L.; Di Palma, M.; Delaloge, S. New oral targeted therapies for metastatic breast cancer disrupt the traditional patients' management-A healthcare providers' view. *Eur. J. Cancer Care* **2016**, *26*, e12624. [CrossRef] [PubMed]
3. Yu, J.; Hu, T.; Chen, Y. Small-arc volumetric-modulated arc therapy: A new approach that is superior to fixed-field IMRT in optimizing dosimetric and treatment-relevant parameters for patients undergoing whole-breast irradiation following breast-conserving surgery. *Medicine* **2016**, *95*, e4609. [CrossRef] [PubMed]
4. Blaschke, S.-M.; Gough, K.C.; Chua, B.H.; Francis, P.A.; Cockerell, R.; Drosdowsky, A.F.; Sheeran, L.; Krishnasamy, M. Implementation of a Multidisciplinary Model of Care for Women with Metastatic Breast Cancer: Challenges and Lessons Learned. *Clin. Breast Cancer* **2019**, *19*, e327–e336. [CrossRef]
5. Di Paolo, A.; Sarkozy, F.; Ryll, B.; Siebert, U. Personalized medicine in Europe: Not yet personal enough? *BMC Health Serv. Res.* **2017**, *17*, 1–9. [CrossRef] [PubMed]
6. Burock, S.; Meunier, F.; Lacombe, D. How can innovative forms of clinical research contribute to deliver affordable cancer care in an evolving health care environment? *Eur. J. Cancer* **2013**, *49*, 2777–2783. [CrossRef]
7. Duburs, G.; Neibecker, D.; Žarković, N. Chemistry and personalized medicine–the research and development future of Europe. *Croat. Med. J.* **2012**, *53*, 291–293. [CrossRef]
8. Thall, P.F. Ethical issues in oncology biostatistics. *Stat. Methods Med. Res.* **2002**, *11*, 429–448. [CrossRef] [PubMed]

9. Meldolesi, E.; Van Soest, J.; Damiani, A.; Dekker, A.; Alitto, A.R.; Campitelli, M.; DiNapoli, N.; Gatta, R.; Gambacorta, M.A.; Lanzotti, V.; et al. Standardized data collection to build prediction models in oncology: A prototype for rectal cancer. *Future Oncol.* **2016**, *12*, 119–136. [CrossRef]
10. Lambin, P.; Roelofs, E.; Reymen, B.; Velazquez, E.R.; Buijsen, J.; Zegers, C.M.; Carvalho, S.; Leijenaar, R.T.; Nalbantov, G.; Oberije, C.; et al. 'Rapid Learning health care in oncology'—An approach towards decision support systems enabling customised radiotherapy. *Radiother. Oncol.* **2013**, *109*, 159–164. [CrossRef]
11. Lambin, P.; Zindler, J.; Vanneste, B.; Van De Voorde, L.; Jacobs, M.; Eekers, D.; Peerlings, J.; Reymen, B.; LaRue, R.T.H.M.; Deist, T.M.; et al. Modern clinical research: How rapid learning health care and cohort multiple randomised clinical trials complement traditional evidence based medicine. *Acta Oncol.* **2015**, *54*, 1289–1300. [CrossRef]
12. Guihard, S.; Thariat, J.; Clavier, J.-B. Métadonnées et leurs applications possibles en radiothérapie. *Bull. Cancer* **2017**, *104*, 147–156. [CrossRef] [PubMed]
13. Aristei, C.; Kaidar-Person, O.; Arenas, M.; Coles, C.; Offersen, B.V.; Bourgier, C.; Frezza, G.; Leonardi, M.C.; Valentini, V.; Poortmans, P.M.P. The 2016 Assisi Think Tank Meeting on breast cancer: White paper. *Breast Cancer Res. Treat.* **2016**, *160*, 211–221. [CrossRef] [PubMed]
14. Meldolesi, E.; Van Soest, J.; DiNapoli, N.; Dekker, A.; Damiani, A.; Gambacorta, M.A.; Valentini, V. An umbrella protocol for standardized data collection (SDC) in rectal cancer: A prospective uniform naming and procedure convention to support personalized medicine. *Radiother. Oncol.* **2014**, *112*, 59–62. [CrossRef] [PubMed]
15. Meldolesi, E.; Van Soest, J.; Alitto, A.R.; Autorino, R.; DiNapoli, N.; Dekker, A.; Gambacorta, M.A.; Gatta, R.; Tagliaferri, L.; Damiani, A.; et al. VATE: VAlidation of high TEchnology based on large database analysis by learning machine. *Colorectal Cancer* **2014**, *3*, 435–450. [CrossRef]
16. Alitto, A.R.; Gatta, R.; Vanneste, B.; Vallati, M.; Meldolesi, E.; Damiani, A.; Lanzotti, V.; Mattiucci, G.C.; Frascino, V.; Masciocchi, C.; et al. PRODIGE: PRediction models in prOstate cancer for personalized meDIcine challenGE. *Futur. Oncol.* **2017**, *13*, 2171–2181. [CrossRef]
17. Wilson, G. Gantt charts: A centenary appreciation. *Eur. J. Oper. Res.* **2003**, *149*, 430–437. [CrossRef]
18. National Comprehensive Cancer Network. *NCCN Clinical Practice Guidelines in Oncology (NCCN Guidelines) Breast Cancer*; NCCN: Plymouth Meeting, PA, USA, 2020.
19. Smith, B.D.; Bellon, J.R.; Blitzblau, R.; Freedman, G.; Haffty, B.; Hahn, C.; Halberg, F.; Hoffman, K.; Horst, K.; Moran, J.; et al. Radiation therapy for the whole breast: Executive summary of an American Society for Radiation Oncology (ASTRO) evidence-based guideline. *Pr. Radiat. Oncol.* **2018**, *8*, 145–152. [CrossRef]
20. *GRUPPO DI COORDINAMENTO AIRO MAMMELLA Triennio 2017–2019, Best Clinical Practice Nella Radioterapia dei Tumori Della Mammella*; Sede Legale: Milano, Italy, 2019. Available online: radioterapiaitalia.it (accessed on 1 February 2021).
21. Baumann, B. Create and Modify Case Report Forms (CRFs). 24 March 2014. Available online: https://docs.openclinica.com/3.1/study-setup/build-study/create-case-report-forms-crfs (accessed on 10 June 2016).
22. Guidelines 2/2019 on the Processing of Personal Data under Article 6(1)(b) GDPR in the Context of the Provision of Online Services to Data Subjects-Version Adopted after Public Consultation. Available online: https://edpb.europa.eu/our-work-tools/our-documents/guidelines/guidelines-22019-processing-personal-data-under-article-61b_en (accessed on 31 October 2018).
23. Article 32, EU GDPR, "Security of Processing". Available online: http://www.privacy-regulation.eu/en/32.htm (accessed on 31 October 2018).
24. Liou, D.-M.; Chang, W.-P. Applying Data Mining for the Analysis of Breast Cancer Data. *Methods Mol. Biol.* **2014**, *1246*, 175–189. [CrossRef]
25. Melo, M.T.D.; Gonçalves, V.H.L.; Costa, H.D.R.; Braga, D.S.; Gomide, L.B.; Alves, C.S.; Brasil, L.M. OntoMama: An Ontology Applied to Breast Cancer. *Stud. Health Technol. Inform.* **2015**, *216*, 1104.
26. Zhu, Q.; Tao, C.; Shen, F.; Chute, C.G. Exploring the Pharmacogenomics Knowledge Base (Pharmgkb) for Repositioning Breast Cancer Drugs by Leveraging Web Ontology Language (Owl) and Cheminformatics Approaches. In *Pac Symp Biocomputing*; World Scientific: Singapore, 2013; pp. 172–182.
27. Papatheodorou, I.; METABRIC Group; Crichton, C.; Morris, L.; Maccallum, P.; Davies, J.; Brenton, J.D.; Caldas, C. A metadata approach for clinical data management in translational genomics studies in breast cancer. *BMC Med. Genom.* **2009**, *2*, 1–10. [CrossRef] [PubMed]
28. Abidi, S.R.; Abidi, S.S.; Hussain, S.; Shepherd, M. Ontology-based Modeling of Clinical Practice Guidelines: A Clinical Decision Support System for Breast Cancer Follow-up Interventions at Primary Care Settings. *Stud. Health Technol. Inform.* **2007**, *129*, 845–849. [PubMed]
29. Wu, S.-G.; Li, H.; Tang, L.-Y.; Sun, J.-Y.; Zhang, W.-W.; Li, F.-Y.; Chen, Y.-X.; He, Z.-Y. The effect of distant metastases sites on survival in de novo stage-IV breast cancer: A SEER database analysis. *Tumor Biol.* **2017**, *39*, 101042831770508. [CrossRef] [PubMed]
30. Murthy, V.; Pawar, S.; Chamberlain, R.S. Disease Severity, Presentation, and Clinical Outcomes Among Adolescents With Malignant Breast Neoplasms: A 20-Year Population-Based Outcomes Study From the SEER Database (1973–2009). *Clin. Breast Cancer* **2017**, *17*, 392–398. [CrossRef]
31. Liu, J.; Su, M.; Hong, S.; Gao, H.; Zheng, X.; Wang, S. Nomogram predicts survival benefit from preoperative radiotherapy for non-metastatic breast cancer: A SEER-based study. *Oncotarget* **2017**, *8*, 49861–49868. [CrossRef]

32. Plasilova, M.L.; Hayse, B.; Killelea, B.K.; Horowitz, N.R.; Chagpar, A.B.; Lannin, D.R. Features of triple-negative breast cancer. *Medicine* **2016**, *95*, e4614. [CrossRef]
33. Diwanji, T.P.; Molitoris, J.K.; Chhabra, A.M.; Snider, J.W.; Bentzen, S.M.; Tkaczuk, K.H.; Rosenblatt, P.Y.; Kesmodel, S.B.; Bellavance, E.C.; Cohen, R.J.; et al. Utilization of hypofractionated whole-breast radiation therapy in patients receiving chemotherapy: A National Cancer Database analysis. *Breast Cancer Res. Treat.* **2017**, *165*, 445–453. [CrossRef]
34. Marazzi, F.; Tagliaferri, L.; Masiello, V.; Moschella, F.; Colloca, G.F.; Corvari, B.; Sanchez, A.M.; Capocchiano, N.D.; Pastorino, R.; Iacomini, C.; et al. GENERATOR Breast DataMart—The Novel Breast Cancer Data Discovery System for Research and Monitoring: Preliminary Results and Future Perspectives. *J. Pers. Med.* **2021**, *11*, 65. [CrossRef] [PubMed]
35. Montero-Luis, A.; Aristei, C.; Meattini, I.; Arenas, M.; Boersma, L.; Bourgier, C.; Coles, C.; Cutuli, B.; Falcinelli, L.; Kaidar-Person, O.; et al. The Assisi Think Tank Meeting Survey of post-mastectomy radiation therapy in ductal carcinoma in situ: Suggestions for routine practice. *Crit. Rev. Oncol.* **2019**, *138*, 207–213. [CrossRef]
36. Arenas, M.; Selek, U.; Kaidar-Person, O.; Perrucci, E.; Luis, A.M.; Boersma, L.; Coles, C.; Offersen, B.; Meattini, I.; Bölükbaşı, Y.; et al. The 2018 assisi think tank meeting on breast cancer: International expert panel white paper. *Crit. Rev. Oncol.* **2020**, *151*, 102967. [CrossRef]

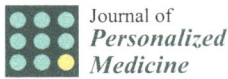

Review

Image-Guided Localization Techniques for Surgical Excision of Non-Palpable Breast Lesions: An Overview of Current Literature and Our Experience with Preoperative Skin Tattoo

Gianluca Franceschini [1,2], Elena Jane Mason [1,*], Cristina Grippo [3], Sabatino D'Archi [1], Anna D'Angelo [4], Lorenzo Scardina [1], Alejandro Martin Sanchez [1], Marco Conti [4], Charlotte Trombadori [4], Daniela Andreina Terribile [1,2], Alba Di Leone [1], Beatrice Carnassale [1], Paolo Belli [4], Riccardo Manfredi [4] and Riccardo Masetti [1,2]

1. Multidisciplinary Breast Centre, Dipartimento Scienze della Salute della Donna e del Bambino e di Sanità Pubblica, Fondazione Policlinico Universitario A. Gemelli IRCCS, 00168 Rome, Italy; gianlucafranceschini70@gmail.com (G.F.); sabatinodarchi@gmail.com (S.D.); lorenzoscardina@libero.it (L.S.); martin.sanchez@hotmail.it (A.M.S.); daniterribile@gmail.com (D.A.T.); albadileone@gmail.com (A.D.L.); carnassale.beatrice@gmail.com (B.C.); riccardo.masetti@policlinicogemelli.it (R.M.)
2. Dipartimento di Scienze Mediche e Chirurgiche, Università Cattolica del Sacro Cuore, 00168 Rome, Italy
3. Dipartimento di Diagnostica per Immagini, Radiologia Terapeutica ed Interventistica, Azienda Ospedaliera Santa Maria Terni, 05100 Terni, Italy; cris.grippo@gmail.com
4. Dipartimento di Diagnostica per Immagini, Radioterapia Oncologica ed Ematologia, Fondazione Policlinico Universitario Agostino Gemelli IRCCS, 00168 Rome, Italy; anna.dangelo05@gmail.com (A.D.); conti.marco87@gmail.com (M.C.); charlotte.trombadori@gmail.com (C.T.); paolo.belli@policlinicogemelli.it (P.B.); riccardo.manfredi@policlinicogemelli.it (R.M.)
* Correspondence: elenajanemason@gmail.com; Tel.: +39-33-5700-4512

Abstract: Breast conserving surgery has become the standard of care and is more commonly performed than mastectomy for early stage breast cancer, with recent studies showing equivalent survival and lower morbidity. Accurate preoperative lesion localization is mandatory to obtain adequate oncological and cosmetic results. Image guidance assures the precision requested for this purpose. This review provides a summary of all techniques currently available, ranging from the classic wire positioning to the newer magnetic seed localization. We describe the procedures and equipment necessary for each method, outlining the advantages and disadvantages, with a focus on the cost-effective preoperative skin tattoo technique performed at our centre. Breast surgeons and radiologists have to consider ongoing technological developments in order to assess the best localization method for each individual patient and clinical setting.

Keywords: breast cancer; breast-conserving surgery; non-palpable breast lesions; image-guided localization; preoperative breast localization; breast ultrasound

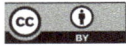

1. Introduction

Breast cancer (BC) is the most commonly diagnosed cancer and the leading cause of cancer-related death among women [1]. A successful BC treatment is based on a multidisciplinary use of surgery, chemotherapy and radiation therapy, with surgery as the central component of treatment for early-stage breast cancer [2,3]. Breast-conserving surgery (BCS) followed by adjuvant radiotherapy, known as breast conservation therapy (BCT), has become the alternative treatment to mastectomy for early stage breast cancer because of equivalent survival and lower morbidity [4–6].

Local recurrence after BCS is strongly correlated to the surgical margin status, as demonstrated by a large number of follow-up studies [7–11]. The main goal of BCS is to fully remove the tumor with clear margins, while avoiding resection of healthy breast tissue in order to achieve better cosmetic results. Image-guided preoperative localization is mandatory for guiding surgery of non-palpable lesions or surgically relevant extension of palpable lesions to improve both oncological and cosmetic outcomes [12,13]. Over the last decade, methods for preoperative localization of breast lesions for BCS have evolved rapidly due to innovative techniques and discovery of novel agents. However, cooperation and communication between breast surgeons and radiologists still play a crucial role.

Different image guided localization techniques are variably used in different institutions depending on personal choices, skills and available technologies. As a general rule, the method chosen should be the most precise to localize the lesion or marker left after biopsy, thus improving free margin rates and decreasing operative time, and possibly cause little to no discomfort to the patient. Preoperative breast lesions localization techniques currently available are wire localization, carbon marking, radio-guided occult lesion localization (ROLL), radioactive seed localization (RSL), magnetic seed localization and non-radioactive radar localization, intraoperative ultrasound and preoperative skin tattoo localization (Table 1). In this article, we provide an overview of current literature of all commercially available techniques. The aim of this review is to educate practicing radiologists and breast surgeons so they can knowingly select new techniques to improve patient care.

Table 1. Comparison of different localization techniques. Abbreviations: ROLL = radio-guided occult lesion localization; RSL = radioactive seed localization; Magseed = magnetic seed localization; IOUS = intraoperative ultrasound; Skin tattoo = preoperative localization with skin tattoo; OR = operating room; US = ultrasound; MRI = magnetic resonance imaging. * Success is defined as removal of target lesion. ** Authors' experience.

Technique	Materials/Procedures	Advantages	Disadvantages	Success * Rate	Clear Margins Rate
Wire localization	Wire Preloaded needle introducer	Simple Cost-effective Different kinds of image-guidance	Wire migration Scheduling difficulties Limits surgical decisions	97.5% [14]	70.8–87.4% [15]
Carbon marking	Diluted charcoal powder	Simple Different kinds of image-guidance Cost-effective Cannot dislodge Scheduling flexibility	Carbon can distort or obscure lesion Unfit for large breasts Unfit for multifocal or extensive lesions	99% [16]	61–85% [17,18]
ROLL	Nuclear radiotracer Technetium 99 Gamma ray probe	Different kinds of image-guidance Does not limit surgeon	Scheduling difficulties Radiation Cost	95–99% [19]	92% [20,21]
RSL	Iodine 125 seed Preloaded needle introducer Gamma probe set for I-125	Scheduling flexibility Does not limit surgeon Different kinds of image-guidance	Radiation Not repositionable after deployment	100% [22,23]	73.5–96.7% [22,23]
Magseed	Paramagnetic seed Preloaded needle introducer	Scheduling flexibility No radiation Does not limit surgeon	Cost Not repositionable after deployment Non magnetizable surgical equipment MRI artifacts	99.86% [24–27]	88.75% [24]
Radiofrequency identification tags	Radiofrequency reflector Needle introducer Detector	Scheduling flexibility No radiation Does not limit surgeon	Cost Depth limit Not repositionable after deployment Interference with halogen lights in the OR	97–100% [28,29]	85–100% [28–30]
IOUS	Portable or OR-stationed US machine and sterile transducer cover	Scheduling flexibility No radiation Does not limit surgeon Non-invasive	Unemployable in US-invisible lesions Surgeon learning curve Interference with air during dissection	100% [31–35]	81–97% [32,34]

Table 1. Cont.

Technique	Materials/Procedures	Advantages	Disadvantages	Success * Rate	Clear Margins Rate
Skin tattoo	Dermographic marker Lead markers	Simple and safe Cost-effective Non-invasive Different kinds of image-guidance Does not limit surgeon	Scheduling difficulties Inability to depict marker	99.5% **	95.9% **

2. Wire Guided Localization

Wire localization (WL) was introduced in the 1970s and for many years has served as the only method for preoperative breast localization [36]. Initially, mammography was the only imaging modality used to guide wire placement. Currently, wire localization can be performed under different kinds of image-guidance (mammographic, sonographic and magnetic resonance imaging). WL is the most commonly used method for non-palpable breast lesions, with clear margins reported in a range of 70.8%–87.4% of cases [15]. Different types of wires are available, ranging in length (from 3 to 15 cm), shape (hook, barb or pigtail), materials and numbers of thickened segments [12,13,15,36,37]. Wires are preloaded in a 16–21 G needle introducer: when the tip is just beyond the target, the hook is deployed by fixing the needle firmly with one hand and gently advancing the wire with the other. The needle is then removed over the wire and the thread extending from the tip of the hookwire is secured on the skin surface. Routinely, post-procedural CC and ML mammograms were obtained to confirm accurate placement (Figure 1). The depth of the wire tip from the skin surface is also recorded. In case of extensive disease wires can be placed in multiple numbers, allowing targeted localization in a procedure known as "bracketing wire localization" [38]. WL remains the most widely adopted approach due to the long-term data supporting its effectiveness [39], although success is strongly dependent upon the surgeon's mental reconstruction of the images, perceived intraoperative position of the lesion and wire trajectory [40]. Approximately 2.5% of wire localizations are unsuccessful; factors associated with an increased risk of unsuccessful localization are multiple lesions, small lesions, lesions containing extensive microcalcifications and small surgical specimens [14]. Established advantages of WL are the widespread availability and the moderate price, with one study estimating the cost of a needle at $22.50 [41].

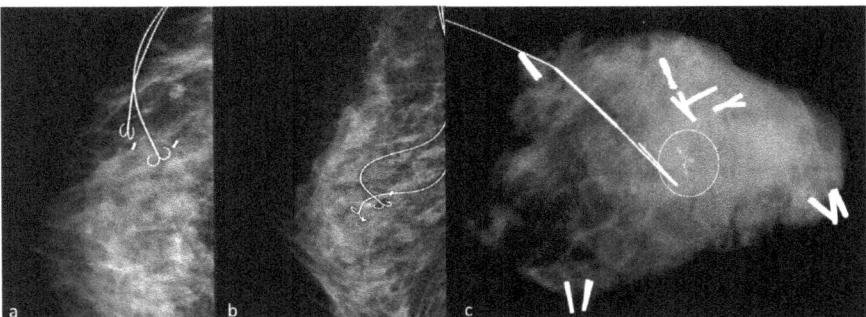

Figure 1. Wire-guided localization. Craniocaudal (**a**) and mediolateral (**b**) oblique mammograms taken after hookwires insertion show optimal wires positioning, with the wires at the biopsy markers site. A specimen radiograph (**c**) contains the hookwire and the residual calcifications (circle).

Moreover, wires emit no ionizing radiation and can be stored safely within the imaging department. This approach also allows localizations of breast lesions under different kinds of image guidance (US, mammography/tomosynthesis or MRI). Although WL is highly effective, it still yields several disadvantages. The procedure is in itself unpleasant and causes patient discomfort; vasovagal reactions are reported in up to 7–10% of patients, although less frequent for US than for mammography guided procedures [12]. Wire migration within the breast, and more infrequently outside the breast, has also been reported [42,43]. The hookwire can be transected during the surgery, with pieces being retained in the breast post-operatively [44,45]. Finally, this localization approach requires adequate coordination between trained breast radiologists and surgeons because the wire placement has to occur on the day of surgery to avoid displacement. This limitation can lead to inconvenience and delay in the operating room or suboptimal localization. Moreover, wire localization could limit the surgical approach and cause a potential worse cosmetic outcome; the placement route of the wire, chosen by the radiologist, often dictates incision choice for the surgeon who then has to follow the wire's course during dissection.

3. Carbon Marking

Carbon marking (CM) is an alternative method for non-palpable breast lesion localization first reported by Svane in 1983, consisting of an injection of sterile charcoal powder diluted with saline solution in close proximity to the lesion [46]. The injection can be performed under either sonographic or mammographic guidance, depending on how the target lesion has been biopsied [17]. A dark trail is created from the lesion to the skin, leaving a visible track that guides the surgeon during the operation. As the carbon track is immobile in breast tissue, it cannot dislodge. In contrast, hookwires can migrate when the patient changes position or when traction is applied during surgery. The main advantages of CM are logistics, patient comfort and cost. As CM and biopsies could be concurrent, the patient may be spared an extra invasive procedure. Moreover, surgery may be planned up to 1 month after the carbon injection, making operative planning easier for surgeons and sparing radiologists the pressure to place hookwires immediately before or during an operating session. The success rate using carbon marking is very high, with failure to remove targeted lesion occurring in about 1 in every 100 procedures [16]. However, there are cases in which CM presents technical difficulties. If the lesion is close to the chest wall, particularly in a large breast, or for extensive or multifocal lesions, long and several carbon tracks will be difficult for the surgeon to follow and a hookwire may be preferable. For extensive or multifocal lesions several carbon tracks are difficult to follow, and WL may be preferable [46]. The disadvantages are that the carbon tracks resist slicing, thus the carbon can distort or obscure the lesion. To avoid this, the carbon should be injected only as far as the edge of the lesion. Another possible, although uncommon, complication of CM is the incomplete surgical removal of the injected charcoal, which can cause a late-onset granuloma that may mimic malignant lesions in postoperative controls [47,48]. In terms of missed lesions and clear margin rates, CL shows similar results as WG: the proportion of cases with close or involved margins ranges between 15% (for invasive cancer) and 39% (in situonly lesions) [17,18].

4. Radio-Guided Occult Lesion Localization

Radio-guided occult lesion localization (ROLL) involves intratumoral injection of a small amount (0.2–0.3 mL) of human serum albumin marked with nuclear radiotracer technetium 99 [49] (Figure 2). This localization technique can be performed either by ultrasonography, stereotactic mammography or MRI.

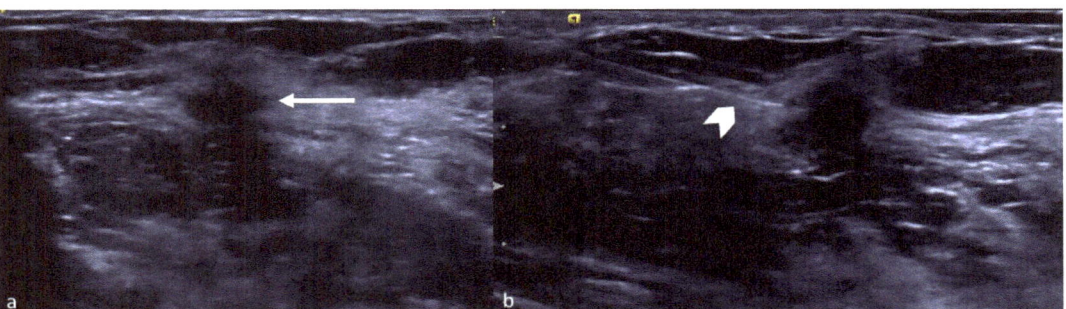

Figure 2. Radio-guided occult lesion localization (ROLL) technique: (**a**) invasive ductal cancer (arrow) in the left upper outer quadrant in a 77-year-old woman. (**b**) Intratumoral injection (arrow head) of a small amount (0.2–0.3 mL) of human serum albumin marked with nuclear radiotracer technetium 99 in order to perform radio-guided occult lesion localization.

The radiation dose is of about 7–10 MBq, equivalent to 1–2% of the dose used for a whole-body bone scintigraphy [50]. A handheld gamma ray detection probe is used by the surgeon to locate the lesion, guide the removal and verify the removed specimen and the surgical bed. To allow an adequate detection, surgery has to be performed no later than 24 h after the injection of the radiotracer. ROLL has gained popularity on account of several advantages associated with a reduced excision volume, more accurate centricity of a lesion within the surgical specimen, better cosmetic results and a higher percentage of tumor-free margins, around 92% of cases [20,21]. There are no serious complications related to ROLL, even though experience in the injection is needed to avoid failure of lesion identification, described only in 1–5% of the cases [19]. ROLL can be performed together with sentinel lymph node identification in the same surgical session, in a procedure known as sentinel node and occult lesion localization (SNOLL), that involves the injection of an additional radiotracer (carried by micromolecules instead of macromolecules used for ROLL) [51,52].

5. Radioactive Seed Localization

Radioactive seed localization (RSL) using Iodine-125 seeds has been proposed in 1999 by Dauway as an attractive alternative to both WL and ROLL. This technique involves targeted placement of a seed, commonly used for brachytherapy, composed of titanium labeled 0.075–0.3 mCi of Iodine-125. Each seed has a half-life (T 1/2) of 59 days and a radioactivity of about 20–30 MBq, a dose equivalent to 3–5% of that used for a whole-body bone scintigraphy [53]. Radioactive seeds can be positioned under different image guidance, ultrasonography, mammography/tomosynthesis or MRI. An 18G needle preloaded or manually loaded with the seed was used, and the tip was occluded by bone wax. Once the needle advanced to the desired location, the seed was deployed through the bone wax by advancing the stilette. At the end of the procedure, regardless of the guidance method, the patient was assessed for radioactivity with a Geiger counter and post-procedural mammograms with two orthogonal images reconfirm proper seed positioning [54]. During surgery a gamma probe set for I-125 guides the surgeon. The different energy peak of technentium-99 and iodine-125 allows one to differentiate the isotope used for sentinel node biopsy. Radioactive seed localization could potentially be performed weeks before the scheduled surgery because of the long half-life (59 days) of I 125; however, according to Nuclear Regulatory Commission guidelines the procedure should be carried out no more than 7 days before surgery in order to minimize radiation exposure [55]. In fact, one of the potential drawbacks of RSL is the presence of radioactivity. Although the activity levels of the seeds are low and considered safe for human exposure, patients are advised to avoid interactions with children and pregnant women to mitigate any potential risk. Moreover, a strict local protocol for quality assurance must be followed in order to guarantee that all implanted seeds are actually removed and recovered by the local Nuclear Medicine

Department. An undeniable benefit of both ROLL and RSL is that the surgeon is no longer impeded by the guidewire when planning breast incision and can use the feedback from the gamma probe to reorientate the surgical approach in real time.

Given oncoplastic breast techniques, this allows greater choice of cosmetically sensitive approaches, such as periareolar, lateral or inframammary fold incisions [56]. Current literature comparing RSL and WL margin status achievements shows variable results, with some studies favoring RSL and more recent studies, including three randomized control trials, suggesting no difference between the two methods [40,57,58]. Due to the real-time intraoperative monitoring of the detected gamma counts from the seed, RSL allows an accurate lesion localization with lower incidence of positive margins and decreased need for repeat surgery than with wire localization. The success rate using RSL is very high: target lesion is effectively removed in nearly 100% of cases and clear margin rates range from 73.5% to 96.7% [22,23].

6. Magnetic Seed Localization

Magnetic seed is a novel localization technique approved by the FDA in 2016 [24]. This technique shares many similarities with RSL, because it consists in seed placement under sonographic or tomosynthesis guidance, however it does not involve radioactivity. First introduced by Sentimag (Magseed®, London, UK), magnetic seeds are cylindrical markers, measuring approximately 5 mm × 1 mm, made of paramagnetic steel and iron oxide. They can be deployed by an 18 G preloaded needle of different length according to different breast sizes (Figure 3). Following insertion, mammograms in double projection are acquired to confirm correct positioning of the seed. The Sentimag probe employed in the operating room generates an alternating magnetic field that temporarily magnetizes the Magseed, and subsequently measures its magnetic field. The surgical technique is therefore similar to that adopted after ROLL or RSL, involving a live numerical feedback that guides surgical direction and reveals the remaining distance from lesion. A final assessment is conducted by probing the specimen and the surgical cavity, and potentially verified with specimen X-ray confirming excision of seed. While sharing with ROLL and RSL the important benefit of granting maximum liberty in the choice of incision, this technique has the further benefit of avoiding exposure to radiation. It also eases coordination between Radiology and Surgery Departments, because seed placement, initially approved for up to 30 days prior to surgery, has now been extended in Europe and USA for long-term implantation [25]. However, while this seed could be potentially implantable during biopsies and even before neoadjuvant treatment, one major drawback is that it interferes with MR imaging by creating artifacts as wide as 4 cm [12]. Another challenge with this technique is that during surgery all ferromagnetic instruments will interfere with the signal. A dedicated set of non-ferromagnetic surgical instruments is therefore always necessary, and weighs on cost-effectiveness [13]. Studies on the efficacy of this technique in terms of successful excision, clear margins and optimal volume of resection are few and include relatively small populations of patients, however preliminary data is encouraging, with a successful placement rate of 94.42%, a successful localization rate of 99.86% and a percentage of clear margins of 88.75% [24,26,27,59].

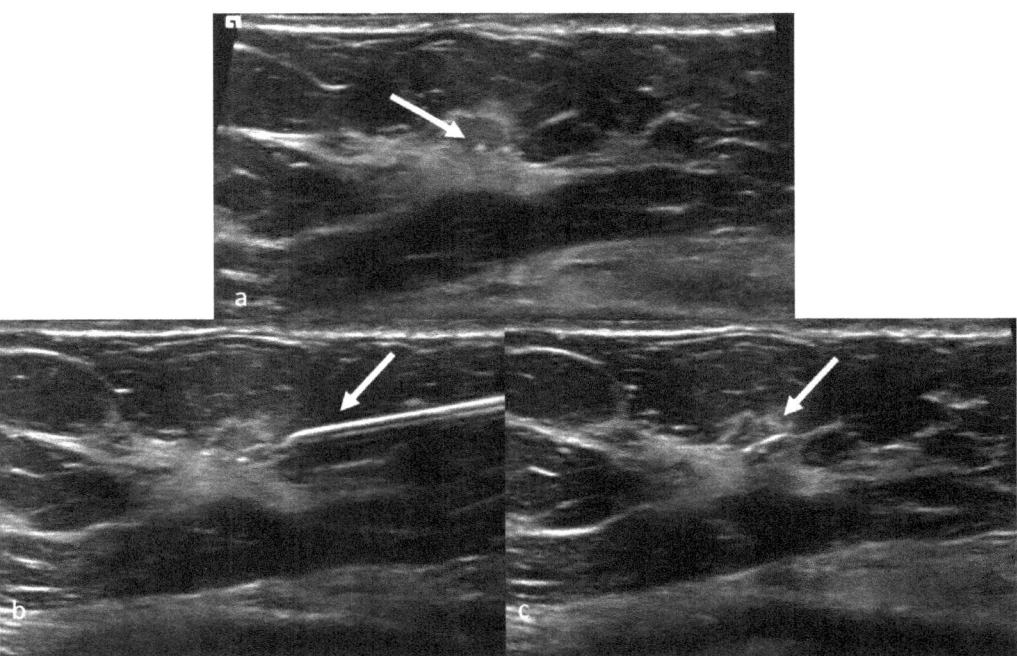

Figure 3. Magseed positioning in a 49-year-old woman with ductal carcinoma in situ. Ultrasound images of the right upper outer quadrant. Biopsy marker is visible in the lesion (**a**, arrow). Magseed magnetic marker is placed under ultrasound guidance (**b**, arrow shows the needle). Magseed® marker is clearly seen in the lesion (**c**, arrow).

7. Radiofrequency Identification Tags

Radio frequency reflector (RFR) is a non-ionizing electromagnetic wave tagging device for localizing non-palpable breast lesions approved in the United States by FDA in 2014 [28]. The identification tag, as any biopsy clip marker, can be placed by radiologists under mammographic, tomosynthesis or ultrasound guidance. The injection can take place up to 30 days preoperatively. During surgery, the surgeon activates the reflector with the hand piece and follows the signal to guide the excision. The audible and numerical signals change with increasing proximity to the lesion. Once the tissue is removed, the reader console can be used to confirm that all tags have been removed from the tissue cavity. RFRs differ in size and shape from vendor to vendor. One of the first available RFR is SAVI SCOUT (Cianna Medical, Aliso Viejo, CA, USA) and another more recent device is the LOCalizer (Faxitron, Tucson, AZ, USA). The SAVI SCOUT reflector has been rated as MR conditional and be considered safe to image in a static magnetic field of 3 Tesla or less and a maximum spatial gradient magnetic field of 3000 G or less [29]. Whereas metallic interference from nearby surgical instruments can interfere with detection of magnetic seeds, metal does not interfere with detection of radiofrequency signals during surgery [59]. Radiofrequency identification tag is an effective technique: data from the literature report success rates of 97–100% and clear margin rates ranging between 85% and 100% [30,31]. The main advantage of RFR localization over wire localization is the decoupling of the radiology and surgery schedules; moreover, it avoids the risk of complications associated with an external wire component. Compared to RSL, RFR is a non-ionizing system and does not require extensive multidisciplinary coordination or regulatory compliance. Disadvantages of localization with the SAVI SCOUT device include its relatively large size (12 mm), especially for small subcentimetric lesions. The LOCalizer overcomes the size hurdle since it is smaller. Other limitations include the inability to reposition the reflector once deployed and the maximum lesion detection depth, as studies have reported problems in intraoperative detection of the reflector in women with large breasts and lesions located >6 cm from the overlying skin surface [30].

8. Intraoperative Ultrasound

Intraoperative ultrasound (IOUS) was first described by Schwartz et al. in 1988 and has gradually spread and evolved with other techniques due to growing experience and technological advances. A sterile-gowned ultrasound probe has to be available in the operating room. The procedure begins at the operating table before incision, once painting and draping procedures have been carried out. The surgeon locates the tumor by ultrasonography and measures its diameter and distance from surrounding hallmarks, such as skin surface, nipple–areolar complex (NAC) and fascia. The surgical approach is then planned in full liberty, and after incision the dissection is carried out by repeatedly reassessing the tumor's position and the distance between the surgical plane and its margins. Once the excision has been completed, specimen ultrasound is performed at the operating table to assess margins, and additional shaving excisions can be acquired if necessary. This technique is highly effective, with identification rates close to 100% [31–35], and studies focusing on margin status have shown that IOUS guided surgeries yield less positive resection margins compared to WGL [32], with free-margin percentages ranging from 81% to 97% [33–35]. Free margin rates are enhanced by IOUS even in resection of palpable lesions [60]. A study by James et al. has instead shown no significant differences in margin status between IOUS and mammographic WGL in patients undergoing surgery for carcinoma in situ, although the authors still recommend performing IOUS as it is more cost-effective [61]. Compared to other techniques, IOUS yields several practical advantages: it does not increase patient presurgery psychological stress, as it is non-invasive compared to techniques involving breast compression or puncture; it grants full liberty to the surgeon in choosing the most convenient oncoplastic surgical approach; it does not aggravate organizational problems and coordination between several departments, as it takes place directly in the operating room and can be carried out completely by the surgeon himself [62]. To this regard, the learning curve of specialists not necessarily familiar with manipulating ultrasounds, such as surgeons, could potentially pose an issue, however a study by Krekel et al. suggests that performance of eight procedures is enough for the surgeon to acquire the expertise necessary to combine ultrasounds to palpation-guided surgery [63]. Drawbacks include technical problems resulting from combining ultrasound with surgery, such as air infiltration beneath the probe that can impede visualization, and refraction issues that can arise when scanning tissue that is irregular in shape [32]. The major, insurmountable issue of this technique is however represented by its inability to localize sonographically invisible tumors. To overcome this problem, some authors have described this technique in combination with hematoma-guided surgery after MRI- or stereotactically-guided biopsies, with mixed results [64].

9. Preoperative Localization with a Skin Tattoo

Preoperative localization with a skin tattoo is a simple and safe technique amply utilized in our centre, as it is easily performed, extremely well tolerated by patients and effective in terms of successful excision and clear margin rates. This method can be carried out by acquiring either sonographic or mammographic images, depending on the type of lesion, but ultrasounds are employed whenever possible because the procedure is easier. In this case, patients lie in the supine position with their arms extended to mimic the position held during surgery. The tumor is located, and its distance from the skin surface is measured taking care not to apply pressure with the probe, so as to report accurately the depth of the tumor in relation to the skin surface [65]. The distance between the lesion, the nipple and the pectoralis major muscle is also measured, as is the distance between separate lesions in case of multifocal or multicentric disease [44,66]. Radiologists with experience in this technique visualize the tumors at their largest diameter to achieve the optimal correspondence between the lesion and the skin markers. The tumor's projection on the skin surface is pinpointed with a dermographic skin marker and the drawing is covered to avoid accidental erasure (Figure 4). The whole procedure, performed by an experienced radiologist, takes 5–10 min and provides minimum patient discomfort. Limitations include poor results in case of sonographically invisible lesions, microcalcifications or biopsy markers, but are easily overcome by implementing this technique with a mammographic approach. Stereotactic-guided skin marking is also a non-invasive technique, albeit it provides a little more discomfort to the patient due to breast compression. Mammograms are acquired in double projection and measurements are performed on the images to determine the distance between the lesion and the nipple, the skin surface and the fascia.

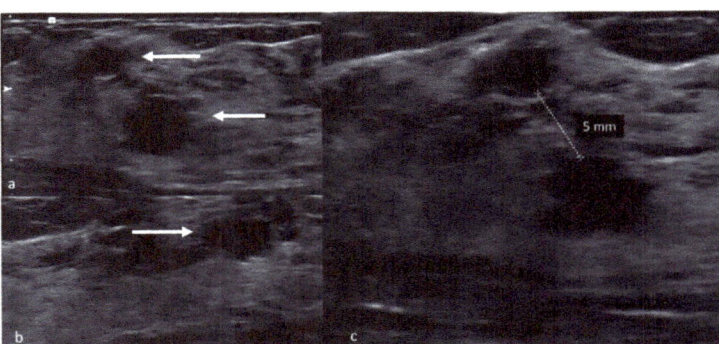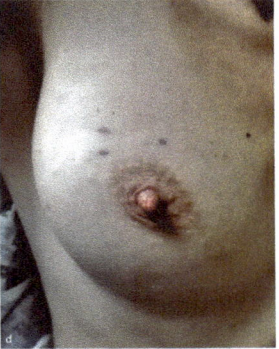

Figure 4. Preoperative skin tattoo. Transverse sonogram showing hypoechoic, round shaped multifocal masses with indistinct margins in the upper outer quadrant of the right breast (**a**,**b**, arrows). The distance between separate lesions is measured (**c**). The dermographic skin markers of the tumor's projection on the skin surface (**d**).

The radiologist then estimates the projection of the tumor on the skin surface and positions a lead marker in the corresponding spot. In case of bigger lesions, such as extensive microcalcifications, or multifocal disease, multiple lead markers can be employed to determine lesion margins. A second stereotactic pair of images is acquired to confirm the correct localization, and in case of inaccurate positioning, the lead markers can be repositioned more accurately and confirmed by a further mammogram [67] (Figure 5). At the end of the procedure the lead markers are removed, and the skin tattoo is drawn in their place. In the operating room, the mark is exposed and retraced with a specific marker resistant to antiseptic solutions, and painting and draping procedures are carried out carefully without wiping out the ink. Our centre strongly advocates pursuit of the maximum aesthetic result achievable with oncological safety, and because this localization technique employs only a temporary skin tattoo, the surgeon is granted total liberty in choice of incision and oncoplastic technique. The skin flap is dissected in the direction of the tattoo, then the incision is deepened and a lumpectomy is carried out taking into account tumor depth measured during the preoperative localization. In some cases, a non-palpable lesion becomes palpable after dissection of the skin flap, allowing the surgeon to easily complete the excision, however in most cases the excision has to be conducted by reassessing the original position of the skin mark from time to time. Once the excision is completed, metallic clips are placed on the orienting sutures in different numbers, so as to recognize margins in the specimen X-ray. The sample is then placed into a transparent plastic bag and sent to the Radiology Department, and mammograms are acquired in double projection. The tumor is usually visible as a radiopaque nodule, and its position inside the lumpectomy specimen is described as either well centered or close to one or more surgical margins, and reported to the operating surgeon. In dense, glandular specimens the nodule can be difficult to distinguish from the surrounding mammary parenchyma: in these cases, the exam can be completed with a specimen ultrasound [68] (Figure 6). If close margins are detected in either technique the surgeon can acquire further cavity shave margins on the affected border.

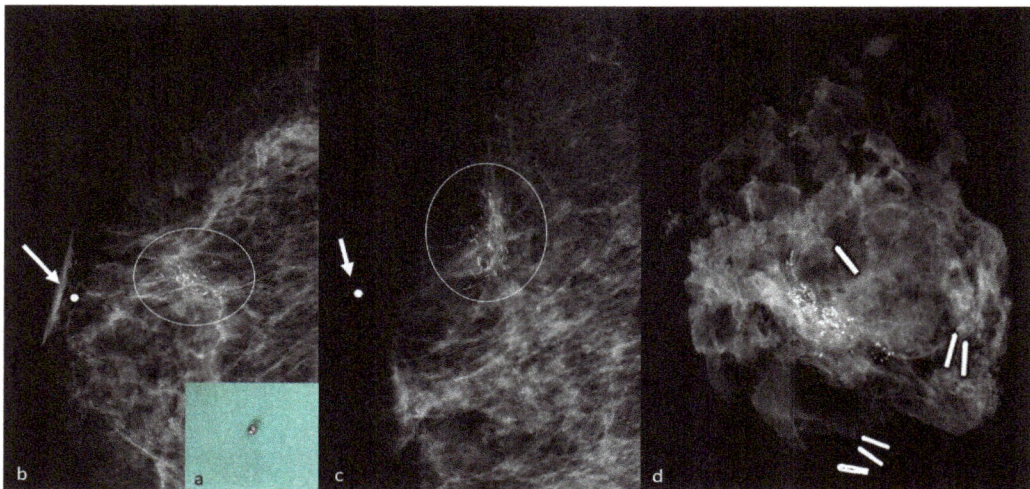

Figure 5. Lead marker positioning during mammographic technique. Metallic marker (**a**). Craniocaudal (**b**) and mediolateral oblique (**c**) views confirm the appropriate marker (arrow) placement on the microcalcifications' (circle) projection on the skin surface. Specimen X-ray contains the microcalcifications (**d**).

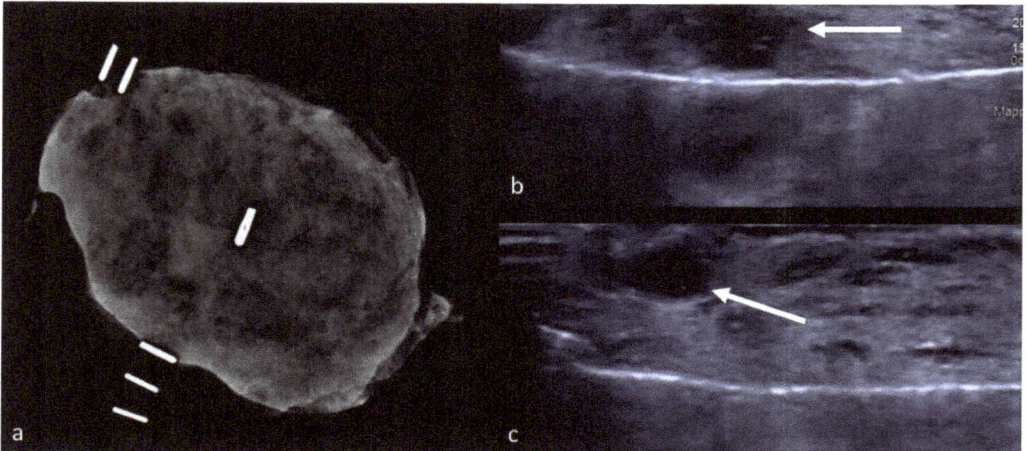

Figure 6. Radiograph of a dense, glandular specimen with scarcely recognizable nodules (**a**). Subsequent specimen ultrasound demonstrates successful removal of two masses (arrows) (**b**,**c**).

This technique is quick, easily performed by breast radiologists and extremely cost-effective. It does not require equipment that is not normally present in any breast surgery department, and is therefore feasible even with scarce resources. Limitations include accurate scheduling to time the procedure before surgery thus avoiding accidental mark erasure, and a certain degree of experience by the surgeon in reassessing the tumor's position based on the skin mark during dissection. Reports on this technique are widely deficient in the literature, however a preliminary analysis of the data from our high-volume centre examining the outcome of 199 lumpectomies performed for non-palpable breast tumors between August and December 2019 identified a global success rate of 99.5% (198/199) and a clear margins rate of 95.9% (192/199). As these rates did not differ significantly from other localization techniques, this method appears safe and especially ideal in the case of limited resources or spending reviews.

10. Conclusions

Image-guided preoperative localization of breast lesions is a common procedure that has rapidly evolved throughout the last decades. Continuous technological developments and results from new clinical trials have provided growing insight and new possibilities for breast specialists to select upon various effective techniques. However, to date, no single perfect method exists. Therefore, the optimal approach should be tailored on each patient by taking into account preoperative disease characterization (both radiologic and histologic) and consulting all stakeholders, including surgeons, radiologists and pathologists.

Author Contributions: Conceptualization: C.G., E.J.M., S.D., A.D.; data curation, E.J.M., S.D.; writing—original draft preparation, C.G., E.J.M.; writing—review and editing, C.G., E.J.M., G.F., S.D., A.D., D.A.T., P.B.; visualization, A.D., P.B., M.C.; supervision, A.M.S., A.D.L., R.M. (Riccardo Masetti); project administration, L.S., B.C., R.M. (Riccardo Manfredi), C.T. All authors have read and agreed to the published version of the manuscript.

Funding: This research received no external funding.

Institutional Review Board Statement: Not applicable.

Informed Consent Statement: Informed consent was obtained from all subjects involved in the study.

Conflicts of Interest: The authors declare no conflict of interest.

References

1. Sharma, R. Breast cancer incidence, mortality and mortality-to-incidence ratio (MIR) are associated with human development, 1990–2016: Evidence from Global Burden of Disease Study 2016. *Breast Cancer* **2019**, *26*, 428–445. [CrossRef] [PubMed]
2. Moo, T.-A.; Sanford, R.; Dang, C.; Morrow, M. Overview of breast cancer therapy. *PET Clin.* **2018**, *13*, 339–354. [CrossRef] [PubMed]
3. Franceschini, G.; Terribile, D.; Fabbri, C.; Magno, S.; D'Alba, P.; Chiesa, F.; Di Leone, A.; Masetti, R. Management of locally advanced breast cancer. Mini-review. *Minerva Chir.* **2007**, *62*, 249–255. Available online: http://europepmc.org/abstract/MED/17641585 (accessed on 8 November 2020). [PubMed]
4. Fisher, B.; Anderson, S.; Bryant, J.; Margolese, R.G.; Deutsch, M.; Fisher, E.R.; Jeong, J.-H.; Wolmark, N. Twenty-year follow-up of a randomized trial comparing total mastectomy, lumpectomy, and lumpectomy plus irradiation for the treatment of invasive breast cancer. *N. Engl. J. Med.* **2002**, *347*, 1233–1241. [CrossRef] [PubMed]
5. Veronesi, U.; Cascinelli, N.; Mariani, L.; Greco, M.; Saccozzi, R.; Luini, A.; Aguilar, M.; Marubini, E. Twenty-year follow-up of a randomized study comparing breast-conserving surgery with radical mastectomy for early breast cancer. *N. Engl. J. Med.* **2002**, *347*, 1227–1232. [CrossRef] [PubMed]
6. Sanchez, A.M.; Franceschini, G.; D'Archi, S.; De Lauretis, F.; Scardina, L.; Di Giorgio, D.; Accetta, C.; Masetti, R. Results obtained with level II oncoplastic surgery spanning 20 years of breast cancer treatment: Do we really need further demonstration of reliability? *Breast J.* **2020**, *26*, 125–132. [CrossRef]
7. Peterson, M.E.; Schultz, D.J.; Reynolds, C.; Solin, L.J. Outcomes in breast cancer patients relative to margin status after treatment with breast-conserving surgery and radiation therapy: The University of Pennsylvania experience. *Int. J. Radiat. Oncol. Biol. Phys.* **1999**, *43*, 1029–1035. [CrossRef]
8. Singletary, S.E. Surgical margins in patients with early-stage breast cancer treated with breast conservation therapy. *Am. J. Surg.* **2002**, *184*, 383–393. [CrossRef]
9. Corsi, F.; Sorrentino, L.; Bossi, D.; Sartani, A.; Foschi, D. preoperative localization and surgical margins in conservative breast surgery. *Int. J. Surg. Oncol.* **2013**, *2013*, 793819. [CrossRef]
10. Park, C.C.; Mitsumori, M.; Nixon, A.; Recht, A.; Connolly, J.; Gelman, R.; Silver, B.; Hetelekidis, S.; Abner, A.; Harris, J.R.; et al. Outcome at 8 years after breast-conserving surgery and radiation therapy for invasive breast cancer: Influence of margin status and systemic therapy on local recurrence. *J. Clin. Oncol.* **2000**, *18*, 1668–1675. [CrossRef] [PubMed]

11. Franceschini, G.; Sanchez, A.M.; Di Leone, A.; Magno, S.; Moschella, F.; Accetta, C.; Natale, M.; Di Giorgio, D.; Scaldaferri, A.; D'Archi, S.; et al. Update on the surgical management of breast cancer. *Ann. Ital. Chir.* **2015**, *86*, 89–99. [PubMed]
12. Hayes, M.K. Update on preoperative breast localization. *Radiol. Clin. N. Am.* **2017**, *55*, 591–603. [CrossRef]
13. Jeffries, D.O.; Dossett, L.A.; Jorns, J.M. Localization for breast surgery: The next generation. *Arch. Pathol. Lab. Med.* **2017**, *141*, 1324–1329. [CrossRef]
14. Jackman, R.J.; Marzoni, F.A. Needle-localized breast biopsy: Why do we fail? *Radiology* **1997**, *204*, 677–684. [CrossRef]
15. Bick, U.; Trimboli, R.M.; Athanasiou, A.; Balleyguier, C.; Baltzer, P.A.T.; Bernathova, M.; Borbély, K.; Brkljacic, B.; Carbonaro, L.A.; Clauser, P.; et al. Image-guided breast biopsy and localisation: Recommendations for information to women and referring physicians by the European Society of Breast Imaging. *Insights Imaging* **2020**, *11*, 1–18. [CrossRef]
16. Riedl, C.C.; Pfarl, G.; Helbich, T.H.; Memarsadeghi, M.; Wagner, T.; Rudas, M.; Fuchsjäger, M. Comparison of wire versus carbon localization of non-palpable breast lesions. *RöFo* **2002**, *174*, 1126–1131. [CrossRef]
17. Rose, A.; Collins, J.; Neerhut, P.; Bishop, C.; Mann, G.B. Carbon localisation of impalpable breast lesions. *Breast* **2003**, *12*, 264–269. [CrossRef]
18. Tran, Q.; Mizumoto, R.; Tran, M.; Reintals, M.; Gounder, V. Carbon-track localisation as an adjunct to wire-guided excision of impalpable breast lesions: A retrospective cohort study. *Int. J. Surg. Open* **2019**, *21*, 7–11. [CrossRef]
19. Öcal, K.; Dag, A.; Turkmenoglu, M.O.; Günay, E.C.; Yücel, E.; Duce, M.N. Radioguided occult lesion localization versus wire-guided localization for non-palpable breast lesions: Randomized controlled trial. *Clinics* **2011**, *66*, 1003–1007. [CrossRef] [PubMed]
20. De Cicco, C.; Pizzamiglio, M.; Trifirò, G.; Luini, A.; Ferrari, M.; Prisco, G.; Galimberti, V.; Cassano, E.; Viale, G.; Intra, M.; et al. Radioguided occult lesion localisation (ROLL) and surgical biopsy in breast cancer. Technical aspects. *Q. J. Nucl. Med.* **2002**, *46*, 145–151. [PubMed]
21. Luini, A.; Zurrida, S.; Paganelli, G.; Galimberti, V.; Sacchini, V.; Monti, S.; Veronesi, P.; Viale, G. Comparison of radioguided excision with wire localization of occult breast lesions. *BJS* **1999**, *86*, 522–525. [CrossRef] [PubMed]
22. Gray, R.J.; Salud, C.; Nguyen, K.; Dauway, E.; Friedland, J.; Berman, C.; Peltz, E.; Whitehead, G.; Cox, C.E. Randomized prospective evaluation of a novel technique for biopsy or lumpectomy of nonpalpable breast lesions: Radioactive seed versus wire localization. *Ann. Surg. Oncol.* **2001**, *8*, 711–715. [CrossRef] [PubMed]
23. Rao, R.; Moldrem, A.; Sarode, V.; White, J.; Amen, M.; Rao, M.; Andrews, V.; Euhus, D.; Radford, L.; Ulissey, M. Experience with seed localization for nonpalpable breast lesions in a public health care system. *Ann. Surg. Oncol.* **2010**, *17*, 3241–3246. [CrossRef] [PubMed]
24. Gera, R.; Tayeh, S.; Al-Reefy, S.; Mokbel, K. Evolving role of magseed in wireless localization of breast lesions: Systematic review and pooled analysis of 1,559 procedures. *Anticancer. Res.* **2020**, *40*, 1809–1815. [CrossRef]
25. Endomag. Available online: https://www.endomag.com/ (accessed on 11 November 2020).
26. Zacharioudakis, K.; Down, S.; Bholah, Z.; Lee, S.; Khan, T.; Howe, M.; Maxwell, A.; Harvey, J. Is the future magnetic? Magseed localisation of non palpable breast cancer—A multicentre comparative cohort study. *Breast* **2019**, *44*, S112. [CrossRef]
27. Thekkinkattil, D.; Kaushik, M.; Hoosein, M.; Al-Attar, M.; Pilgrim, S.; Gvaramadze, A.; Hyklova, L.; Jibril, A. A prospective, single-arm, multicentre clinical evaluation of a new localisation technique using non-radioactive Magseeds for surgery of clinically occult breast lesions. *Clin. Radiol.* **2019**, *74*, 974.e7–974.e11. [CrossRef]
28. Mango, V.L.; Wynn, R.T.; Feldman, S.; Friedlander, L.; Desperito, E.; Patel, S.N.; Gomberawalla, A.; Ha, R. Beyond wires and seeds: Reflector-guided breast lesion localization and excision. *Radiology* **2017**, *284*, 365–371. [CrossRef]
29. Mango, V.; Ha, R.; Gomberawalla, A.; Wynn, R.; Feldman, S. Evaluation of the SAVI SCOUT surgical guidance system for localization and excision of nonpalpable breast lesions: A feasibility study. *Am. J. Roentgenol.* **2016**, *207*, W69–W72. [CrossRef]
30. Cox, C.E.; Garcia-Henriquez, N.; Glancy, M.J.; Whitworth, P.; Cox, J.M.; Themar-Geck, M.; Prati, R.; Jung, M.; Russell, S.; Appleton, K.; et al. Pilot study of a new nonradioactive surgical guidance technology for locating nonpalpable breast lesions. *Ann. Surg. Oncol.* **2016**, *23*, 1824–1830. [CrossRef]
31. Jadeja, P.H.; Mango, V.; Patel, S.; Friedlander, L.; Desperito, E.; Ayala-Bustamante, E.; Wynn, R.; Chen-Seetoo, M.; Taback, B.; Feldman, S.; et al. Utilization of multiple SAVI SCOUT surgical guidance system reflectors in the same breast: A single-institution feasibility study. *Breast J.* **2018**, *24*, 531–534. [CrossRef]
32. Colakovic, N.; Zdravkovic, D.; Skuric, Z.; Mrda, D.; Gacic, J.; Ivanovic, N. Intraoperative ultrasound in breast cancer surgery—from localization of non-palpable tumors to objectively measurable excision. *World J. Surg. Oncol.* **2018**, *16*, 1–7. [CrossRef] [PubMed]
33. Haid, A.; Knauer, M.; Dunzinger, S.; Jasarevic, Z.; Köberle-Wührer, R.; Schuster, A.; Toeppker, M.; Haid, B.; Wenzl, E.; Offner, F. Intra-operative sonography: A valuable aid during breast-conserving surgery for occult breast cancer. *Ann. Surg. Oncol.* **2007**, *14*, 3090–3101. [CrossRef] [PubMed]
34. Fortunato, L.; Penteriani, R.; Farina, M.; Vitelli, C.E.; Piro, F. Intraoperative ultrasound is an effective and preferable technique to localize non-palpable breast tumors. *Eur. J. Surg. Oncol. (EJSO)* **2008**, *34*, 1289–1292. [CrossRef]

35. Ramos, M.; Díaz, J.C.; Ramos, T.; Ruano, R.; Aparicio, M.; Sancho, M.; González-Orús, J.M. Ultrasound-Guided Excision Combined with Intraoperative Assessment of Gross Macroscopic Margins Decreases the Rate of Reoperations for Non-Palpable Invasive Breast Cancer. *Breast* **2012**, *22*, 520–524. Available online: https://www.unboundmedicine.com/medline/citation/23110817/Ultrasound_guided_excision_combined_with_intraoperative_assessment_of_gross_macroscopic_margins_decreases_the_rate_of_reoperations_for_non_palpable_invasive_breast_cancer_ (accessed on 30 October 2020). [CrossRef]
36. Hall, F.; Kopans, D.B.; Sadowsky, N.L.; Homer, M.J. Development of wire localization for occult breast lesions: Boston remembrances. *Radiology* **2013**, *268*, 622–627. [CrossRef]
37. Homer, M.J.; Pile-Spellman, E.R. Needle localization of occult breast lesions with a curved-end retractable wire: Technique and pitfalls. *Radiology* **1986**, *161*, 547–548. [CrossRef]
38. Liberman, L.; Kaplan, J.; Van Zee, K.J.; Morris, E.A.; LaTrenta, L.R.; Abramson, A.F.; Dershaw, D.D. Bracketing wires for preoperative breast needle localization. *Am. J. Roentgenol.* **2001**, *177*, 565–572. [CrossRef] [PubMed]
39. Chan, B.K.; Wiseberg-Firtell, J.A.; Jois, R.H.; Jensen, K.; Audisio, R.A. Localization techniques for guided surgical excision of non-palpable breast lesions. *Cochrane Database Syst. Rev.* **2015**, CD009206. [CrossRef]
40. Lovrics, P.J.; Cornacchi, S.; Vora, R.; Goldsmith, C.; Kahnamoui, K. Systematic review of radioguided surgery for non-palpable breast cancer. *Eur. J. Surg. Oncol. (EJSO)* **2011**, *37*, 388–397. [CrossRef]
41. Loving, V.A.; Edwards, D.B.; Roche, K.T.; Steele, J.R.; Sapareto, S.A.; Byrum, S.C.; Schomer, D.F. Monte Carlo simulation to analyze the cost-benefit of radioactive seed localization versus wire localization for breast-conserving surgery in fee-for-service health care systems compared with accountable care organizations. *Am. J. Roentgenol.* **2014**, *202*, 1383–1388. [CrossRef] [PubMed]
42. Van Susante, J.; Barendregt, W.; Bruggink, E. Migration of the guide-wire into the pleural cavity after needle localization of breast lesions. *Eur. J. Surg. Oncol. (EJSO)* **1998**, *24*, 446–448. [CrossRef]
43. Azoury, F.M.; Sayad, P.; Rizk, A. Thoracoscopic management of a pericardial migration of a breast biopsy localization wire. *Ann. Thorac. Surg.* **2009**, *87*, 1937–1939. [CrossRef]
44. Volders, J.H.; Haloua, M.H.; Krekel, N.M.A.; Meijer, S.; Van Den Tol, P.M. Current status of ultrasound-guided surgery in the treatment of breast cancer. *World J. Clin. Oncol.* **2016**, *7*, 44–53. [CrossRef]
45. Bronstein, A.D.; Kilcoyne, R.F.; Moe, R.E. Complications of needle localization of foreign bodies and nonpalpable breast lesions. *Arch. Surg.* **1988**, *123*, 775–779. [CrossRef]
46. Svane, G. A Stereotaxic technique for preoperative marking of non-palpable breast lesions. *Acta Radiol. Diagn.* **1983**, *24*, 145–151. [CrossRef]
47. Ruiz-Delgado, M.L.; López-Ruiz, J.A.; Sáiz-López, A. Abnormal mammography and sonography associated with foreign-body giant-cell reaction after stereotactic vacuum-assisted breast biopsy with carbon marking. *Acta Radiol.* **2008**, *49*, 1112–1118. [CrossRef]
48. Salvador, G.L.O.; Barbieri, P.P.; Maschke, L.; Nunes, A.L.A.; Louveira, M.H.; Budel, V.M. Charcoal granuloma mimicking breast cancer: An emerging diagnosis. *Acta Radiol. Open* **2018**, *7*, 2058460118815726. [CrossRef]
49. Luini, A.; Zurrida, S.; Galimberti, V.; Paganelli, G. Radioguided surgery of occult breast lesions. *Eur. J. Cancer.* **1998**, *34*, 204–205. [CrossRef]
50. Grüning, T.; Brogsitter, C.; Jones, I.W.; Heales, J.C. Resolution recovery in planar bone scans: Diagnostic value in metastatic disease. *Nucl. Med. Commun.* **2012**, *33*, 1307–1310. Available online: https://journals.lww.com/nuclearmedicinecomm/Fulltext/2012/12000/Resolution_recovery_in_planar_bone_scans__.11.aspx (accessed on 27 October 2020). [CrossRef]
51. Monti, S.; Galimberti, V.; Trifirò, G.; De Cicco, C.; Peradze, N.; Brenelli, F.; Fernandez-Rodriguez, J.; Rotmensz, N.; Latronico, A.; Berrettini, A.; et al. Occult breast lesion localization plus Sentinel Node Biopsy (SNOLL): Experience with 959 patients at the European Institute of Oncology. *Ann. Surg. Oncol.* **2007**, *14*, 2928–2931. [CrossRef] [PubMed]
52. Follacchio, G.A.; Monteleone, F.; Anibaldi, P.; De Vincentis, G.; Iacobelli, S.; Merola, R.; D'Orazi, V.; Monti, M.; Pasta, V. A modified sentinel node and occult lesion localization (SNOLL) technique in non-palpable breast cancer: A pilot study. *J. Exp. Clin. Cancer Res.* **2015**, *34*, 1–7. [CrossRef] [PubMed]
53. Pavlicek, W.; Walton, H.A.; Karstaedt, P.J.; Gray, R.J. Radiation safety with use of I-125 seeds for localization of nonpalpable breast lesions. *Acad. Radiol.* **2006**, *13*, 909–915. [CrossRef]
54. Goudreau, S.H.; Joseph, J.P.; Seiler, S.J. Preoperative radioactive seed localization for nonpalpable breast lesions: Technique, pitfalls, and solutions. *Radiographics* **2015**, *35*, 1319–1334. [CrossRef]
55. Jakub, J.W.; Gray, R.J.; Degnim, A.C.; Boughey, J.C.; Gardner, M.; Cox, C.E. Current status of radioactive seed for localization of non palpable breast lesions. *Am. J. Surg.* **2010**, *199*, 522–528. [CrossRef]
56. Sharek, D.; Zuley, M.L.; Zhang, J.Y.; Soran, A.; Ahrendt, G.M.; Ganott, M.A. Radioactive seed localization versus wire localization for lumpectomies: A comparison of outcomes. *Am. J. Roentgenol.* **2015**, *204*, 872–877. [CrossRef]
57. Bloomquist, E.V.; Ajkay, N.; Patil, S.; Collett, A.E.; Frazier, T.G.; Barrio, A.V. A randomized prospective comparison of patient-assessed satisfaction and clinical outcomes with radioactive seed localization versus wire localization. *Breast J.* **2016**, *22*, 151–157. [CrossRef]
58. Langhans, L.; Tvedskov, T.F.; Klausen, T.L.; Jensen, M.-B.; Talman, M.-L.; Vejborg, I.; Benian, C.; Roslind, A.; Hermansen, J.; Oturai, P.S.; et al. Radioactive seed localization or wire-guided localization of nonpalpable invasive and in situ breast cancer: A randomized, multicenter, open-label trial. *Ann. Surg.* **2017**, *266*, 29–35. [CrossRef]

59. Harvey, J.R.; Lim, Y.; Murphy, J.; Howe, M.; Morris, J.; Goyal, A.; Maxwell, A.J. Safety and feasibility of breast lesion localization using magnetic seeds (Magseed): A multi-centre, open-label cohort study. *Breast Cancer Res. Treat.* **2018**, *169*, 531–536. [CrossRef]
60. Haloua, M.H.; Volders, J.H.; Krekel, N.M.; Lopes Cardozo, A.M.F.; De Roos, W.K.; De Widt-Levert, L.M.; Van Der Veen, H.; Rijna, H.; Bergers, E.; Jóźwiak, K.; et al. Intraoperative ultrasound guidance in breast-conserving surgery improves cosmetic outcomes and patient satisfaction: Results of a Multicenter Randomized Controlled Trial (COBALT). *Ann. Surg. Oncol.* **2016**, *23*, 30–37. [CrossRef]
61. James, T.A.; Harlow, S.; Sheehey-Jones, J.; Hart, M.; Gaspari, C.; Stanley, M.; Krag, D.; Ashikaga, T.; McCahill, L.E. Intraoperative ultrasound versus mammographic needle localization for ductal carcinoma in situ. *Ann. Surg. Oncol.* **2009**, *16*, 1164–1169. [CrossRef]
62. Gerrard, A.D.; Shrotri, A. Surgeon-led intraoperative ultrasound localization for nonpalpable breast cancers: Results of 5 years of practice. *Clin. Breast Cancer* **2019**, *19*, e748–e752. [CrossRef] [PubMed]
63. Krekel, N.M.; Cardozo, A.L.F.; Muller, S.; Bergers, E.; Meijer, S.; van den Tol, M. Optimising surgical accuracy in palpable breast cancer with intra-operative breast ultrasound—Feasibility and surgeons' learning curve. *Eur. J. Surg. Oncol. (EJSO)* **2011**, *37*, 1044–1050. [CrossRef] [PubMed]
64. Dogan, B.E.; Whitman, G.J. Intraoperative breast ultrasound. *Semin. Roentgenol.* **2011**, *46*, 280–284. [CrossRef]
65. Carlino, G.; Rinaldi, P.; Giuliani, M.; Rella, R.; Bufi, E.; Padovano, F.; Ciardi, C.; Romani, M.; Belli, P.; Manfredi, R. Ultrasound-guided preoperative localization of breast lesions: A good choice. *J. Ultrasound* **2019**, *22*, 85–94. [CrossRef] [PubMed]
66. Franceschini, G.; Visconti, G.; Sanchez, A.M.; Di Leone, A.; Salgarello, M.; Masetti, R. Oxidized regenerated cellulose in breast surgery: Experimental model. *J. Surg. Res.* **2015**, *198*, 237–244. [CrossRef]
67. Madeley, C.; Kessell, M.; Madeley, C.; Taylor, D.B. A comparison of stereotactic and tomosynthesis-guided localisation of impalpable breast lesions. *J. Med. Radiat. Sci.* **2019**, *66*, 170–176. [CrossRef]
68. Fusco, R.; Petrillo, A.; Catalano, O.; Sansone, M.; Granata, V.; Filice, S.; D'Aiuto, M.; Pankhurst, Q.; Douek, M. Procedures for location of non-palpable breast lesions: A systematic review for the radiologist. *Breast Cancer* **2012**, *21*, 522–531. [CrossRef]

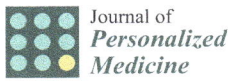

Article

GENERATOR Breast DataMart—The Novel Breast Cancer Data Discovery System for Research and Monitoring: Preliminary Results and Future Perspectives

Fabio Marazzi [1], Luca Tagliaferri [1], Valeria Masiello [1,*], Francesca Moschella [2], Giuseppe Ferdinando Colloca [1], Barbara Corvari [1], Alejandro Martin Sanchez [2], Nikola Dino Capocchiano [3], Roberta Pastorino [4], Chiara Iacomini [4], Jacopo Lenkowicz [3], Carlotta Masciocchi [4], Stefano Patarnello [4], Gianluca Franceschini [2,5], Maria Antonietta Gambacorta [1,3], Riccardo Masetti [2,5] and Vincenzo Valentini [1,3]

1 Dipartimento di Diagnostica per Immagini, Radioterapia Oncologica ed Ematologia, UOC di Radioterapia Oncologica, Fondazione Policlinico Universitario "A. Gemelli" IRCCS, 00186 Rome, Italy; fabio.marazzi@policlinicogemelli.it (F.M.); luca.tagliaferri@policlinicogemelli.it (L.T.); giuseppeferdinando.colloca@policlinicogemelli.it (G.F.C.); barbara.corvari@policlinicogemelli.it (B.C.); mariaantonietta.gambacorta@policlinicogemelli.it (M.A.G.); vincenzo.valentini@policlinicogemelli.it (V.V.)
2 Dipartimento di Scienze della Salute della Donna e del Bambino e di Sanità Pubblica, UOC di Chirurgia Senologica, Fondazione Policlinico Universitario "A. Gemelli" IRCCS, 00186 Roma, Italy; francesca.moschella@policlinicogemelli.it (F.M.); martin.sanchez@policlinicogemelli.it (A.M.S.); gianluca.franceschini@policlinicogemelli.it (G.F.); riccardo.masetti@policlinicogemelli.it (R.M.)
3 Istituto di Radiologia, Università Cattolica del Sacro Cuore, 00186 Rome, Italy; nikoladino.capocchiano@unicatt.it (N.D.C.); jacopo.lenkowicz@gmail.com (J.L.)
4 Fondazione Policlinico Universitario "A. Gemelli" IRCCS, 00186 Roma, Italy; roberta.pastorino@policlinicogemelli.it (R.P.); chiara.iacomini@guest.policlinicogemelli.it (C.I.); carlotta.masciocchi@guest.policlinicogemelli.it (C.M.); stefano.patarnello@guest.policlinicogemelli.it (S.P.)
5 Istituto di Semeiotica Chirurgica, Università Cattolica del Sacro Cuore, 00186 Rome, Italy
* Correspondence: valeria.masiello@guest.policlinicogemelli.it

Citation: Marazzi, F.; Tagliaferri, L.; Masiello, V.; Moschella, F.; Colloca, G.F.; Corvari, B.; Sanchez, A.M.; Capocchiano, N.D.; Pastorino, R.; Iacomini, C.; et al. GENERATOR Breast DataMart—The Novel Breast Cancer Data Discovery System for Research and Monitoring: Preliminary Results and Future Perspectives. *J. Pers. Med.* **2021**, *11*, 65. https://doi.org/10.3390/jpm11020065

Academic Editor: Enrico Capobianco
Received: 30 December 2020
Accepted: 20 January 2021
Published: 22 January 2021

Publisher's Note: MDPI stays neutral with regard to jurisdictional claims in published maps and institutional affiliations.

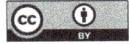

Copyright: © 2021 by the authors. Licensee MDPI, Basel, Switzerland. This article is an open access article distributed under the terms and conditions of the Creative Commons Attribution (CC BY) license (https://creativecommons.org/licenses/by/4.0/).

Abstract: Background: Artificial Intelligence (AI) is increasingly used for process management in daily life. In the medical field AI is becoming part of computerized systems to manage information and encourage the generation of evidence. Here we present the development of the application of AI to IT systems present in the hospital, for the creation of a DataMart for the management of clinical and research processes in the field of breast cancer. Materials and methods: A multidisciplinary team of radiation oncologists, epidemiologists, medical oncologists, breast surgeons, data scientists, and data management experts worked together to identify relevant data and sources located inside the hospital system. Combinations of open-source data science packages and industry solutions were used to design the target framework. To validate the DataMart directly on real-life cases, the working team defined tumoral pathology and clinical purposes of proof of concepts (PoCs). Results: Data were classified into "Not organized, not 'ontologized' data", "Organized, not 'ontologized' data", and "Organized and 'ontologized' data". Archives of real-world data (RWD) identified were platform based on ontology, hospital data warehouse, PDF documents, and electronic reports. Data extraction was performed by direct connection with structured data or text-mining technology. Two PoCs were performed, by which waiting time interval for radiotherapy and performance index of breast unit were tested and resulted available. Conclusions: GENERATOR Breast DataMart was created for supporting breast cancer pathways of care. An AI-based process automatically extracts data from different sources and uses them for generating trend studies and clinical evidence. Further studies and more proof of concepts are needed to exploit all the potentials of this system.

Keywords: breast cancer; DataMart; real world data; predictive model; healthcare

1. Background

In the last few years, breast cancer (BC) curability has been highly improved thanks to implementation of treatments and technologies [1]. In oncology, clinical research is usually supported through prospective clinical trials in which collected records are usually codified by an ontological system [2] and electronic case report forms (CRFs) [3]. However, prospective clinical trials require a considerable number of resources and time to obtain statistically meaningful outcomes. In addition, the results obtained after 5–10 years from a clinical trial often cannot reflect up-to-date technical needs and can be overtaken by new therapeutic choices [4]. Alongside the high-quality data from clinical trials, low-quality but high-quantity data generated by clinical practice are often not used because they are difficult to collect and analyze [5]. Real-world data (RWD) studies represent a possibility for obtaining evidence from clinical practice, because they are considered to be more representative of the patients and trends that are currently being treated. RWD are stored and potentially available inside hospital informatic systems, both in structured and unstructured formats, and carry truly relevant information applicable for different scopes (research, monitoring, alert, etc.).

The use of automated data discovery and Artificial Intelligence (AI) in medical research has also increased exponentially in recent years, and the continuous development of improved computer science and machine learning tools helps raise the efficiency of research by automating various processes that are usually either performed manually or in a suboptimal way [6]. Additionally, even more thriving applications of data discovery and AI in oncological sciences have led to the development of systems capable of substantially improving diagnostic and therapeutic choices [6–8]. Thanks to the automated process of AI, RWD extraction and analysis could become even more feasible without manual work, but, even more, the system could learn from RWD to predict trends and improve processes [9].

The primary aim of this work is to show an integrated, highly replicable approach where the use of modern technologies (e.g., data discovery, transformation, and AI-based technologies) is leveraged in order to extract, validate, and organize RWD data. This approach is applied to the domain of breast cancer and will allow doctors to organize information for patients' treatment history in a time-effective manner, by centralizing such data from different archives distributed in the hospital healthcare systems into a single standardized repository for breast cancer real-world data (called Breast DataMart). This procedure will, in turn, enable focused studies to be much more effective in their aims. In this work, we also highlight how this DataMart can be exploited through machine learning, to obtain models for outcome prediction and development of guardian systems set up to monitor the clinical flow of patients (pts) and provide supporting info for corrective actions, e.g., in time-sensitive treatment schedules. We describe the architectural structure of the Breast DataMart, and two proof-of-concept designs intended to show the potential of the guardian systems and the automated data-extraction procedures.

2. Materials and Methods

2.1. Domain-Specific Ontology

At the very start of the project, we focused on the definition of a terminology dictionary aligned to the requirements of the clinician team, in terms of completeness of patients' data, accuracy in the description of clinical workflow, and relationships among entities. This phase of the ontology definition was developed jointly among clinical experts and data scientists, to make sure that the mapping into the target IT framework was accurate and viable.

2.2. Multidisciplinary Team and Rapid Requirement Definition

The goal of building a framework that can be extensively leveraged across multiple studies and trials has naturally led to organize a team which could offer a comprehensive view of the needs from a clinical research side, tightly connected with the technology experts for the technical design and architectural builds. A multidisciplinary team of experts was formed by radiation oncologists, epidemiologists, medical oncologists, and breast surgeons, to approach breast cancer RWD from a clinical perspective. To develop a system able to collect, transform, and organize data from different archives within the hospital IT system, data scientists and data management experts worked to capture requirements from clinical teams and translate them into fast prototypes and implementation. Combinations of open-source data science packages and industry solutions (SAS® Viya framework) were used to design the target framework. To validate the DataMart directly on real-life cases, the working team defined tumoral pathology and clinical purposes of proof of concepts (PoCs). The PoCs were immensely helpful for a user-oriented approach to select, classify, and organize data in the DataMart. From the project-management perspective, the working group adopted a rapid development strategy, where the clinical team (i.e., end users) and technology staff were highly integrated in designing, prototyping, and validating intermediate and final outcomes.

2.3. Breast Cancer DataMart Architecture

The working team chose breast cancer as the initial pathology to be investigated for the DataMart creation process. Besides the expertise of the working team, breast cancer was properly chosen for its high range of possible variables and different archives with relevant information in the hospital IT infrastructure. The approach to extract, transform, and organize information in the target DataMart is based on a multilayer approach: The first layer is based on the hospital IT platform, in which the retrospective data are centralized and structured in accordance with the ontology defined, and prospective data items are collected daily from physicians, analysis laboratories, and electromedical devices, to then be stored and protected with the strictest physical and logical security criteria. The working team also classified sources or "Channel Doors" from which to import data. The second layer is the DataMart structured dataset; the interchange between the first and second layer is handled with a set of IT tools: automated procedures to feed a real-time flow of data stemming from the daily clinical practice; connectors to electromedical devices (e.g., to extract radiomic data); text-mining techniques, which transform unstructured text (e.g., consultancies, exam reports, and diagnoses) into clinically relevant structured data. Raw data from production repositories are extracted in pseudo-anonymized form, to protect patients' privacy. The third layer is the discovery one, where analytics, machine learning, and AI methods are applied to perform the studies (in our case, the PoC). The output of this semi-automated AI layer can be represented in formats which are relevant for the clinical staff through the development of easy-to-use graphical user interfaces or different forms based on the specific study (production of synthetic data, out-come-related risk scoring, etc.).

With this approach, the Breast Cancer DataMart was defined and structured as the shared global archive of all available breast cancer data inside the hospital IT system of Fondazione Policlinico Gemelli IRCCS, which will be continuously updated through the scheduled procedures (Figure 1).

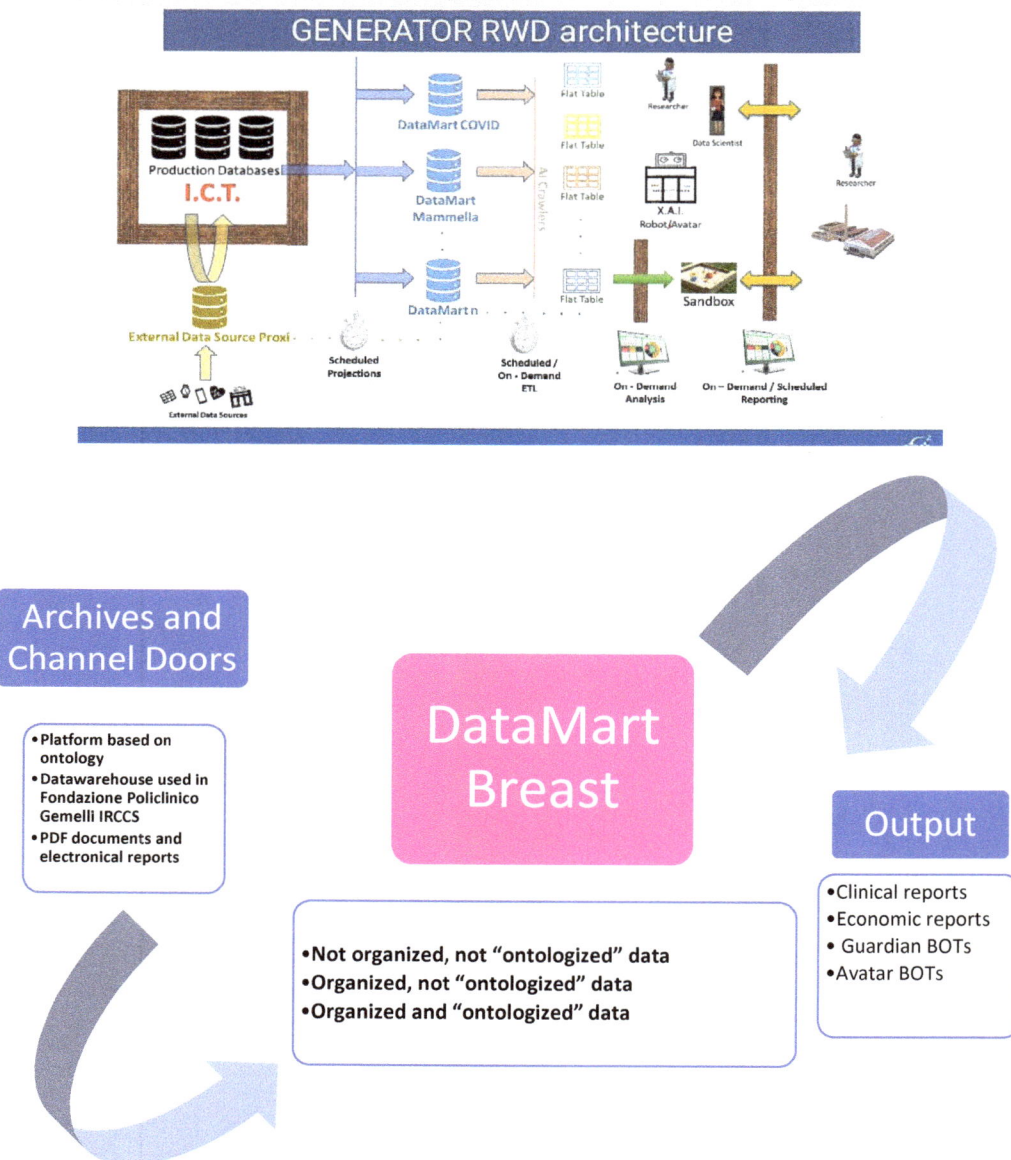

Figure 1. GENERATOR Breast DataMart architecture. In this figure, architecture of GENERATOR Breast DataMart is described. On the left, the sources are reported (a description is provided in Table 1). Thanks to Artificial Intelligence (AI) automatism, connection, and procedures, it is feasible to extract these data sources and deposit them inside Breast DataMart. An external server support Breast DataMart. Data extracted are available for further elaboration, such as creation of robots (or BOTs) for implementation of clinical research.

Table 1. Data definition and classification, according to their availability.

Data Definition and Classification		
Definition	Description	Example
Not organized, not "ontologized" data	Data to be constructed from other records and not captured by a pre-existing ontology system	For example, "Therapeutic indications from a Tumor Board"
Organized, not "ontologized" data	Records constructed but not captured by a pre-existing ontology system from begin	For example, "Data of radiotherapy beginning" or ICD9 code for diagnosis
Organized and "ontologized" data	Data captured by a pre-existing ontology system that can be directly recovered or is deposited in another software system	For example, data collected by data manager and data entry on dedicated web or hub systems

Finally, to program the DataMart implementation, the working group (WG) divided future processes into 3 distinct phases:

Phase 1: proof of concept;
Phase 2: internal consent with multidisciplinary contribution;
Phase 3: dynamic DataMart with data access for monitored and authorized internal and external requests.

To verify the usability and effectiveness of the DataMart and the overall framework, the team proposed two proofs of concept (PoCs) for testing purposes. The first one was identified as a "waiting time" calculation test from surgery to radiotherapy beginning. The second PoC was set up to calculate and test a series of key performance indicators (KPIs) based on diagnostic and therapeutic performance markers. Each end-product of the two PoCs was defined as a robot (BOT) in accordance with the AI-related features, in terms of AI data governance, automated procedures, and end-user output.

For each PoC, the definition of specific methodology and development pathways were required: DataMart access and usage (including variables selection and definition, archives and channel doors identifications, and data extraction processes), modeling phase (BOT construction), and end-user testing (BOT clinical validation).

3. Results

Starting from October 2019, the working team organized meetings on a regular basis, in order to keep the workflow initially defined. Meetings were both live and online. All the tasks planned for phase one of the DataMart development were completed.

Data definition: The WG defined data on the basic of their availability. Results are resumed in Table 1.

Archives and channel doors definition: Based on data definition, Multidisciplinary Team then defined where to find data for filling Breast Cancer DataMart and for capture them different "channel door" were identified. "Channel door" identified are reported in Table 2.

Waiting Time Bot: As already mentioned, this PoC addresses the waiting-time calculation from surgery to the start of radiotherapy. We believe this is a relevant testbed for two purposes: as a process BOT, to identify areas to improve and accelerate patients' clinical paths; and as a supporting platform for interventional studies, to track the evolution of the selected cohorts. The team identified pathways for data extraction and elaboration.

ICD9 codes for diagnosis and surgery were selected for identifying pts with breast cancer who underwent surgery. We evaluated 10 main variables to extract by the text-mining technology the time lapses in which the RT was performed: Seven were structured variable, such as the date of birth or the kind of surgery, and three were unstructured variables (multidisciplinary board indication to chemotherapy, radiotherapy, or both). Text mining selected patients with multidisciplinary indication to adjuvant chemotherapy and radiotherapy. Waiting-time interval was calculated as the interval between surgery and the first day of treatment.

Table 2. Archives and channels doors definitions.

Definition	Description	Type of Data Extraction	AI Technologies and Automatisms Performed
Platform based on ontology	Platform in use in our hospital for standardized data collection (BLADE, RedCAP, etc.). In this platform it is integrated a shared ontology that codifies data in unique, non-ambiguous way.	Organized and "ontologized" data	NEURAL NETWORKS
Datawarehouse used in Fondazione Policlinico Gemelli IRCCS	Data warehouses in use in our hospital for clinical assistance (SI, Aria, Speed (advanced evolution of Spider [10], Armonia, TrackCare, etc.). In these systems, data are codified based on clinical practice (e.g., Hb value, date of surgery, etc.), and are data validated by conventional clinical use	Organized, not "ontologized" data	NEURAL NETWORKS
Text mining extraction from PDF documents or electronic reports	All the electronic documents present in previous archives in which a procedure of text-mining extraction was applied to recover non-structured data. This is a very relevant part of data extraction, because we can recover a big quantity of granular information and translate it into structured data for usage in clinical practice and research.	Not organized, not "ontologized" data	TEXT MINING AUTOLEARN NEURAL NETWORKS

From January 2017 till December 2019, a cohort of 2074 patients underwent surgery for breast cancer. Between them, 655 pts were addressed to adjuvant RT alone, 113 to adjuvant chemotherapy alone, and 153 to both. Of this cohort, 1023 underwent RT in our hospital. Mean waiting time was 119 days (31–345). They were divided into three groups, based on waiting-time interval: 154 patients underwent RT within 60 days from the surgery; 407 patients, starting from 60 days after the index breast surgery and up to 90 days; and 462 patients who were treated after 90 days from surgery. Patients who came from other regions, and so, far from our center, experienced a wider delay in the beginning of RT.

The Wating Time BOT showed that it is feasible to extract data from different data sources inside the hospital system, to obtain an output for monitoring real-time pts' waiting time for radiotherapy treatments (Figure 2). Output of this evaluation needs to be implemented and integrated inside the hospital system, to have an alert for managing patients' waiting-time delay. Specific further prospective studies are needed to highlight predictive factors that can influence the timing of RT.

KPIs Bot: The goal of this PoC is to create, through data clustering, a group of Key Performance Indicators (KPIs) based on diagnostic and therapeutic performance [11]. Among other potential exploitations, this is a simplified example of how the DataMart can be used for rule-based patients' recruitment. ICD9 codes for diagnosis and surgery were chosen for selecting pts with breast cancer who underwent surgery. In accordance with the aim of the study, we selected nine KPIs to be extracted (Table 3). For each KPI, variables for its definition were selected and divided in structured and not structured. The last one was extracted by text mining. Artificial Intelligence automated pathway of extraction identified 2144 patients. Five different data sources were used for data extraction.

Nine structured (age, ICD9 diagnosis, ICD9 surgery, ICD9 diagnostic exams, data of beginning chemotherapy and/or radiotherapy, data of recovery and dismissal, and data of pathology exam) and four not-structured variables by text-mining elaboration (subtypes, staging, and multidisciplinary board therapeutic indications) for KPIs' calculation were identified. Extraction populated all KPIs, and mean rate of data extraction in text-mining elaboration was 78% and 88.3%, respectively, for staging and subtypes' characterization. KPIs' performance was, respectively, (1) 20.91%, (2) 17.88%, (3) 26.9%, (4) 0.25%, (5) 1.72%, (6) 44.6%, (7) 92.2%, (8) 95%, and (9) 67.3%.

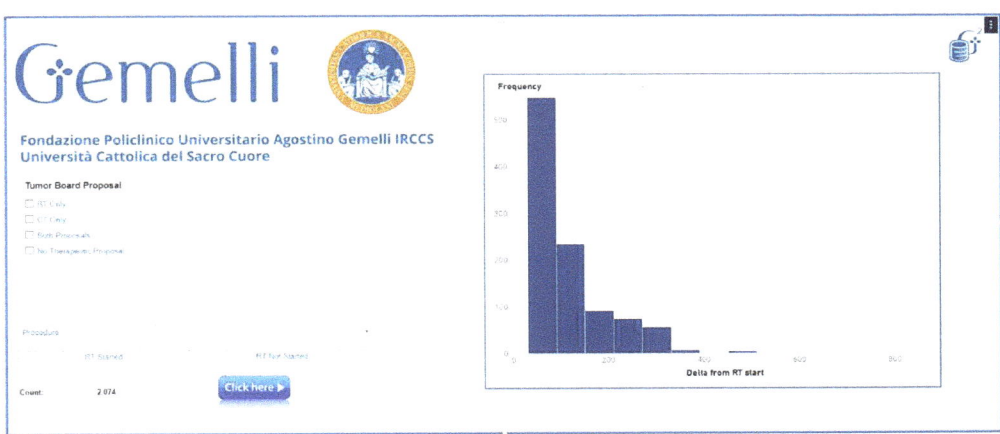

Figure 2. Waiting Time BOT platform.

Table 3. KPIs description.

KPI Name	KPI Description
KPI pre-surgery	percentage of stage I and II breast cancer patients who underwent at least one radiological exam in the 60 days prior to the breast surgery
KPI post-surgery	percentage of stage I and II breast cancer patients who underwent at least one radiological exam within the 60 days after the surgery
KPI follow-up	percentage of stage I and II breast cancer patients who underwent at least one radiological exam from 60 days after the index breast surgery and up to 365 days after this surgery
KPI Subsequent Breast Reconstruction/Axillary dissection	percentage of patients with BC who underwent subsequent surgery
KPI subsequent breast surgery	percentage of patients with BC who underwent subsequent surgery following a partial resection
KPI chemotherapy timing	percentage of patients with BC who, as candidates for chemotherapy, initiated adjuvant treatment within 60 days of the index breast surgery
KPI radiotherapy timing	Percentage of patients who initiated radiotherapy within 180 days of the last surgery
KPI time of recovery	Percentage of patients who presented a recovery time in less than 7 days
KPI pathology exam	Percentage of patients who received a pathology exam in less than 15 days

KPI, Key Performance Indicator.

KPIs' extraction was feasible, even if further validation is necessary to implement data extraction and optimize quality of data, to create a simultaneous evaluation of them, integrated inside the hospital system.

4. Discussion

Artificial Intelligence (AI) is the ability of technology applications to accomplish any cognitive task, at least as humans [12]. Even more than ever, AI is transforming our lives and job-automating processes, and it is becoming an indispensable tool for research and development of technology. Creation of a system based on AI requires the use of neural network replications that are capable of answering some questions, identifying specific patterns of data, and learning from them. For this, it is fundamental to create algorithm connections on which system AI technologies need to run. It has been already reported by Carter et al. that breast cancer care was always supported by AI applications since the 1970s, and now it is even more integrated in diagnostic systems [13], for example, in mammography implementation [12,14]. There are many single experiences of AI application in breast cancer care. An example of this issue is reported by Schaffter et al., in a study in which AI was applied to build algorithms for interpretation of screening mammography [15]. Another study by Pantanowitz L et al. reported application of AI to pathology activity of quantifying mitotic figures in digital images of invasive breast carcinoma with implementation of accuracy and overall time savings, respectively, in 87.5% and in 27.8% of cases [16].

Moreover, it is demonstrated that, thanks to AI application, it is possible to save time, lower costs, and raise efficacy [12].

In our experience, we created an AI connection to allow not only storage of all data repository of breast cancer patients who were treated in our hospital, but also a system that is capable of being interrogated for different purposes. In fact, data stored in our Breast DataMart were analyzed and used to create two systems: Waiting Time BOT for monitoring waiting time from surgery to radio-therapy, and KPIs' BOT for evaluating different aspects of breast unit performance. In both cases, BOT were comparable with clinical practice and the literature. In fact, waiting time in breast cancer represents a key point of treatments, and its delay can lead to reduced efficacy in terms of breast cancer outcomes [17–20]. In particular, a waiting time of 12 weeks or more from surgery to the start of radiation (for patients who are not candidate to adjuvant chemotherapy) and a waiting time of six weeks or more from completion of chemotherapy to start of radiation (for patients who are candidate to adjuvant chemotherapy) are associated with worse event-free survival after a median follow-up of seven years [17]. Given that radiotherapy should be started as soon as reasonably possible, a monitoring system such as Waiting Time BOT could allow not only to track possible delays in pts' pathway of care, but also to learn to predict factors that can be associated to this delay and can be prevented. On the other hand, the KPIs BOT, which allows users to track the performance of breast tumor pathway of care, is based on a system of indicators published by Altini et al. [11] in 2019. In this system, multidisciplinary evaluation is fundamental, but in the hospital system, services provided by the various departments can be reported on different informatic platforms or archives. This usually requires a data entry or data manager to report the folder manually inside CRFs for data collection [21]. In the literature, systems for tracking breast unit performance are reported, for example, EUSOMA, which is used for quality assurance [22]. However, the GENERATOR Breast DataMart does not want to replace these already established systems, but rather offers the possibility to search for data sources automatically for any type of analysis and can therefore be integrated with them.

Beyond the individual project with AI application, there is a multitude of data that could be analyzed by different prospective for implement patterns of care by the following:

- GUARDIAN ROBOT: an instrument that is able to alert the physician on determined items, capable to learn by data implementation.
- PREDICTIVE ROBOT: an instrument capable to predict trend of outcomes capable to learn by data implementation.
- DESCRIPTIVE ROBOT: an instrument capable to describe determined trends that can be used for cost/effectiveness purposes.
- AUTHOMATED ROBOT: an instrument that is linked to some diagnostic and therapeutic procedure, to reduce time of elaboration and lead physicians to more precise results.

Breast DataMart is a dynamic system based on AI, with the purpose of connecting data patterns from different sources, answer specific questions, and learn from data analyses, to implement outputs. The PoCs we performed in this study demonstrate that it is feasible to achieve this purpose for breast cancer care, using simple pathways. We interrogate the system about waiting-time data, the system returns data of interest, and it learns from them, constructing a "guardian system" to predict waiting time of patients and surgery data. On the other side, we created a second system of data elaboration by KPIs analysis. DataMart system was trained to find and return data of interest for analysis. Final elaboration allows clinicians to have a system integrated in the hospital system for on-line contemporary analysis. DataMart goals are not only to obtain a single PoC, but to have an entire data repository for breast cancer continually analyzed and processed, with the possibility to perform unlimited queries. Results of these queries can be integrated in the Hospital System for Guardian or Avatar robot system. Future application of Breast DataMart system in breast cancer care is addressed to reduce biases in patterns of care, manage heterogeneity of disease, and create algorithms for implement cost/effectiveness.

Standardized Data Collection (SDC) is a recent methodology for extract and use of real-world data. It is based on the concept that, besides structured data available by clinical trials, we have a multitude of low-quality big data inside electronic and paper folders, from which evidences can be generated, also closer to clinical practice [23–26]. AI introduction leads to the evolution concept that modern oncology not necessarily needs to be built only on SDC, but here AI application allows us to use real-world data to obtain data classificatory, predictive model, or guardian for clinical practice also in a not-time-consuming process. In this way, a system such as Breast DataMart, which we developed, becomes a dynamic application of SDC-captured data, with automated possibility of on-line queries. Moreover, DataMart AI technology, thanks to neural networks applied to building unstructured data and retrieving data through text mining, ensures that otherwise lost data are included in its system. In fact, it is possible to also recover from the hospital system PDF documents and electronic reports. The guarantee that the data contained in them are certified is linked to the officiality of these reports. Finally, since the DataMart is linked to the hospital system, its outputs can be integrated, in turn, into clinical practice, as alert systems, to obtain predictions or simply to describe useful trends to manage cost/effectiveness items.

5. Conclusions

GENERATOR Breast DataMart was created for supporting breast cancer pathways of care. An AI-based process automatically extracts data from different sources and uses them for generating trend studies and clinical evidence. For testing its use, two proof of concepts on waiting time and KPIs' calculations were built and validated. Further steps will include DataMart population with all data online in the hospital system and to start queries to implement clinical practice. Further studies and more proof of concepts are needed to exploit all the potentials of this system.

Author Contributions: Conceptualization, F.M. (Fabio Marazzi), L.T., V.M. and S.P.; Data curation, N.D.C., J.L. and C.M.; Funding acquisition, V.V.; Investigation, N.D.C., R.P., G.F. and V.V.; Methodology, N.D.C., R.P. and C.M.; Project administration, L.T., S.P. and V.V.; Software, C.I. and J.L.; Validation, F.M. (Francesca Moschella), A.M.S., M.A.G., R.M. and V.V.; Visualization, G.F.C. and B.C.; Writing—original draft, V.M. All authors have read and agreed to the published version of the manuscript.

Funding: This research received no external funding.

Institutional Review Board Statement: Not applicable.

Informed Consent Statement: Not applicable.

Data Availability Statement: The data presented in this study are available on request from the corresponding author.

Conflicts of Interest: The authors declare no conflict of interest.

References

1. Harbeck, N.; Penault-Llorca, F.; Cortes, J.; Gnant, M.; Houssami, N.; Poortmans, P.; Ruddy, K.; Tsang, J.; Cardoso, F. Breast cancer. *Nat. Rev. Dis. Primers* **2019**, *5*, 66. [CrossRef] [PubMed]
2. Tagliaferri, L.; Budrukkar, A.; Lenkowicz, J.; Cambeiro, M.; Bussu, F.; Guinot, J.L.; Hildebrandt, G.; Johansson, B.; Meyer, J.E.; Niehoff, P.; et al. ENT COBRA ONTOLOGY: The covariates classification system proposed by the Head & Neck and Skin GEC-ESTRO Working Group for interdisciplinary standardized data collection in head and neck patient cohorts treated with interventional radiotherapy (brachytherapy). *J. Contemp. Brachytherapy* **2018**, *10*, 260–266. [CrossRef]
3. Tagliaferri, L.; Gobitti, C.; Colloca, G.F.; Boldrini, L.; Farina, E.; Furlan, C.; Paiar, F.; Vianello, F.; Basso, M.; Cerizza, L.; et al. A new standardized data collection system for interdisciplinary thyroid cancer management: Thyroid COBRA. *Eur. J. Intern. Med.* **2018**, *53*, 73–78. [CrossRef] [PubMed]

4. Meldolesi, E.; van Soest, J.; Alitto, A.R.; Autorino, R.; Dinapoli, N.; Dekker, A.; Gambacorta, M.A.; Gatta, R.; Tagliaferri, L.; Damiani, A.; et al. VATE: VAlidation of high TEchnology based on large database analysis by learning machine. *Colorectal Cancer* **2014**, *3*, 435–450. [CrossRef]
5. Lambin, P.; Roelofs, E.; Reymen, B.; Velazquez, E.R.; Buijsen, J.; Zegers, C.M.; Carvalho, S.; Leijenaar, R.T.; Nalbantov, G.; Oberije, C.; et al. Rapid Learning health care in oncology'—An approach towards decision support systems enabling customised radiotherapy. *Radiother. Oncol.* **2013**, *109*, 159–164. [CrossRef]
6. Weidlich, V.; Weidlich, G.A. Artificial Intelligence in Medicine and Radiation Oncology. *Cureus* **2018**, *10*. [CrossRef]
7. Wolberg, W.H.; Street, W.N.; Mangasarian, O.L. Machine learning techniques to diagnose breast cancer from image-processed nuclear features of fine needle aspirates. *Cancer Lett.* **1994**, *77*, 163–171. [CrossRef]
8. Yang, M.; Jaaks, P.; Dry, J.; Garnett, M.; Menden, M.P.; Saez-Rodriguez, J. Stratification and prediction of drug synergy based on target functional similarity. *NPJ Syst. Biol. Appl.* **2020**, *6*. [CrossRef]
9. Holzinger, A.; Haibe-Kains, B.; Jurisica, I. Why imaging data alone is not enough: AI-based integration of imaging, omics, and clinical data. *Eur. J. Nucl. Med. Mol. Imaging* **2019**, *46*, 2722–2730. [CrossRef]
10. Valentini, V.; Maurizi, F.; Tagliaferri, L.; Balducci, M.; Cellini, F.; Gambacorta, M.A.; Lanzotti, V.; Manfrida, S.; Mantini, G.; Mattiucci, G.C.; et al. Spider: Managing clinical data of cancer patients treated through a multidisciplinary approach by a palm based system. *Public Health* **2008**, *5*, 11.
11. Altini, M.; Balzi, W.; Maltoni, R.; Falcini, F.; Foca, F.; Ioli, G.M.; Ricotti, A.; Bertetto, O.; Mistrangelo, M.; Amunni, G.; et al. Key performance indicators for monitoring the integrated care pathway in breast cancer: The E.Pic.A. project. *AboutOpen* **2019**, *6*, 31–38. [CrossRef]
12. Carter, S.M.; Rogers, W.; Win, K.T.; Frazer, H.; Richards, B.; Houssami, N. The ethical, legal and social implications of using artificial intelligence systems in breast cancer care. *Breast* **2020**, *49*, 25–32. [CrossRef] [PubMed]
13. Zhao, Z.; Pi, Y.; Jiang, L.; Xiang, Y.; Wei, J.; Yang, P.; Zhang, W.; Zhong, X.; Zhou, K.; Li, Y.; et al. Deep neural network based artificial intelligence assisted diagnosis of bone scintigraphy for cancer bone metastasis. *Sci. Rep.* **2020**, *10*, 17046. [CrossRef]
14. Xing, L.; Goetsch, S.; Cai, J. Artificial Intelligence should be part of medical physics graduate program curriculum. *Med. Phys.* **2020**. [CrossRef] [PubMed]
15. Schaffter, T.; Buist, D.S.; Lee, C.I.; Nikulin, Y.; Ribli, D.; Guan, Y.; Lotter, W.; Jie, Z.; Du, H.; Wang, S.; et al. Evaluation of Combined Artificial Intelligence and Radiologist Assessment to Interpret Screening Mammograms. *JAMA Netw. Open* **2020**, *3*, e200265. [CrossRef]
16. Pantanowitz, L.; Hartman, D.; Qi, Y.; Cho, E.Y.; Suh, B.; Paeng, K.; Dhir, R.; Michelow, P.; Hazelhurst, S.; Song, S.Y.; et al. Accuracy and efficiency of an artificial intelligence tool when counting breast mitoses. *Diagn. Pathol.* **2020**, *15*, 80. [CrossRef]
17. Raphael, M.J.; Saskin, R.; Singh, S. Association between waiting time for radiotherapy after surgery for early-stage breast cancer and survival outcomes in Ontario: A population-based outcomes study. *Curr. Oncol.* **2019**, *27*. [CrossRef]
18. Fisher, B.; Bauer, M.; Margolese, R.; Poisson, R.; Pilch, Y.; Redmond, C.; Fisher, E.; Wolmark, N.; Deutsch, M.; Montague, E.; et al. Five-year results of a randomized clinical trial comparing total mastectomy and segmental mastectomy with or without radiation in the treatment of breast cancer. *N. Engl. J. Med.* **1985**, *312*, 665–673. [CrossRef]
19. Recht, A.; Come, S.E.; Henderson, I.C.; Gelman, R.S.; Silver, B.; Hayes, D.F.; Shulman, L.N.; Harris, J.R. The Sequencing of Chemotherapy and Radiation Therapy after Conservative Surgery for Early-Stage Breast Cancer. *N. Engl. J. Med.* **1996**, *334*, 1356–1361. [CrossRef]
20. Clark, R.M.; Whelan, T.; Levine, M.; Roberts, R.; Willan, A.; McCulloch, P.; Lipa, M.; Wilkinson, R.H.; Mahoney, L.J. Randomized Clinical Trial of Breast Irradiation Following Lumpectomy and Axillary Dissection for Node-Negative Breast Cancer: An Update. *J. Natl. Cancer Inst.* **1996**, *88*, 1659–1664. [CrossRef]
21. Schnapper, G.; Marotti, L.; Casella, D.; Mano, M.P.; Mansel, R.E.; Ponti, A.; EUSOMABreast Centers Network Data Managers; Baldini, V.; Bassani, L.G.; Bissolotti, E.; et al. Data managers: A survey of the European Society of Breast Cancer Specialists in certified multi-disciplinary breast centers. *Breast J.* **2018**, *24*, 811–815. [CrossRef] [PubMed]
22. Biganzoli, L.; Marotti, L.; Hart, C.D.; Cataliotti, L.; Cutuli, B.; Kühn, T.; Mansel, R.E.; Ponti, A.; Poortmans, P.; Regitnig, P.; et al. Quality indicators in breast cancer care: An update from the EUSOMA working group. *Eur. J. Cancer* **2017**, *86*, 59–81. [CrossRef] [PubMed]
23. Tagliaferri, L.; Kovács, G.; Autorino, R.; Budrukkar, A.; Guinot, J.L.; Hildebrand, G.; Johansson, B.; Monge, R.M.; Meyer, J.E.; Niehoff, P.; et al. ENT COBRA (Consortium for Brachytherapy Data Analysis): Interdisciplinary standardized data collection system for head and neck patients treated with interventional radiotherapy (brachytherapy). *J. Contemp. Brachytherapy* **2016**, *4*, 336–343. [CrossRef] [PubMed]
24. Tagliaferri, L.; Pagliara, M.M.; Masciocchi, C.; Scupola, A.; Azario, L.; Grimaldi, G.; Autorino, R.; Gambacorta, M.A.; Laricchiuta, A.; Boldrini, L.; et al. Nomogram for predicting radiation maculopathy in patients treated with Ruthenium-106 plaque brachytherapy for uveal melanoma. *J. Contemp. Brachytherapy* **2017**, *9*, 540–547. [CrossRef]
25. Damiani, A.; Masciocchi, C.; Boldrini, L.; Gatta, R.; Dinapoli, N.; Lenkowicz, J.; Chiloiro, G.; Gambacorta, M.; Tagliaferri, L.; Autorino, R.; et al. Preliminary data analysis in healthcare multicentric data mining: A privacy-preserving distributed approach. *J. E-Learn. Knowl. Soc.* **2018**, *14*, 71–81.
26. Damiani, A.; Onder, G.; Valentini, V. Large databases (Big Data) and evidence-based medicine. *Eur. J. Intern. Med.* **2018**, *53*. [CrossRef]

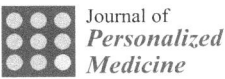

Journal of Personalized Medicine

Review

Is It Possible to Personalize the Diagnosis and Treatment of Breast Cancer during Pregnancy?

Petra Tesarova [1],*, David Pavlista [2] and Antonin Parizek [2]

[1] Department of Oncology, 1st Faculty of Medicine Charles University and General University Hospital, 128 08 Prague, Czech Republic

[2] Department of Gynecology and Obstetrics, 1st Faculty of Medicine Charles University and General University Hospital, 128 08 Prague, Czech Republic; david.pavlista@vfn.cz (D.P.); antonin.parizek@vfn.cz (A.P.)

* Correspondence: petra.tesarova@lf1.cuni.cz; Tel.: +420-224966751

Abstract: The main goal of precision medicine in patients with breast cancer is to tailor the treatment according to the particular genetic makeup and the genetic changes in the cancer cells. Breast cancer occurring during pregnancy (BCP) is a complex and difficult clinical problem. Although it is not very common, both maternal and fetal outcome must be always considered when planning treatment. Pregnancy represents a significant barrier to the implementation of personalized treatment for breast cancer. Tailoring therapy mainly takes into account the stage of pregnancy, the subtype of cancer, the stage of cancer, and the patient's preference. Results of the treatment of breast cancer in pregnancy are as yet not very satisfactory because of often delayed diagnosis, and it usually has an unfavorable outcome. Treatment of patients with pregnancy-associated breast cancer should be centralized. Centralization may result in increased experience in diagnosis and treatment and accumulated data may help us to optimize the treatment approaches, modify general treatment recommendations, and improve the survival and quality of life of the patients.

Keywords: breast cancer; pregnancy; chemotherapy; tailoring; personalization

1. Introduction

The need to protect the fetus from the adverse events associated with the treatment of cancer represents a significant barrier to the implementation of genomic and molecular biological personalization of treatment in a subgroup of pregnant patients with breast cancer. Pregnancy-associated breast cancer (PABC) is defined as breast cancer diagnosed during pregnancy (BCP) or in the first postpartum year or at any time during lactation. BCP is a special situation of concomitant pregnancy and cancer and, due to different subtypes of breast cancer, tumor detection at different stages and diagnosis confirmed at different trimesters of pregnancy does not allow the application of only one standard treatment approach. The reason is also the fact that despite the increasing experience with the treatment of such patients, the published data on PABC are still limited. Prospective studies of breast cancer during pregnancy are almost lacking, and we must rely on data from retrospective case series [1,2].

The development of personalized precision medicine as the ultimate aim of the treatment of PABC is dependent on a better understanding of the pathogenesis of PABC [3].

The advent of big genomic data has shifted our attention from examining single genes to whole exome and transcriptome analysis with the aim of identifying new predictive factors, biomarkers, and therapeutic targets although until now, still only some more frequently mutated genes are tested to achieve better cost-effectiveness, i.e., genes that seem to be associated with better cost-effectiveness, enhanced data analysis, and rapid availability for the immediate clinical decisions [4]. Unfortunately, pregnant patients with breast cancer do not yet benefit from these advances in precision medicine.

Tailoring the treatment of breast cancer in pregnancy must primarily adapt to the course of pregnancy. Due to the young age, the disease is more often associated with hereditary mutations of risk genes. Cancer is more likely to have a high histological risk profile and is diagnosed at a more advanced stage. Therefore, in clinical practice we are more often faced with the need to treat patients with a very advanced stage of cancer, frequently with the presence of metastases in the skeleton or visceral organs.

2. Epidemiology

Increasing incidence of PABC is associated with an overall increase of breast cancer in the population and increasing age at conception. PABC is still, however, relatively uncommon (with an incidence of 15 to 35 per 100,000 deliveries, more frequently occurring during the first postpartum year rather than during the pregnancy) although breast cancer is the most common type of cancer in pregnancy [5]. PABC is very rare (one per 1000 pregnancies annually, i.e., 0.07% to 0.1% of all malignant tumors, only) [6].

Pregnancy generally has a lifelong protective effect on breast cancer risk, but it increases the risk of breast cancer for several years after pregnancy with the highest risk at 6 years after delivery and significantly higher risk in older primiparas. There are important differences (in terms of diagnosis, treatment, and outcome) between PABC and breast cancer after pregnancy [2].

3. Pathophysiology

The pathogenesis of PABC is not fully understood [7]. Pregnancy and lactation are associated with increased levels of estrogens with the impairment of their normal cyclical pattern resulting in resultant molecular and histological changes in the breast gland. Increased estrogen levels may also promote the formation of metastases. Other factors, e.g., immune changes and inflammation [8], also promote carcinogenesis, especially in women with occult disease at conception (more frequent during the involution of the mammary gland) [9]. It should also be stressed that late diagnosis of breast cancer in pregnancy may also contribute to the more frequent presence of metastatic disease.

Pregnancy-associated plasma protein A (PAPP-A) may also play an important role in the development of metastatic PABC (by its collagen-modifying properties) and may help to identify patients at risk of metastatic disease [10].

4. Pathology

As in non-pregnant women, the most common form of PABC is infiltrating ductal adenocarcinoma. PABC is, however, less differentiated and (as already stressed) diagnosed at more advanced stage. Inflammatory breast cancer is also more frequent in pregnancy than in non-pregnant women [11]. The molecular pattern of PABC is different, namely in terms of more frequent mutations of the mucin gene family, mismatch repair deficiencies, and other non-silent mutations [12].

Estrogen and progesterone receptor expression seems to be decreased in PABC compared to that in non-pregnant patients with breast cancer (25% vs. 55% to 60%) [13] probably with no significant difference in overexpression of human epidermal growth factor receptor 2 (HER2) ([14,15], Table 1). Despite many differentially expressed genes, there seems to be no correlation between genetic changes and histopathological and clinical characteristics of BCP. Further studies in search of putative novel biomarkers that could identify the subpopulation of women in childbearing age at risk of PABC are warranted [16].

Table 1. Tailoring treatment according to the type of breast cancer.

Tumor Subtype	Luminal A	Luminal B	HER2+	Triple Negative
Preferred approach	Surgery, postponement of hormone therapy, and radiotherapy after delivery	Surgery, adjuvant/neoadjuvant chemotherapy, depending on the stage, postponement of hormone therapy, and radiotherapy after delivery	Surgery, adjuvant/neoadjuvant chemotherapy depending on the stage, postponement of anti-HER2 treatment, and radiotherapy after delivery	Surgery, adjuvant/neoadjuvant chemotherapy depending on the stage, postponement of radiotherapy after delivery

HER2, human epidermal growth factor receptor 2.

5. Precision Medicine in Breast Cancer

Precision medicine involves the identification of molecular signature, biomarkers, and clinical phenotype and the evaluation of their impact in combination with lifestyle and environmental factors on the prevention and treatment of the disease [17]. Cancer biomarkers may be diagnostic, prognostic, predictive, or used to monitor treatment responses. Prognostic biomarkers provide information about a patient's overall cancer outcome, irrespective of therapy [18]. They can identify high-risk patients who may benefit from more aggressive treatment but provide no information on which patients will most likely derive a clinical benefit from any specific therapy. Conversely, modifiable predictive markers responding to the treatment can indicate the probability of a patient gaining a therapeutic benefit from a specific treatment [19].

Breast cancer can be classified based on gene expression and histology including the expression of estrogen receptor (ER), progesterone receptor (PgR), and human epidermal growth factor receptor 2 (HER2) into several subtypes, characterized as luminal, normal-like, HER2-overexpressing, and triple negative breast cancer (TNBC) [20]. Gene expression profiling is more in-depth and provides more detailed stratification of breast cancer compared to histology itself. Based on these analyses, breast cancer was shown to be very heterogeneous with substantial variability in biological behavior, pathogenesis, response to treatment, and outcome [21].

Analysis based on microarray gene expression is already available, but its cost prevents its broader use in routine clinical practice with more focused analysis aimed at smaller gene sets (breast cancer index, Endopredict, the Oncotype DX 21-gene recurrence score, the BreastOncPx 14-gene distant metastasis signature, 50-gene signature called PAM50 (Prosigna), and the MammaPrint 70-gene prognosis signature) used for breast cancer stratification may emerge as more cost-effective and help clinicians to pinpoint the use of endocrine treatment and adjuvant chemotherapy [22].

To overcome the need to obtain biopsy samples from primary or metastatic lesions, great attention is paid to the blood-based biomarkers, e.g., circulating tumor cells (CTCs), exosomes and circulating tumor DNA (ctDNA), sometimes called liquid biopsy. CTCs are released from the primary tumor and are related to the propensity of the cancer to form distant metastases [23].

Genomic instability, which is common in cancer, results in genetic and epigenetic heterogeneity, and so the outcomes of patients with the same histologic type of cancer may be different in terms of response to treatment and outcome [24].

Epigenetic modification, e.g., DNA methylation and histone acetylation, is instrumental in the early phase of carcinogenesis. Recently, the role of different types of non-coding RNAs (ncRNAs) regulating gene expression and working as epigenetic modifiers has been uncovered [25].

Evaluation of the expression of both estrogen (ER) and progesterone (PR) receptors is indispensable before the introduction of hormonal treatment, and similarly, evaluation of HER2 amplification is necessary for the prediction of the response to anti-HER2 treatment. Mutation of the gene for the estrogen receptor (ESR1) predicts the risk of resistance to aromatase inhibitors. Similar markers predicting the response to radiotherapy and different modes of chemotherapy are warranted [26].

Analysis of some of these biomarkers in clinical practice may refine the search for suitable clinical trials with drugs aimed at the identified targets, but pregnant patients, unfortunately, cannot be recruited to the clinical trials. In the treatment of pregnant women, we can use neither standard, breast-cancer-specific immunohistochemical targets, such as hormone receptor or HER2 antigen positivity, nor targets derived from genomic analysis, such as PIK3 (phosphatidylkinase 3) or ESR1 (gene for estrogen receptor 1) mutations, nor those found by pathologists (TILs (tumor infiltrating lymphocytes)). Off-label treatment aimed at molecular targets not typical for breast cancer (KRas, BRAF, EGFR, etc.) cannot be used in the treatment of PABC.

Pregnancy and concomitantly diagnosed breast cancer are currently a major barrier to the use of precision medicine in the treatment of breast cancer. Its inclusion in treatment plans must be postponed until after delivery or modified so that the questions we specifically address in these situations can be answered. Due to the small number of patients and the fetuses, there are currently no (and will hardly be any in the future) clinical studies in this breast cancer subpopulation.

6. Clinical Presentation

Common signs and symptoms of cancer (lump, thickening, change in the size, shape, inverted nipple, etc.) may be hidden because of the pregnancy-associated physiological changes of the breast gland. This can delay diagnosis and adequate care. Patients with the presence of metastases may develop general symptoms, fatigue, back pain, dyspnea, pain and pressure in the right ribs, etc.

7. Diagnosis

Physical examination of the breast gland in pregnancy in search for putative cancer is difficult because of pregnancy-associated changes of the breast gland and also the utility of mammography may be limited resulting often in delayed diagnosis of PABC [27]. Any persisting (for more than two weeks) mass should be examined although 80% of the findings in breast biopsies in pregnant women are benign [28]. Mammography is not contraindicated in pregnancy with abdominal shielding (although the decrease of fetal radiation exposure with shielding remains uncertain). The sensitivity of mammography may be decreased due to higher density of the breast gland during pregnancy and lactation, but it still remains useful as a diagnostic tool. Breast ultrasonography can determine whether a breast mass is a simple or complex cyst or a solid tumor without the risk of fetal radiation exposure and may be used to guide the diagnostic biopsy. Gadolinium-enhanced MRI should be (if possible) avoided during pregnancy [29]. Needle core biopsy is the preferred method in any clinically suspicious breast mass and can be safely done during pregnancy, preferably under local anesthesia [30]. Possible infiltration of the lymph nodes by cancer cells should be further evaluated with ultrasound and fine needle aspiration biopsy for cytologic confirmation [31].

8. Staging

Modifications of the standard staging work-up should be implemented to protect the fetus (Table 2). Chest radiographs to evaluate for lung metastases should be performed with appropriate fetal shielding and limited late in gestation when the gravid uterus is pressing against the diaphragm. Computed tomography (CT) scans should be avoided during pregnancy because of the radiation exposure. Abdominal ultrasound for the evaluation of liver metastases is safe, but in pregnant women, significantly less sensitive than CT or MRI. MRI without gadolinium can be considered only if needed, especially in the first trimester, since there is a limited experience assessing safety during organogenesis [32]. Bone scans must not be used in pregnant patients for the evaluation of bone disease in the absence of signs or symptoms of bone abnormality. As an alternative, skeletal MRI may be considered (without contrast). Increases in tumor markers CA (cancer antigen) 15.3 and CEA (Carcinoembryonic antigen) always give rise to the suspicion of metastasis [33]. Locally advanced-stage disease and/or suspicious symptoms should prompt a complete radiographic staging evaluation with modifications and shielding to protect the fetus. Since the therapeutic approach to patients with early or metastatic breast cancer is not usually changed during pregnancy (neither targeted nor hormonal treatment is considered), it is possible to safely leave staging of early breast cancer examinations after delivery, preferably using PET-CT or CT scans [34].

Table 2. Tailoring treatment according to the stage of breast cancer.

Stage	Local	Local Advanced	Metastatic
Treatment approach	Surgery with subsequent adjuvant chemotherapy, hormone therapy, targeted therapy, and radiotherapy must be postponed after delivery	Neoadjuvant chemotherapy, subsequent surgery usually after delivery, hormone therapy, targeted therapy, and radiotherapy must be postponed after delivery	Palliative chemotherapy in pregnancy, targeted treatment, hormone therapy, must be postponed after delivery

9. Hereditary Breast Cancer and PABC

Genetic predisposition to breast cancer is more frequent among pregnant women with cancer. The protective effect of multiparity and breastfeeding may be lost in women who inherit BRCA2 (but not BRCA1) mutations. *BRCA1* (Breast cancer antigen 1) or *BRCA2* (Breast cancer antigen 2) mutations confer the women with a 50–80% lifetime risk of breast cancer and 16–65% lifetime risk of ovarian cancer. These risks far exceed those of breast (13%) and ovarian (1.5%) cancer in the general population [35].

Most cases of breast cancer related to BRCA1 and BRCA2 are diagnosed in young women, and the probability of pregnancy in young women is high. At present, several other genes that increase the risk of breast cancer (*PALB2, CHECK2, CDH1*, etc.) are being identified in genetic screening panels. Genetic counseling is recommended for all patient with PABC [36]. Carriers of BRCA/2 not only have a higher risk of developing PABC but also have probably poorer outcomes with higher probability of developing distant metastases [37].

If a pregnant woman carries a BRCA1/2 mutation, this information may influence the decision on the type of surgery but does not allow the use of PARP (poly-ADP ribose polymerase) inhibitors in pregnancy in case of metastatic spread.

10. Monitoring of the Pregnancy

The pregnant woman with breast cancer requires careful and continuous monitoring of her pregnancy by her obstetrician and her oncologist. Confirmation of gestational age and expected date of delivery are important, as both are significant factors in treatment planning. For this reason, follow-up should take place at the center with experience in the care of patients with BCP and the gynecologist/obstetrician should be the part of the multidisciplinary team [38]. Breast-feeding should be discontinued immediately after delivery. Since, according to clinical studies, a properly selected cancer treatment does not compromise the cognitive function of the newborn as opposed to its immaturity, it is optimal to complete pregnancy until physiological delivery, if this is possible in terms of the severity of the disease course [39].

11. Prognosis

Based on smaller studies, maternal outcome may be worse in women with breast cancer diagnosed in pregnancy [40]. The largest cohort study in women treated for PABC, however, demonstrated similar disease-free survival and overall survival comparable to those of the general population [41].

In the registry study that compared over 300 women with breast cancer during pregnancy with almost 870 women who were not pregnant at the time of diagnosis, there was no significant difference in either progression-free survival (PFS, hazard ratio (HR) 1.34, 95% CI 0.93–1.91) or overall survival (OS, HR 1.19, 95% CI 0.73–1.93) [42]. In another smaller study that included 75 women who received standard chemotherapy during the second and third trimesters, women who were pregnant had a significantly improved five-year disease-free survival (72% vs. 57%) and OS (77% vs. 71%) [43].

A 2012 meta-analysis comprising over 3000 cases of gestational breast cancer and 37,100 controls found that gestational breast cancer was associated with a higher risk of death (HR 1.44, 95% CI 1.27–1.63), however, the association appeared to be limited primarily to women diagnosed in the postpartum period (HR 1.84, 95% CI 1.28–2.65) rather than during pregnancy (HR 1.29, 95% CI 0.72–2.24) [44].

12. Treatment of BCP

Pregnant women with breast cancer should be treated according to the guidelines for non-pregnant patients, with some modifications to protect the fetus (Table 3) [42,45].

Table 3. Personalization of breast cancer treatment in pregnancy with regard to its stage (adapted according to [46–48]).

Stage	Early First Trimester Conception—4 Weeks	First Trimester 4—14 Weeks	Second Trimester 14 Weeks—28 Weeks	Third Trimester 28 Weeks—Delivery
Surgery	1–2% increased risk of miscarriage	1–2% increased risk of miscarriage	Premature delivery	Premature delivery
Radiotherapy	All or none	Gross malformation, microcephaly, mental retardation	Mental and growth retardation, cataracts, microcephaly, sterility, secondary malignancies	Growth retardation, sterility, cataracts, secondary malignancies
Gamma Knife stereotactic radiosurgery (GKSRS)	Lack of data	Lack of data	Probably safe by a conservative treatment of patients with multiple brain metastases	Probably safe by a conservative treatment of patients with multiple brain metastases
Chemotherapy	All or none	High risk of severe fetal malformation. Increased risk of miscarriage	Growth restriction, low birth weight, preterm labor, myelosuppression, need for neonatal intensive care unit admission	Growth restriction low birth weight, preterm labor, myelosuppression, need for neonatal intensive care unit admission
Anti-HER2	Fetus unaffected in review of limited case reports	Fetus unaffected in review of limited case reports	Oligohydramnios/ anhydramnios	Oligohydramnios/ anhydramnios
Hormonal therapy	Possible increased risk of miscarriage	Facial malformations, ambiguous genitalia, possible increased risk of miscarriage, some cases with no adverse effects observed, data limited to animal studies and case reports	Insufficient data	Insufficient data

Table 3. *Cont.*

Stage	Early First Trimester Conception—4 Weeks	First Trimester 4—14 Weeks	Second Trimester 14 Weeks—28 Weeks	Third Trimester 28 Weeks—Delivery
Immunotherapy	Increased risk of miscarriage	Increased risk of miscarriage	Increased risk of stillbirth, premature delivery, infant mortality	Increased risk of stillbirth, premature delivery, infant mortality
Anti-VEGF/VEGFR (Vascular endothelial growth factor/Vascular endothelial growth factor receptor)	All or none	Increased risk of miscarriage, skeletal malformations, abnormal vascular development of the skin, pancreas, kidney, and lung	Intrauterine growth restriction, preeclampsia, hypertension	Intrauterine growth restriction, preeclampsia, hypertension
PARP inhibitors	Lack of data in pregnant women	Potential to cause embryo-fetal harm, but lack of data	Potential to cause embryo-fetal harm, but lack of data	Potential to cause embryo-fetal harm, but lack of data

12.1. Surgery

Either breast-conserving surgery or mastectomy are a reasonable option for the pregnant woman with breast cancer. A choice between them is guided by tumor characteristics and the result of the genetic test and patient preferences [49]. Women with breast cancer during pregnancy should undergo an axillary node evaluation. While axillary lymph node dissection is preferred, there are increasing data on the safety and efficacy of sentinel lymph node dissection [50].

The best cosmetic results and the least complications are achieved by surgery on a hormonally unstimulated breast preferably after childbirth after lactation arrest.

12.2. Radiotherapy

If the breast-conserving surgery is performed, the adjuvant radiotherapy (RT) should be postponed after delivery. The threshold for adverse radiation effects in fetuses is less than 100 mGy. Given the high dosage of fetal radiation, radiation therapy for breast cancer in pregnancy is still considered an absolute contraindication, although this may change in coming years with improving technologies [51].

As methods of stereotactic radiation and improved modalities of delivery are developed, radiation therapy may be an option for more women during pregnancy [46].

12.3. Systemic Antitumor Therapy

- **Pharmacokinetics and Distribution of Drugs in Pregnancy**

Alterations in drug distribution are expected due to the physiologic changes that occur in pregnancy. Pregnancy leads to 40–60% increase in plasma volume even as early as 6 weeks after gestation. Increased fluid volume is associated with decreased plasma albumin, which may interfere with plasma concentration of some protein-bound drugs, e.g., taxanes, but this effect may be counterbalanced by high levels of estrogens, which increase other plasma proteins. Drug clearance by the kidney and liver increases, which may again reduce plasma levels of cytotoxic drugs. Diminished gastric motility may impact the absorption of orally administered drugs. "Third space" of the amniotic sac may play a role as well. The multidrug-resistance p-glycoprotein has been detected in fetal tissues and in the gravid endometrium and may offer some degree of protection to the fetus. However, currently it is not clear how these physiologic changes impact upon active drug concentrations and their resulting efficacy and toxicity. Moreover, pregnant women receive similar body surface-area based chemotherapy doses as non-pregnant women, which are adjusted according to continuing weight gains [52].

- **Chemotherapy**

    Patients indicated to chemotherapy during pregnancy may only start treatment after the first trimester. Data are available namely for anthracycline-based chemotherapy, often on an every-three-week schedule. Anthracyclines, more specifically doxorubicin, have not been found to significantly affect the cardiac function of children exposed in utero [53]. However, at least four cases of neonatal adverse cardiac effects have been reported after in utero exposure to anthracyclines, and there are several cases of in utero fetal death after exposure to idarubicin or epirubicin. Largely because of these reports, doxorubicin is preferred to idarubicin or epirubicin for the use in pregnancy [54]. Cyclophosphamide also has not been demonstrated to increase neonatal morbidity. In a prospective single-arm study, 87 pregnant breast cancer patients were treated with FAC (5-fluorouracil, adriamycine (doxorubicine), cyclophosphamide) in the adjuvant or neoadjuvant setting [55]. No stillbirths, miscarriages, or perinatal deaths occurred in the cohort of patients who received FAC chemotherapy during their second and/or third trimester. Most of the children did not have any significant neonatal complications. Three children were born with congenital abnormalities: one each with Down syndrome, ureteral reflux, or clubfoot. The rate of congenital abnormalities in the cohort was similar to the national average of 3%.

    Taxanes, specifically paclitaxel, have not been found to be teratogenic when administered in the third trimester. Paclitaxel is preferred over docetaxel due to the better transplacental transfer of docetaxel. Taxanes were administered in the second and third trimesters in 38 patients and for the treatment of breast cancer in 27 patients. Despite the limitations and bias inherent in case reports, the use of taxanes appears feasible and safe during the second and third trimesters of pregnancy, with minimal maternal, fetal, or neonatal toxicity [56]. Although taxanes have promising treatment outcomes, we still have information about their safety only from case reports and small case series, and therefore, we must use them with caution [57]. Platinum derivatives may play a role in the treatment of triple negative breast cancer. They are highly protein bound, but the unbound fraction may cross the placenta. Carboplatin may be associated with the derangements of trophoblast invasion and disrupting placental development, which is not complete until 20 weeks of gestation. Although the data regarding the safety of platinum in pregnancy are limited, a systematic review of the use of carboplatin and cisplatin in pregnancy found that no malformation or toxicity was reported in seven carboplatin-exposed neonates [58]. Although only limited case reports are available, anthracycline chemotherapy administered on a dose-dense schedule (i.e., treatment every two weeks) does not appear to increase the risks of maternal or fetal complications compared with treatment administered every three weeks [59]. Chemotherapy should be avoided for three to four weeks before delivery whenever possible to avoid transient neonatal myelosuppression and potential complications, including sepsis and death. Weekly regimens with low hematotoxicity are an exception [60].

- **Targeted Treatment**

    The use of trastuzumab during pregnancy is relatively contraindicated. Exposure to trastuzumab during pregnancy can result in oligohydramnios, which in some cases may lead to pulmonary hypoplasia, skeletal abnormalities, and neonatal death. Women exposed to trastuzumab during pregnancy require ongoing monitoring of amniotic fluid volume, which is a marker of fetal renal status, throughout the pregnancy [61,62]. In a case report of maternal exposure to lapatinib for 11 weeks during the first and second trimester of pregnancy, there was an uneventful delivery of a healthy female infant, who was developmentally normal at 18 months of age [63].

    However, until more information is available, we recommend against the use of lapatinib during pregnancy and lactation. There are currently no significant data on the safety of other anti-HER2 agents such as pertuzumab and ado-trastuzumab emtansine (TDM-1), and therefore, we do not recommend these agents until after delivery. However accidental short-term exposure to these agents during the first trimester does not appear to be associated with increased risk of fetal malformation, which is different compared to the risk from chemotherapy [64].

Currently we have not enough information on the safety of using bevacizumab, PARP inhibitors, and immunotherapy (PD-1 (Programmed death-1) and PDL-1 (Programmed death ligand-1) inhibitors) during pregnancy.

- **Endocrine Treatment**

The use of selective estrogen receptor modulators (SERMs) such as tamoxifen during pregnancy should be generally avoided. They have been associated with vaginal bleeding, ambiguous genitalia, miscarriage, congenital malformations (spinal abnormalities, absent ears, craniofacial abnormalities, and cardiac malformation seen in Goldenhar's syndrome), and fetal death [65]. Aromatase inhibitors (AIs) and luteinizing hormone-releasing hormone (LHRH) agonists are both contraindicated in pregnancy. AIs are not used in premenopausal women, but AIs combined with ovarian suppression by LHRH agonists may be used following term delivery.

- **Supportive Care**

Antiemetics, including selective serotonin (5-HT) and neurokinin 1 (NK1) antagonists, are used to treat severe nausea and vomiting in pregnant women and are generally considered safe. However, long-term dexamethasone therapy should be avoided, if possible, because of potential maternal and fetal risks. Safe use of G-CSF (Granulocyte-colony stimulating factor) (and recombinant erythropoietin) in human pregnancy has been reported. Although there are no prospective trials evaluating the use of G-CSF or granulocyte-macrophage colony-stimulating factor (GM-CSF) in pregnant women, these agents are safe in the treatment of neonatal neutropenia and/or sepsis, but more caution is needed considering the very limited data. Hence, dose-dense chemotherapy is not the optimal strategy in pregnant patients [66].

12.4. Postponement of Treatment

If a malignant tumor is diagnosed in the first trimester, it is possible to terminate the pregnancy prematurely or postpone treatment until the second trimester. Delay can mean the risk of progression and generalization of the disease depending on the type of cancer and its staging at the time of diagnosis and may worsen prognosis (Table 4) [67]. If the patient has a lower-grade hormone-dependent cancer limited to the breast itself, the risk of delay is lower than in triple-negative cancer with nodal involvement. Delaying chemotherapy by 3–6 months may increase the risk of metastases by 5–10% [68].

Table 4. Personalization according to patient preference.

Patient Preference	Request	A Possible Solution
Staging	Avoid all imaging methods with radiation	Tumor markers, abdominal ultrasonography, MRI without contrast, until after delivery complete staging using PET-CT (Positron emission tomography—computed tomography) or CT(Computed tomography)
Termination of pregnancy	To prioritize the life of the mother over the life of the child	Does not bring any benefits in terms of overall survival, subsequent pregnancy is possible but uncertain, interruption must be considered in the first trimester of pregnancy, if the initiation of anticancer treatment cannot be delayed
Anticancer treatment in pregnancy	Avoid anticancer treatment during pregnancy due to concerns about the baby	Treatment can be delayed with varying degrees of risk of progression and generalization depending on the type of cancer, the patient must be informed of the risks of delay and the fact that properly timed surgery and chemotherapy do not pose a serious risk to the fetus
Spontaneous vaginal delivery	Avoid a planned cesarean delivery	The reason for the planned delivery is the risk of severe neonatal life-threatening neutropenia of the fetus after chemotherapy, in pregnant women treated with a weekly chemotherapy regimen (e.g., taxol), it is possible to consider spontaneous delivery

12.5. The Course of Pregnancy, Fetal Monitoring, and Childbirth

Based on the available evidence, chemotherapy in BC patients may be safe during the second and third trimesters, with cessation of treatment three weeks prior to expected delivery. The most common complications of pregnancy associated with the application of chemotherapy are intrauterine growth retardation, prematurity, low birth weight, and bone marrow toxicity. Prematurity is generally associated with worse neonatal and long-term outcomes and, thus, should be avoided. Fetal condition can be well monitored by regular ultrasound biometrics and Doppler flowmetry. If premature birth is necessary, induction of fetal pulmonary maturity by corticoid administration is indicated. Most women expect vaginal delivery at term, but due to chemotherapy, delivery must be planned and induced, and immediately after delivery, lactation must be stopped.

13. Infant Outcome

Data suggest that early development among children born to women with cancer appears similar to that of children of the same gestational age, irrespective of in utero exposure to radiation or chemotherapy.

In a study of 129 children born to mothers diagnosed with cancer during pregnancy (over half of whom had breast cancer), cardiac, cognitive, and general development after a median of 22 months was equivalent with controls matched for gestational age [69]. In a subgroup analysis of children exposed to anticancer therapy in utero, similar outcomes were reported for the 96 children exposed to chemotherapy after the first trimester and the 11 children exposed to radiation compared with gestational-age-matched controls. There was a non-significant trend toward higher rates of small for gestational age at birth infants born to women with cancer (22% vs. 15%), particularly if exposed to chemotherapy or radiation. While the median gestational age of the children born to women with cancer was 36 weeks and, thus late preterm, it is unclear whether these children were born early because of early induction given their mothers' diagnosis of cancer.

In the cohort study of 1170 pregnant women with all types of cancer treated at multiple institutions, 39% of whom had breast cancer, 88% of pregnancies resulted in live births [70]. Half of these deliveries were preterm, almost 90% of which were iatrogenic. These studies suggest that low neonatal complication rates are associated with in utero exposure to chemotherapy, but long-term data are limited. Moreover, studies may be limited by the fact that treatment providers may sometimes opt for early delivery induction, even when pregnancy does not affect treatment. One study reported 40% mortality among patients with advanced BCP who received chemotherapy when studied over a 13-year period (1991–2004) [71]. For women with breast cancer during pregnancy, the risk of cancer to the unborn is unknown, although there are no reported cases of childhood cancer arising in children exposed to chemotherapy of their mothers for breast cancer in utero.

14. Termination of Pregnancy

Early termination of pregnancy does not improve the outcome of BCP. In fact, some series suggest decreased survival in pregnant women who electively terminate their pregnancies compared with that in those who continue the pregnancy. However, these studies are retrospective case reviews and possible bias cannot be excluded; women with more advanced disease or poorer prognostic features possibly were more likely to be counseled to have an abortion [71]. The decision to terminate pregnancy for health reasons is difficult and should always be comprehensively considered in terms of the risk of fetal cancer treatment, the patient's prognosis, and the impact of cancer therapy on the mother's fertility. Although this situation is quite ambiguous, many physicians recommend to the patients with BCP to end pregnancy and so often deprive the patient of their only chance of having a child (Table 4).

15. Metastatic BCP

During pregnancy we can also diagnose patients with de novo metastatic breast cancer, and some patients with early breast cancer treated in a neo/adjuvant setting later metastasize. The main problem of the care of the metastatic breast cancer in pregnancy is limited treatment options with respect to the fetus. The main goal of therapy is to prolong the patient's life, maintain its quality, not to damage the fetus, and for mother to spend as much time as possible with the child. This situation is extremely physically and psychologically demanding for the patient and affects the whole extended family [72].

16. Tailoring Treatment of Breast Cancer in Pregnancy

Personalized medicine has changed our approach from a "one size fits all" to the treatment of patients in a more individually tailored way. The goal of clinical research programs with a personalized approach to patients with breast cancer is to evaluate the unique code of RNA and DNA of cancer, enabling individualization of the treatment plan [73].

During pregnancy, tailoring to immunohistochemical markers such as hormone receptors, HER2 or PDL-1 expression, cannot be used at present, due to the risk of fetal harm. Genome testing and the use of next-generation sequencing (NGS) could, in the future, refine the prognosis of cancer and its sensitivity to chemotherapy, as the only acceptable systemic treatment in pregnancy.

From 2010 to 2020, 53 patients with BCP were treated at the Department of Oncology of the First Faculty of Medicine and the General Hospital in Prague. The number and proportion of patients has been influenced by the fact that in our comprehensive cancer center we have a program dedicated to young patients under 35 years of age and pregnant patients with breast cancer are referred to us from almost all over the Czech Republic (Table 5).

Table 5. Patients with breast cancer occurring during pregnancy (BCP) were treated at the Department of Oncology of the First Faculty of Medicine and the General Hospital in Prague (2010–2020).

N	Termination Pregnancy	BRCA1+/ BRCA2+	Local Recurrence	De Novo Metastatic	Systemic Recurrence	Median Age
53	3	4/2	1	7	14	31 years

17. Conclusions

BCP is an example of cancer where individualization of the treatment approach could significantly improve the results of treatment and the hope of patients with concomitant breast cancer and pregnancy to prolong survival. The therapeutic plan must be adapted to the clinical parameters, the degree of pregnancy, the type and stage of the tumor, and the patient's preference. The current options for a personalized treatment approach are not yet widely used in this subgroup of patients, although, in the future it would certainly be possible to focus molecular biology, NGS, and liquid biopsy methods to refine staging, estimate tumor chemosensitivity, and cancer prognosis to assess possible postponement of treatment to the postpartum period. Physicians treating patients with breast cancer in pregnancy have increased responsibility because they are trying to save two lives. While information and data on BCPs are increasing, it is necessary to centralize the treatment of BCP in the hands of experienced oncologists and obstetricians with praxis in this type of high-risk pregnancy and personalized access to each pregnant patient.

Author Contributions: P.T. prepared the draft of the paper which was then extensively consulted with both of them and D.P. and A.P. added valuable information from the gynecologist's point view. All authors collaborated on the analysis of available data and their interpretation and contributed significantly to the final version of the manuscript. All authors have read and agreed to the published version of the manuscript.

Funding: The work on the paper was supported by the research initiative the Ministry of Health of the Czech Republic Progress Q28/LF1 and DRO VFN 64165.

Conflicts of Interest: No potential conflict of interest is to be disclosed.

References

1. Peccatori, F.A.; Lambertini, M.; Scarfone, G.; Del Pup, L.; Codacci-Pisanelli, G. Biology, staging, and treatment of breast cancer during pregnancy: Reassessing the evidences. *Cancer Biol. Med.* **2018**, *15*, 6–13. [CrossRef] [PubMed]
2. Borges, V.F.; Schedin, P.J. Pregnancy-associated breast cancer: An entity needing refinement of the definition. *Cancer* **2012**, *118*, 3226–3228. [CrossRef]
3. Hanahan, D.; Weinberg, R.A. Hallmarks of cancer: The next generation. *Cell* **2011**, *144*, 646–674. [CrossRef] [PubMed]
4. Low, S.K.; Zembutsu, H.; Nakamura, Y. Breast cancer: The translation of big genomic data to cancer precision medicine. *Cancer Sci.* **2018**, *109*, 497–506. [CrossRef] [PubMed]
5. Parazzini, F.; Franchi, M.; Tavani, A.; Negri, E.; Peccatori, F.A. Frequency of pregnancy related cancer: A population based linkage study in Lombardy, Italy. *Int. J. Gynecol. Cancer* **2017**, *27*, 613–619. [CrossRef] [PubMed]
6. Litton, J.K. Gestational Breast Cancer: Epidemiology and Diagnosis. 2020. Available online: https://www.uptodate.com/contents/gestational-breast-cancer-epidemiology-and-diagnosis (accessed on 19 November 2020).
7. Wohlfahrt, J.; Andersen, P.K.; Mouridsen, H.T.; Melbye, M. Risk of late-stage breast cancer after childbirth. *Am. J. Epidemiol.* **2001**, *153*, 1079–1084. [CrossRef] [PubMed]
8. Ruiz, R.; Herrero, C.; Strasser-Weippl, K.; Touya, D.; St Louis, J.; Bukowski, A.; Goss, P.E. Epidemiology and pathophysiology of pregnancy-associated breast cancer: A review. *Breast* **2017**, *35*, 136–141. [CrossRef]
9. Schedin, P. Pregnancy-associated breast cancer and metastasis. *Nat. Rev. Cancer* **2006**, *6*, 281–291. [CrossRef]
10. Slocum, E.; Craig, A.; Villanueva, A.; Germain, D. Parity predisposes breasts to the oncogenic action of PAPP-A and activation of the collagen receptor DDR2. *Breast Cancer Res.* **2019**, *21*, 56. [CrossRef]
11. Callihan, E.G.; Gao, D.; Jindal, S.; Lyons, T.R.; Manthey, E.; Edgerton, S.; Urquhart, A.; Schedin, P.; Borges, V.F. Postpartum diagnosis demonstrates a high risk for metastasis and merits an expanded definition of pregnancy-associated breast cancer. *Breast Cancer Res. Treat.* **2013**, *138*, 549–559. [CrossRef]
12. Nguyen, B.; Venet, D.; Azim, H.A., Jr.; Brown, D.; Desmedt, C.; Lambertini, M.; Majjaj, S.; Pruneri, G.; Peccatori, F.; Piccart, M.; et al. Breast cancer diagnosed during pregnancy is associated with enrichment of non-silent mutations, mismatch repair deficiency signature and mucin mutations. *NPJ Breast Cancer* **2018**, *4*, 23. [CrossRef] [PubMed]
13. Middleton, L.P.; Amin, M.; Gwyn, K.; Theriault, R.; Sahin, A. Breast carcinoma in pregnant women: Assessment of clinicopathologic and immunohistochemical features. *Cancer* **2003**, *98*, 1055–1060. [CrossRef] [PubMed]
14. Reed, W.; Hannisdal, E.; Skovlund, E.; Thoresen, S.; Lilleng, P.; Nesland, J.M. Pregnancy and breast cancer: A population-based study. *Virchows Arch.* **2003**, *443*, 44–50. [CrossRef] [PubMed]
15. Collins, L.C.; Gelber, S.; Marotti, J.D.; White, S.; Ruddy, K.; Brachtel, E.F.; Schapira, L.; Come, S.E.; Borges, V.F.; Schedin, P.; et al. Molecular phenotype of breast cancer according to time since last pregnancy in a large cohort of young women. *Oncologist* **2015**, *20*, 713–718. [CrossRef] [PubMed]
16. Korakiti, A.-M.; Moutafi, M.; Zografos, E.; Dimopoulos, M.A.; Zagouri, F. The genomic profile of pregnancy-associated breast cancer: A systematic review. *Front. Oncol.* **2020**, *10*, 1773. [CrossRef]
17. Ghasemi, M.; Nabipour, I.; Omrani, A.; Alipour, Z.; Assadi, M. Precision medicine and molecular imaging: New targeted approaches toward cancer therapeutic and diagnosis. *Am. J. Nuclear Med. Mol. Imaging* **2016**, *6*, 310–327.
18. Mandrekar, S.J.; Sargent, D.J. Clinical trial designs for predictive biomarker validation: Theoretical considerations and practical challenges. *J. Clin. Oncol.* **2009**, *27*, 4027–4034. [CrossRef]
19. Polley, M.Y.C.; Freidlin, B.; Korn, E.L.; Conley, B.A.; Abrams, J.S.; McShane, L.M. Statistical and practical considerations for clinical evaluation of predictive biomarkers. *J. Natl. Cancer Inst.* **2013**, *105*, 1677–1683. [CrossRef]
20. Sotiriou, C.; Neo, S.Y.; McShane, L.M.; Korn, E.L.; Long, P.M.; Jazaeri, A.; Martiat, P.; Fox, S.B.; Harris, A.L.; Liu, E.T. Breast cancer classification and prognosis based on gene expression profiles from a population-based study. *Proc. Natl. Acad. Sci. USA* **2003**, *100*, 10393–10398. [CrossRef]
21. Wang, Y.; Yin, Q.; Yu, Q.; Zhang, J.; Liu, Z.; Wang, S.; Lv, S.; Niu, Y. A retrospective study of breast cancer subtypes: The risk of relapse and the relations with treatments. *Breast Cancer Res. Treat.* **2011**, *130*, 489–498. [CrossRef]
22. Meehan, J.; Gray, M.; Martínez-Pérez, C.; Kay, C.; Pang, L.Y.; Fraser, J.A.; Poole, A.V.; Kunkler, I.H.; Langdon, S.P.; Argyle, D.; et al. Precision Medicine and the Role of Biomarkers of Radiotherapy Response in Breast Cancer. *Front Oncol.* **2020**, *10*, 628. [CrossRef] [PubMed]
23. Pantel, K.; Speicher, M.R. The biology of circulating tumor cells. *Oncogene* **2016**, *35*, 1216–1224. [CrossRef]
24. Burrell, R.A.; McGranahan, N.; Bartek, J.; Swanton, C. The causes and consequences of genetic heterogeneity in cancer evolution. *Nature* **2013**, *501*, 338–345. [CrossRef] [PubMed]
25. Pasculli, B.; Barbano, R.; Parrella, P. Epigenetics of breast cancer: Biology and clinical implication in the era of precision medicine. *Semin Cancer Biol.* **2018**, *51*, 22–35. [CrossRef]
26. Nicolini, A.; Ferrari, P.; Duffy, M.J. Prognostic and predictive biomarkers in breast cancer: Past, present and future. *Semin Cancer Biol.* **2018**, *52*, 56–73. [CrossRef] [PubMed]

27. Lethaby, A.E.; O'Neill, M.A.; Mason, B.H.; Holdaway, I.M.; Harvey, V.J. Overall survival from breast cancer in women pregnant or lactating at or after diagnosis. Auckland Breast Cancer Study Group. *Int. J. Cancer* **1996**, *67*, 751–755. [CrossRef]
28. Byrd, B.F., Jr.; Bayer, D.S.; Robertson, J.C.; Stephenson, S.E., Jr. Treatment of breast tumors associated with pregnancy and lactation. *Ann. Surg.* **1962**, *155*, 940–947. [CrossRef]
29. Yang, W.T.; Dryden, M.J.; Gwyn, K.; Whitman, G.J.; Theriault, R. Imaging of breast cancer diagnosed and treated with chemotherapy during pregnancy. *Radiology* **2006**, *239*, 52–60. [CrossRef]
30. Collins, J.C.; Liao, S.; Wile, A.G. Surgical management of breast masses in pregnant women. *J. Reprod. Med.* **1995**, *40*, 785–788. [CrossRef]
31. Annane, K.; Bellocq, J.P.; Brettes, J.P.; Mathelin, C. Infiltrative breast cancer during pregnancy and conservative surgery. *Fetal. Diagn. Ther.* **2005**, *20*, 442–444. [CrossRef]
32. Case, A.S. Pregnancy-associated Breast Cancer. *Clin. Obstet. Gynecol.* **2016**, *59*, 779–788. [CrossRef] [PubMed]
33. Nicklas, A.H.; Baker, M.E. Imaging strategies in the pregnant cancer patient. *Semin. Oncol.* **2000**, *27*, 623–632. [PubMed]
34. Chen, M.M.; Coakley, F.V.; Kaimal, A.; Laros, R.K., Jr. Guidelines for computed tomography and magnetic resonance imaging use during pregnancy and lactation. *Obstet. Gynecol.* **2008**, *112*, 333–340. [CrossRef] [PubMed]
35. Chen, J.; Prasath, V.; Axilbund, J.; Habibi, M. Concerns of Hereditary Breast Cancer in Pregnancy and Lactation. *Adv. Exp. Med. Biol.* **2020**, *1252*, 129–132. [CrossRef]
36. Cullinane, C.A.; Lubinski, J.; Neuhausen, S.; Ghadirian, P.; Lynch, H.T.; Isaacs, C.; Weber, B.; Moller, P.; Offit, K.; Kim-Sing, C.; et al. Effect of pregnancy as a risk factor for breast cancer in BRCA1/BRCA2 mutation carriers. *Int. J. Cancer* **2005**, *117*, 988–991. [CrossRef]
37. Johansson, O.; Loman, N.; Borg, A.; Olsson, H. Pregnancy-associated breast cancer. *Lancet* **1998**, *352*, 1359–1360. [CrossRef]
38. Azim, H.A., Jr.; Del Mastro, L.; Scarfone, G.; Peccatori, F.A. Treatment of breast cancer during pregnancy: Regimen selection, pregnancy monitoring and more. *Breast* **2011**, *20*, 1–6. [CrossRef]
39. Keyser, E.A.; Staat, B.C.; Fausett, M.B.; Shields, A.D. Pregnancy-associated breast cancer. *Rev. Obstet. Gynecol.* **2012**, *5*, 94–99.
40. Hartman, E.K.; Eslick, G.D. The prognosis of women diagnosed with breast cancer before, during and after pregnancy: A meta-analysis. *Breast Cancer Res. Treat.* **2016**, *160*, 347–360. [CrossRef]
41. Amant, F.; von Mickwitz, G.; Han, S.N.; Bontenbal, M.; Ring, A.E.; Giermek, J.; Wildiers, H.; Fehm, T.; Linn, S.C.; Schlehe, B.; et al. Prognosis of women with primary breast cancer diagnosed during pregnancy: Results from an international collaborative study. *J. Clin. Oncol.* **2013**, *31*, 2532–2539. [CrossRef]
42. Peccatori, F.A.; Azim, H.A., Jr.; Orecchia, R.; Hoekstra, H.J.; Pavlidis, N.; Kesic, V.; Pentheroudakis, G.; ESMO Guidelines Working Group. Cancer, pregnancy and fertility. ESMO Clinical Practice Guidelines for diagnosis, treatment and follow-up. *Ann. Oncol.* **2013**, *24*, vi160–vi170. [CrossRef] [PubMed]
43. Litton, J.K.; Warneke, C.L.; Hahn, K.M.; Palla, S.L.; Kuerer, H.M.; Perkins, G.H.; Mittendorf, E.A.; Barnett, C.; Gonzalez-Angulo, A.M.; Horgobágyi, G.N.; et al. Case control study of women treated with chemotherapy for breast cancer during pregnancy as compared with nonpregnant patients with breast cancer. *Oncologist* **2013**, *18*, 369–376. [CrossRef] [PubMed]
44. Azim, H.A.; Santoro, L., Jr.; Russell-Edu, W.; Pentheroudakis, G.; Pavlidis, N.; Peccatori, F.A. Prognosis of pregnancy-associated breast cancer: A meta-analysis of 30 studies. *Cancer Treat. Rev.* **2012**, *38*, 834–842. [CrossRef] [PubMed]
45. Loibl, S.; Schmidt, A.; Gentilini, O.; Kaufman, B.; Kuhl, C.; Denkert, C.; von Mickwitz, G.; Parokonnaya, A.; Stensheim, H.; Thomssen, C.; et al. Breast cancer diagnosed during pregnancy: Adapting recent advances in breast cancer care for pregnant patients. *JAMA Oncol.* **2015**, *1*, 1145–1153. [CrossRef]
46. Folsom, S.M.; Woodruff, T.K. Good news on the active management of pregnant cancer patients. *F1000 Res.* **2020**, *9*. [CrossRef]
47. Paulsson, K.; Braunstein, S.; Phillips, J.; Theodosopoulos, P.V.; McDermott, M.; Sneed, P.K.; Ma, L. Patient-specific fetal dose determinatioin for multi-target gamma knife radiosurgery: Computational model and case report. *Cureus* **2017**, *9*, e1527.
48. Ringley, J.T.; Moore, D.C.; Patel, J.; Rose, M.S. Poly (ADP-ribose) polymerase inhibitors in the management of ovarian cancer: A drug class review. *Pharm. Ther.* **2018**, *32*, 549–556.
49. Litton, J.K. Gestational Breast Cancer: Treatment. 2020. Available online: https://www.uptodate.com/contents/gestational-breast-cancer-treatment (accessed on 19 November 2020).
50. Khera, S.Y.; Kiluk, J.V.; Hasson, D.M.; Meade, T.M.; Meyers, M.P.; Dupont, E.L.; Berman, C.G.; Cox, C.E. Pregnancy-associated breast cancer patients can safely undergo lymphatic mapping. *Breast J.* **2008**, *14*, 250–254. [CrossRef]
51. Boere, I.; Lok, C.; Vandenbroucke, T.; Amant, F. Cancer in pregnancy: Safety and efficacy of systemic therapies. *Curr. Opin. Oncol.* **2017**, *29*, 328–334. [CrossRef]
52. Wiebe, V.J.; Sipila, P.E. Pharmacology of antineoplastic agents in pregnancy. *Crit. Rev. Oncol. Hematol.* **1994**, *16*, 75–112. [CrossRef]
53. Gziri, M.M.; Hui, W.; Amant, F.; Van Calsteren, K.; Ottevanger, N.; Kapusta, L.; Mertens, L. Myocardial function in children after fetal chemotherapy exposure. A tissue Doppler and myocardial deformation imaging study. *Eur. J. Pediatr.* **2013**, *172*, 163–170. [CrossRef]
54. Cardonick, E.; Iacobucci, A. Use of chemotherapy during human pregnancy. *Lancet Oncol.* **2004**, *5*, 283–291. [CrossRef]
55. Murthy, R.K.; Theriault, R.L.; Barnett, C.M.; Hodge, S.; Ramirez, M.M.; Milbourne, A.; Rimes, S.A.; Hortobagyi, G.N.; Valero, V.; Litton, J.K. Outcomes of children exposed in utero to chemotherapy for breast cancer. *Breast Cancer Res.* **2014**, *16*, 500. [CrossRef]

56. Amant, F.; Deckers, S.; Van Calsteren, K.; Loibl, S.; Halaska, M.; Brepoels, L.; Beijnen, J.; Cardoso, F.; Gentilini, O.; Lagae, L.; et al. Breast cancer in pregnancy: Recommendations of an international consensus meeting. *Eur. J. Cancer* **2010**, *46*, 3158–3168. [CrossRef]
57. Hahn, K.M.; Johnson, P.H.; Gordon, N.; Kuerer, H.; Middleton, L.; Ramirez, M.; Yang, W.; Perkins, G.; Hortobagyi, N.; Theriault, R.L. Treatment of pregnant breast cancer patients and outcomes of children exposed to chemotherapy in utero. *Cancer* **2006**, *107*, 1219–1226. [CrossRef]
58. Mir, O.; Berveiller, P.; Ropert, S.; Goffinet, F.; Goldwasser, F. Use of platinum derivatives during pregnancy. *Cancer* **2008**, *113*, 3069–3074. [CrossRef]
59. Cardonick, E.; Gilmandyar, D.; Somer, R.A. Maternal and neonatal outcomes of dose-dense chemotherapy for breast cancer in pregnancy. *Obstet. Gynecol.* **2012**, *120*, 1267–1272. [CrossRef]
60. Ring, A.E.; Smith, I.E.; Jones, A.; Shannon, C.; Galani, E.; Ellis, P.A. Chemotherapy for breast cancer during pregnancy: An 18-year experience from five London teaching hospitals. *J. Clin. Oncol.* **2005**, *23*, 4192–4197. [CrossRef]
61. Zagouri, F.; Sergentanis, T.N.; Chrysikos, D.; Papadimitriou, C.A.; Dimopoulos, M.A.; Bartsch, R. Trastuzumab administration during pregnancy: A systematic review and meta-analysis. *Breast Cancer Res. Treat.* **2013**, *137*, 349–357. [CrossRef]
62. Lambertini, M.; Martel, S.; Campbell, C.; Guillaume, S.; Hilbers, F.S.; Schuehly, U.; Korde, L.; Azim, H.A.; Di Cosimo, S., Jr.; Tenglin, R.C.; et al. Pregnancies during and after trastuzumab and/or lapatinib in patients with human epidermal growth factor receptor 2–positive early breast cancer: Analysis from the NeoALTTO (BIG 1-06) and ALTTO (BIG 2-06) trials. *Cancer* **2019**, *125*, 307–316. [CrossRef]
63. Kelly, H.; Graham, M.; Humes, E.; Dorflinger, L.J.; Boggess, K.A.; O'Neil, B.H.; Harris, J.; Spector, N.L.; Dees, E.C. Delivery of a healthy baby after first-trimester maternal exposure to lapatinib. *Clin. Breast Cancer* **2006**, *7*, 339–341. [CrossRef]
64. Lambertini, M.; Di Maio, M.; Pagani, O.; Curigliano, G.; Poggio, F.; Del Mastro, L.; Paluch-Shimon, S.; Loibl, S.; Partridge, A.H.; Demeestere, I.; et al. The BCY3/BCC 2017 survey on physicians' knowledge, attitudes and practice towards fertility and pregnancy-related issues in young breast cancer patients. *Breast* **2018**, *4*, 41–49. [CrossRef]
65. Buonomo, B.; Brunello, A.; Noli, S.; Miglietta, L.; Del Mastro, L.; Lambertini, M.; Peccatori, F.A. Tamoxifen exposure during pregnancy: A systematic review and three more cases. *Breast Care* **2020**, *15*, 148–156. [CrossRef]
66. Bilgin, K.; Yaramiş, A.; Haspolat, K.; Taş, M.A.; Gunbey, S.; Derman, O. A randomized trial of granulocyte-macrophage colony-stimulating factor in neonates with sepsis and neutropenia. *Pediatrics* **2001**, *107*, 36–41. [CrossRef]
67. Rojas, K.E.; Bilbro, N.; Manasseh, D.M.; Borgen, P.I.J. A review of pregnancy-associated breast cancer: Diagnosis, local and systemic treatment and prognosis. *Womens Health* **2019**, *28*, 778–784. [CrossRef]
68. Nettleton, J.; Long, J.; Kuban, D.; Wu, R.; Shaeffer, J.; El-Mahdi, A. Breast cancer during pregnancy: Quantifying the risk of treatment delay. *Obstet. Gynecol.* **1996**, *87*, 414–418. [CrossRef]
69. Amant, F.; Vandenbroucke, T.; Verheecke, M.; Fungalli, M.; Halaska, M.J.; Boere, I.; Han, S.; Gziri, M.M.; Peccatori, F.; Rob, L.; et al. Pediatric outcome after maternal cancer diagnosed during pregnancy. *N. Engl. J. Med.* **2015**, *373*, 1824–1834. [CrossRef]
70. de Haan, J.; Verheecke, M.; Van Calsteren, K.; Van Calster, B.; Shmakov, R.G.; Gziri, M.; Halaska, M.J.; Fruscio, R.; Lok, C.A.R.; Boere, I.A.; et al. Oncological management and obstetric and neonatal outcomes for women diagnosed with cancer during pregnancy: A 20-year international cohort study of 1170 patients. *Lancet Oncol.* **2018**, *19*, 337–346. [CrossRef]
71. Rodriguez, A.O.; Chew, H.; Cress, R.; Xing, G.; McElvy, S.; Danielsen, B.; Smith, L. Evidence of poorer survival in pregnancy associated breast cancer. *Obstet. Gynecol.* **2008**, *112*, 71–78. [CrossRef]
72. Tang, T.; Liu, Y.; Yang, C.; Ma, L. Diagnosis and treatment of advanced HER2-positive breast cancer in young pregnant female: A case report. *Medicine* **2020**, *99*, e22929. [CrossRef]
73. Kern, R.; Correa, S.C.; Scandolara, T.B.; Carla da Silva, J.; Pires, B.R.; Panis, C. Current advances in the diagnosis and personalized treatment of breast cancer: Lessons from tumor biology. *Per. Med.* **2020**, *17*, 399–420. [CrossRef] [PubMed]

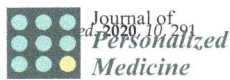 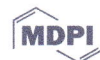

Article

Palbociclib Plus Fulvestrant or Everolimus Plus Exemestane for Pretreated Advanced Breast Cancer with Lobular Histotype in ER+/HER2− Patients: A Propensity Score-Matched Analysis of a Multicenter Retrospective Patient Series [†]

Armando Orlandi [1,*], Elena Iattoni [1], Laura Pizzuti [2], Agnese Fabbri [3], Andrea Botticelli [4], Carmela Di Dio [1], Antonella Palazzo [1], Giovanna Garufi [1], Giulia Indellicati [1], Daniele Alesini [3], Luisa Carbognin [5], Ida Paris [5], Angela Vaccaro [6], Luca Moscetti [7], Alessandra Fabi [2], Valentina Magri [4], Giuseppe Naso [4], Alessandra Cassano [1,8], Patrizia Vici [2], Diana Giannarelli [9], Gianluca Franceschini [8,10], Paolo Marchetti [4], Emilio Bria [1,8,‡] and Giampaolo Tortora [1,8,‡]

1. Comprehensive Cancer Center, UOC di Oncologia Medica,
   Fondazione Policlinico Universitario A. Gemelli IRCCS, 00168 Rome, Italy; elena.iattoni@unicatt.it (E.I.); carmela.didio@unicatt.it (C.D.D.); antonella.palazzo@policlinicogemelli.it (A.P.); giovanna.garufi@unicatt.it (G.G.); giulia.indellicati@unicatt.it (G.I.); alessandra.cassano@unicatt.it (A.C.); emilio.bria@unicatt.it (E.B.); giampaolo.tortora@unicatt.iT (G.T.)
2. Division of Medical Oncology, Regina Elena National Cancer Institute IRCCS, 00128 Rome, Italy; pizzuti8@hotmail.com (L.P.); alessandra.fabi@virgilio.it (A.F.); patrizia.vici@ifo.gov.it (P.V.)
3. Medical Oncology, Central Hospital of Belcolle, 01100 Viterbo, Italy; agnese.fabbri@yahoo.it (A.F.); danielealesini@yahoo.it (D.A.)
4. Clinical and Molecular Medicine Department, Sapienza University of Rome, 00185 Rome, Italy; andreabotticelli@hotmail.it (A.B.); magri.v@hotmail.it (V.M.); Giuseppe.Naso@uniroma1.it (G.N.); paolo.marchetti@uniroma1.it (P.M.)
5. Comprehensive Cancer Center Division of Gynecologic Oncology,
   Fondazione Policlinico Universitario A. Gemelli IRCCS, 00168 Rome, Italy; luisa.carbognin@policlinicogemelli.it (L.C.); ida.paris@policlinicogemelli.it (I.P.)
6. Oncology Department, Ospedale di Frosinone, 03100 Frosinone, Italy; angelavaccaro64@gmail.com
7. Oncology Department, Azienda Ospedaliero-Universitaria Policlinico di Modena, 41125 Modena, Italy; l.moscetti@icloud.com
8. Medical Oncology, Department of Traslational Medicine and Surgery, Università Cattolica del Sacro Cuore, 00168 Rome, Italy; gianluca.franceschini@unicatt.it
9. Biostatistical Unit, Regina Elena National Cancer Institute IRCCS, 00128 Rome, Italy; diana.giannarelli@ifo.gov.it
10. Multidisciplinary Breast Center, Dipartimento Scienze della Salute della donna e del Bambino e di Sanità Pubblica, Fondazione Policlinico Universitario A. Gemelli IRCCS, 00168 Roma, Italy
* Correspondence: armando.orlandi@policlinicogemelli.it; Tel.: +39-0630156318
† Preliminary results of this study were presented at a poster session at ESMO 2019 (339P) Abstract published in Annals of Oncology, 30, Supplement 5, October 2019.
‡ Equally contributors.

Received: 10 November 2020; Accepted: 16 December 2020; Published: 18 December 2020

Abstract: Cyclin-dependent kinase 4/6 inhibitors (CDK4/6i) in combination with endocrine therapy (ET) show meaningful efficacy and tolerability in patients with metastatic breast cancer (MBC), but the optimal sequence of ET has not been established. It is not clear if patients with lobular breast carcinomas (LBC) derive the same benefits when receiving second line CDK4/6i. This retrospective study compared the efficacy of palbociclib plus fulvestrant (PALBO–FUL) with everolimus plus exemestane (EVE–EXE) as second-line ET for hormone-resistant metastatic LBC. From 2013 to 2018, patients with metastatic LBC positivity for estrogen and/or progesterone receptors and HER2/neu negativity, who had relapsed during adjuvant hormonal therapy or first-line hormonal treatment, were enrolled from six centers in Italy in this retrospective study. A total of 74 out of 376 patients (48 treated with PALBO–FUL and 26 with EVE–EXE) with metastatic LBC were eligible for inclusion. Progression-free survival (PFS) was longer in patients receiving EVE–EXE compared with PALBO–FUL (6.1 vs. 4.5 months, univariate HR 0.58, 95% CI 0.35–0.96; p = 0.025). On the propensity score (PS) analysis, PFS was confirmed to be significantly longer for patients treated with EVE–EXE compared to PALBO–FUL (6.0 vs. 4.6 months, p = 0.04). This retrospective analysis suggests that EVE–EXE is more effective than PALBO–FUL for second line ET of metastatic LBC, allowing us to speculate on the optimal therapeutic sequence.

Keywords: advanced breast cancer; mTOR inhibitor; CDK4/6 inhibitor; endocrine resistance

1. Introduction

Invasive lobular breast carcinomas (LBCs), which account for up to 15% of all invasive breast cancers (BC), are almost always estrogen-positive (ER, coded by the ESR1 gene) and lacking HER2 amplification and as such are treated with endocrine therapy (ET) [1]. Options for ET have expanded in the last two decades with the availability of new agents, including selective estrogen receptor modulators (SERM), aromatase inhibitors (AIs), and selective estrogen receptor degrader (SERD) [2,3]. However, resistance to therapy and subsequent disease progression continue to be major problems. More than a third of patients with ER-responsive early-stage BC and almost all of those with metastatic disease become refractory to these treatments during the course of their disease [4–6]. New approaches to treatment are clearly required, and to this end, cyclin-dependent kinase 4/6 inhibitors (CDK4/6i) were developed. CDK4/6i palbociclib, ribociclib, and abemaciclib in combination with ET have shown clinically meaningful efficacy and a good tolerability profile in patients with metastatic breast cancer (MBC), in endocrine sensitive and endocrine resistant disease, within the PALOMA, MONALEESA, and MONARCH trials, respectively [7–12]. The MONALEESA-3, MONALEESA-7, and MONARCH-2 trials showed significantly improved overall survival with a combination of a CDK4/6i and ET [10,13].

While subgroup analysis of the PALOMA 2 trial showed that the combination of palbociclib plus letrozole is effective in first-line treatment both in ductal and lobular histotypes, no evidence is currently available on the efficacy of CDK4/6i exclusively in second-line treatment according to histotype (PALOMA 3, MONARCH 2, and MONALEESA 3) [7,12,13]. Recently, a pooled analysis of seven phase III trials (combining the data of the endocrine sensitive and resistant setting) was made to investigate the benefit of adding CDKIs to endocrine therapy in patients whose tumors might have differing degrees of endocrine sensitivity, such as the lobular histotype [14]. This pooled analysis shows that all subsets, including LBC, of patients derived benefits from the addition of a CDKI to endocrine therapy.

For some time in our clinical practice, we have observed that patients with ER-positive metastatic LBC who had relapsed on adjuvant tamoxifen/AIs or had progressed with first-line hormonal therapy tended to show poor responses, and their disease showed faster progression with CDK4/6i [15]. Interestingly, in some of these patients, the subsequent use of a mTOR inhibitor (everolimus) produced greater clinical benefits and prolonged survival. In light of these considerations, we conducted a multicentric, retrospective study to compare the efficacy of the combination of palbociclib plus fulvestrant (PALBO–FUL) with everolimus plus exemestane (EVE–EXE) as second-line ET for hormone-resistant metastatic LBC.

2. Materials and Methods

This retrospective study enrolled women with metastatic LBC from six Italian oncology centers over a five-year period from 2013 to 2018. Female patients (≥18 years at diagnosis) with metastatic

LBC (confirmed by metastasis biopsy) or with a clinical history of disease, compatible with recurrent lobular carcinoma of the previously diagnosed primary breast cancer, positivity for estrogen and/or progesterone receptors, and HER2/neu negativity, who had relapsed during adjuvant hormonal therapy or a first-line hormonal treatment, were eligible for inclusion. Patients were excluded if they relapsed in a period of more than 12 months from the end of adjuvant hormonal therapy or they had not received prior hormonal treatments. Patients received second line therapy with PALBO–FUL or EVE–EXE according to standard approved administration schedules. All patients enrolled in the study provided written informed consent for their data to be used for future medical research. The study was conducted in accordance with Italian legislation on observational studies (Min. Sal. Circular 6 September 2002). Data from the six participating centers were processed and stored at the coordinating center (Fondazione Policlinico Universitario Agostino Gemelli IRCCS, Rome, Italy) in compliance with local privacy regulations.

The primary endpoint was progression-free survival (PFS) defined as the interval between the treatment start date and the disease progression date. Secondary endpoints were objective response rate (ORR, rate of complete objective responses and partial objective responses of the disease to the treatment evaluated using clinical and/or radiological criteria, according to RECIST 1.1 Criteria) and clinical benefit rate (CBR, rate of complete objective responses, partial objective responses, and stable disease in response to the treatment evaluated with clinical and/or radiological criteria).

All continuous data were expressed as mean ±SD, range, and median value; frequencies and percentages were reported for categorical variables. The clinical, biological, and pathological characteristics of tumors at baseline were determined using Fisher's exact test. PFS and overall survival were estimated by the Kaplan–Meier limit product method. The Cox regression model was applied to multivariate survival analysis, and p values and hazard ratios (HRs) with 95% CI were obtained. All significant variables in the univariate model were used to build the multivariate model of survival. A propensity score (PS) adjustment for baseline characteristics was conducted for survival analysis. The Statistical Package for the Social Sciences (SPSS) 20.0 software, (Chicago, IL, USA) was used for statistical analysis and integrated with Medcalc software V.9.4.2.0 (Mariakerke, Belgium). In all analyses, the significance level was specified as $p < 0.05$. As the study was explorative, an estimate of the sample size was not calculated.

3. Results

3.1. Patient Demographics

Of a total of 376 women screened over the five-year period (2013–2018) in the six centers, 74 were diagnosed with metastatic LBC. Of these, 48 patients received PALBO–FUL and 26 EVE–EXE. Baseline patient characteristics were comparable between the two treatment groups (Table 1). Most patients were post-menopausal (89% and 100% in the PALBO–FUL and EVE–EXE groups, respectively), had non-visceral disease (61 and 68%, respectively), and had less than three sites of metastasis (78 and 79%, respectively). Overall, 43 and 57% of patients in the PALBO–FUL and EVE–EXE groups, respectively, had previously received two lines of endocrine therapy, and 15 and 17% of patients, respectively, had metastatic disease on diagnosis. All patients had received at least one or two lines of endocrine therapy (aromatase inhibitors alone or in combination with tamoxifen, or fulvestrant).

Table 1. Baseline and treatment characteristics ($n = 74$).

Characteristics ($n = 74$)	Palbociclib + Fulvestrant ($n = 46$) (%)	Everolimus + Exemestane ($n = 28$) (%)
Age		
>65	14 (30)	17 (61)
≤65	32 (70)	11 (39)
Menopausal status		
Pre-/Peri-menopausal	5 (11)	0
Post-menopausal	41 (89)	28 (100)
Performance status (ECOG)		
0	23 (50)	12 (43)
1	23 (50)	15 (54)
2	0	1 (3)
Metastatic site		
Bone only	12 (26)	10 (36)
Visceral	18 (39)	9 (32)
Other	16 (35)	9 (32)
Sites of metastasis		
1	19 (41)	15 (54)
2	17 (37)	7 (25)
≥3	10 (22)	6 (21)
Number of previous lines of endocrine therapy		
1	26 (57)	12 (43)
2	20 (43)	16 (57)
Purpose of the most recent treatment		
Adjuvant therapy	13 (28)	1 (3)
Treatment for advanced disease	33 (72)	27 (97)
Disease-free interval		
<12 months	23 (50)	8 (29)
12–24 months	3 (7)	2 (7)
>24 months	13 (28)	9 (32)
Previous endocrine therapies		
Aromatase inhibitors	22 (48)	11 (39)
Tamoxifen	10 (22)	0
Aromatase inhibitors + tamoxifen	14 (30)	7 (25)
Fulvestrant	0	15 (54)
Previous chemotherapy		
Yes	28 (63)	18 (61)
No	18 (37)	10 (39)
Setting of previous chemotherapy		
Neoadjuvant or adjuvant	23 (50)	17 (61)
Advanced disease	5 (13)	1 (3)
Stage at diagnosis		
I	7 (15)	0
II	16 (35)	8 (29)
III	16 (35)	15 (54)
IV	7 (15%)	5 (17)

ECOG: Eastern Cooperative Oncology Group.

3.2. Efficacy and Activity

Median PFS was significantly longer in patients receiving EVE–EXE than in those receiving PALBO–FUL (6.1 vs. 4.5 months, univariate HR 0.58, 95% CI 0.35–0.96; $p = 0.025$ (Figure 1)). Univariate analysis showed that metastatic stage at diagnosis (HR 2.82, 95% CI 1.43–5.56; $p = 0.003$), previous chemotherapy exposure (HR 0.41, 95% CI 0.24–0.72, p = 0.002), and study treatments (HR 0.58, 95% CI 0.35–0.96, p = 0.025), correlated positively with PFS (Table 2). On multivariate analysis, previous chemotherapy exposure was the only factor significantly associated with PFS (HR 0.41, 95% CI 0.24–0.72, p = 0.002).

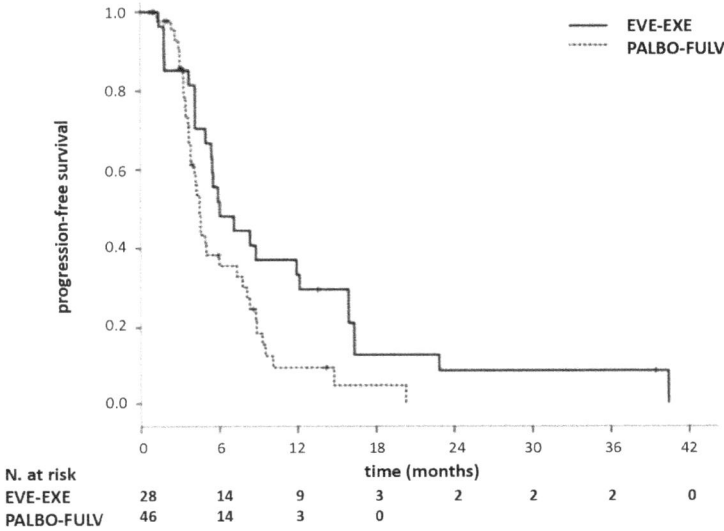

Figure 1. Progression-free survival (PFS). N: number; EVE: everolimus; EXE: exemestane; PALBO: palbociclib; FULV: fulvestrant.

Table 2. Univariate and multivariate analysis for progression-free survival (PFS).

Characteristics	Univariate	Multivariate
Age (≥65 vs. <65 years)	1.11 (0.66–1.85), p = 0.69	-
Menopausal status (post vs. pre)	1.16 (0.42–3.23), p = 0.77	-
Metastatic status (synchronous vs. metachronous)	2.82 (1.43–5.56), p = 0.003	-
Previous chemotherapy (yes vs. no)	0.41 (0.24–0.72), p = 0.002	0.41 (0.24–0.72), p = 0.002
Previous hormonal therapy (yes vs. no)	0.67 (0.40–1.13), p = 0.13	-
Metastatic sites (visceral vs. not visceral)	1.34 (0.80–2.25), p = 0.27	-
Treatment (EVE-EXE vs. Palbo)	0.58 (0.35–0.96), p = 0.025	-

PFS was significantly longer in patients receiving EVE–EXE in comparison with PALBO–FUL (6.0 vs. 4.6 months, p = 0.04) on PS analysis adjusted for prior chemotherapy and synchronous/metachronous metastatic status (Figure 2). Objective response rates in both groups did not significantly differ, with 7 out of 46 patients (ORR 15.2%, 95% CI 4.8–25.6) in the PALBO–FULV group and 9 out of 28 patients (ORR 32.1%, 95% CI 14.8–49.4) in the EVE–EXE group (p = 0.0725). Accordingly, no difference in CBR was found between both groups (PALBO–FULV 65.2%, 95% CI 51.4–78.9 and EVE–EXE 67.8%, 95% CI 50.5–85.1, p = 1.0) (Figure 3). Only 1 patient experienced a complete response (CR) in the PALBO–FULV group (CR 2%, 95% CI < 1–6.3). Stable disease (SD) and progressive disease (PD) were 35.7% (95% CI 17.9–53.4) and 32.1% (95% CI 14.8–49.4), respectively, in the EVE–EXE group, and 50.0% (95% CI 35.5–64.4) and 34.7% (95% CI 21.0–48.5) in the PALO–FULV group, respectively.

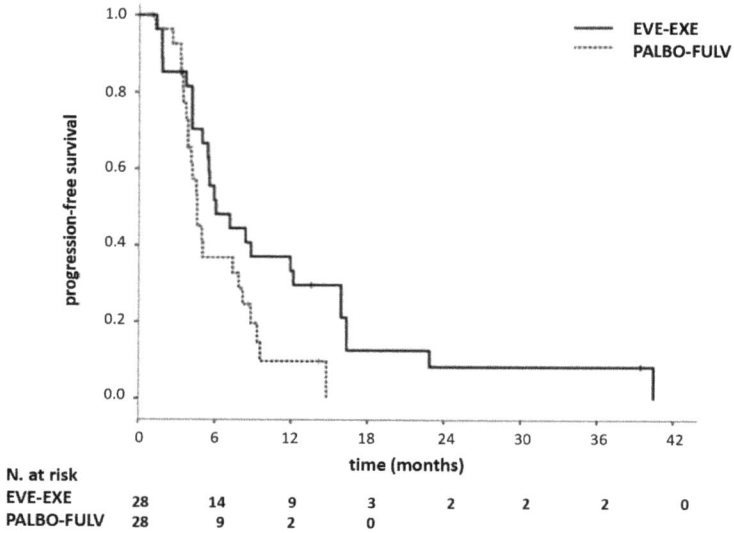

Figure 2. Progression-free survival (PFS) after propensity score adjustment. EVE: everolimus; EXE: exemestane; PALBO: palbociclib; FULV: fulvestrant.

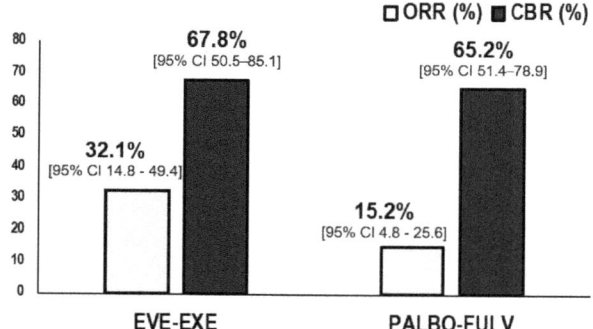

Figure 3. Objective response rate (ORR) according to RECIST 1.1 and clinical benefit rate (CBR). EVE: everolimus; EXE: exemestane; PALBO: palbociclib; FULV: fulvestrant; CI: confidence interval; p-value: chi-square.

3.3. Safety/Adverse Events

In terms of safety and adverse events, both treatments were relatively well tolerated (Table 3). In the PALBO–FUL group, neutropenia (65%) and anemia (41%) were the most commonly reported events, while in the EVE–EXE group, fatigue (64%), stomatitis (35%), and rash (25%) were the most reported adverse events (Table 3). Grades 3 and 4 adverse events (in the main afebrile neutropenia) occurred in 24 patients (52%) in the PALBO–FUL group, and 6 patients (21%) receiving EVE–EXE reported grade 3 adverse events (stomatitis and cutaneous rash and one case of interstitial pneumonitis). Dose reduction was required in 11 (24%) of patients in PALBO–FUL and 12 (43%) in the EVE–EXE group. Treatment discontinuations were all subsequent to disease progression, except in one case—a patient who developed interstitial pneumonitis while receiving EVE–EXE discontinued treatment. No deaths related to study medications were reported.

Table 3. Adverse events for any causes observed during the study period.

Adverse Events from Any Cause	Palbociclib + Fulvestrant (n = 46, %)			Everolimus + Exemestane (n = 28, %)		
	Any Grade	Grade 3	Grade 4	Any Grade	Grade 3	Grade 4
Any adverse event	35 (76)	22 (48)	2 (4)	24 (85)	6 (21)	0
Neutropenia	30 (65)	18 (39)	2 (4)	3 (10)	0	0
Febrile neutropenia	0	0	0	0	0	0
Anemia	19 (41)	2 (4)	0	4 (14)	0	0
Thrombocytopenia	11 (24)	2 (4)	0	2 (7)	0	0
Fatigue	16 (35)	0	0	18 (64)	0	0
Nausea	4 (9)	0	0	5 (18)	0	0
Diarrhea	0	0	0	4 (14)	0	0
Stypsis	4 (9)	0	0	3 (10)	0	0
Headache	1 (2)	0	0	0	0	0
Hot flash	6 (13)	0	0	0	0	0
Stomatitis	1 (3)	0	0	10 (35)	3 (10)	0
Rash	1 (3)	0	0	7 (25)	2 (7)	0
Alopecia	6 (13)	0	0	0	0	0
Myalgia	4 (9)	0	0	2 (7)	0	0
Dyslipidemia and/or Hyperglycemia	0	0	0	4 (14)	0	0
Pneumonitis	0	0	0	6 (21)	1 (4)	0

4. Discussion

Despite the clinically meaningful efficacy and good tolerability profile of the combination of CDK4/6i and ET in patients with MBC, patients eventually experienced disease progression and the emergence of resistance [16]. Resistance to CDK4/6i plus ET represents the next clinical challenge for the breast cancer community to overcome and requires a deep understanding of the mechanism of CDK4/6i resistance in an endocrine sensitive and resistant setting. Furthermore, there are limited data on the efficacy of these treatments in different BC histological types, in particular in patients with LBC who are often not well represented in clinical trials. While a subgroup analysis of PALOMA 2 trial showed that the combination of palbociclib plus letrozole was effective as a first-line treatment both in ductal and lobular histotypes, and in BOLERO-2, everolimus was shown to be effective both in ductal and lobular histotype hormone-refractory patients [17], no evidence is currently available on the efficacy of CDK4/6i as a second-line treatment based on histotype [18]. Thus, the treatment options for this frequent BC subtype are limited if tumors develop resistance to anti-estrogen treatment regimens.

In our clinical experience, the combination of PALBO–FUL in patients with metastatic LBC whose disease relapsed during adjuvant hormonal therapy or progressed after first-line ET for advance disease did meet the expectation. Most patients showed early disease progression and low clinical benefit [15]. We posed the question, why did patients with LBC show lower than reported responses to CDK4/6i? We know that the development and progression of invasive lobular carcinoma (ILC) are characterized by the loss of E-cadherin–E-cadherin binding in normal cells that prevents beta-catenin inhibition of PTEN, thus permitting the inhibition of AKT [19]. As a consequence of the loss of E-cadherin in LBC, the PI3K/AKT pathway is constitutively activated and represents one of the main pathways of proliferation and growth [20,21]. We hypothesized that in patients with metastatic LBC that becomes resistant to endocrine therapy, the hyperactivation of PI3K/AKT signaling may promote an intrinsic resistance to CDK4/6i through the activation of cyclin E/CDK2—amplification of cyclin E is the only factor that showed a correlation with resistance to a CDK 4/6i (palbociclib) in trials [22,23]. Alternatively, inhibition of the AKT pathway could perhaps represent a superior strategy for these patients.

Everolimus is a sirolimus derivative that inhibits mTOR (a key downstream point of the PI3K pathway) through allosteric binding to mTORC1. The results of the BOLERO-2 trial showed that dual-blockade with EVE–EXE more than doubled median PFS versus EXE alone in patients with hormone receptor-positive (HR+)/human epidermal growth receptor 2-negative (HER2−) metastatic BC recurring/progressing on prior non-steroidal aromatase inhibitors (NSAIs) (7.8 versus 3.2 months) [24–26]. In addition, results of an Italian observational study suggest that treatment with EXE–EVE is an active and safe therapeutic option for endocrine-sensitive MBC patients in a real-world clinical setting, regardless of treatment lines [27]. These results were confirmed in the BALLET study that enrolled patients more heavily pretreated, with a safety profile consistent with that observed in BOLERO-2 [28]. These results are important because the treatment pattern of MBC is based on the sequence of multiple lines of therapy, and it is therefore vital to determine the possible additive/cumulative effects of different regimens. The combination regimen of EVE and EXE is the only regimen currently registered with an mTOR inhibitor in this setting and represents a valid alternative to the harmful toxicity profile of cytotoxic chemotherapy [29].

In our real-world analysis, median PFS was significantly longer for patients with metastatic LBC receiving EVE–EXE as second-line hormonal treatment compared with PALBO–FUL. Both treatments were well tolerated and only one patient (in the EVE–EXE group) discontinued therapy due to adverse events. Univariate analysis showed that prognosis may be influenced by disease status (de novo metastatic vs. relapsed disease), previous exposure to chemotherapy, and study treatment (PALBO–FUL or EVE–EXE). In particular, patients who had disease relapse and those who received a neo/adjuvant and/or first-line chemotherapy had shorter median PFS, suggesting that de novo metastatic and relapsed disease are characterized by different molecular background which for relapsed cancer is probably the result of clone selection derived from the exposure to previous treatments. The efficacy of chemotherapy in LBC is the subject of much debate, and it is usually reserved for patients with negative prognostic scores, visceral crisis, or when all possible ET lines have been exhausted. Most of our patients received cytotoxic agents (as neoadjuvant/adjuvant), which may have resulted in a detrimental effect, in particular when used in early lines. The PS analysis adjusted for previous chemotherapy exposure and synchronous/metachronous metastatic status confirmed a longer median PFS for patients receiving EVE–EXE (6.0 vs. 4.6 months, $p = 0.04$). Therefore, the activation of the PI3K/AKT pathway in LBC may result in intrinsic resistance to palbociclib after development of refractory disease to prior ET.

The results of this study allow us to speculate that EVE–EXE as a second-line treatment of metastatic LBC may improve therapeutic outcomes. In terms of optimizing sequential therapy, using a CDK4/6i for the first-line treatment of endocrine sensitive tumors is indicated, while mTOR inhibitors could be considered the preferred option when resistance to adjuvant/first-line ET has occurred. Activation of the PI3K/AKT pathway may not solely explain the lack of effectiveness of palbociclib in LBC, and other factors may drive resistance to Palbociclib [30]. Further studies are needed to explore the potential implications of these pathways in the mechanisms of resistance to CDK4/6i. In the era of personalized medicine, improving molecular characterization of cancer to define the best therapeutic program for each patient is paramount.

This retrospective real-world analysis generates the hypothesis of a potential benefit from EVE–EXE in comparison with PALBO–FUL as a second line hormonal-treatment for metastatic luminal breast cancer with lobular histology, and it allows us to speculate on the best therapeutic sequence. However, the limitations of this study, including its retrospective nature and small sample size, need to be addressed.

5. Conclusions

The results of this retrospective, real-world analysis seem to suggest a potential benefit of EVE–EXE in comparison with PALBO–FUL as a second-line ET of MBC with lobular histology.

Author Contributions: Conceptualization, A.O.; methodology, A.O., E.B., G.T.; writing—review and editing, all authors; supervision, A.O., E.B., G.T., and G.F.; All authors have read and agreed to the published version of the manuscript.

Funding: This research received no external funding.

Acknowledgments: E.B. is currently supported by the Associazione Italiana per la Ricerca sul Cancro (AIRC) under Investigator Grant (IG) No. IG20583. G.T. is supported by AIRC, IG18599, AIRC 5 × 1000 21052. E.B. is currently supported by Institutional funds of Università Cattolica del Sacro Cuore (UCSC-project D1-2018/2019). Medical editorial assistance was provided by Edra S.p.A. Financial support for this assistance was provided by Novartis Farma S.p.A. Authors had full control of the content and made the final decision for all aspects of this article.

Conflicts of Interest: The authors declare no conflict of interest.

References

1. Desmedt, C.; Pingitore, J.; Roth, F.; Marchio, C.; Clatot, F.; Rouas, G.; Richard, F.; Bertucci, F.; Mariani, O.; Galant, C.; et al. ESR1 mutations in metastatic lobular breast cancer patients. *NPJ Breast Cancer* **2019**, *5*, 9. [CrossRef]
2. Kaklamani, V.G.; Gradishar, W.J. Endocrine Therapy in the Current Management of Postmenopausal Estrogen Receptor-Positive Metastatic Breast Cancer. *Oncologist* **2017**, *22*, 507–517. [CrossRef]
3. Rugo, H.S.; Rumble, R.B.; Macrae, E.; Barton, D.L.; Connolly, H.K.; Dickler, M.N.; Fallowfield, L.J.; Fowble, B.; Ingle, J.N.; Jahanzeb, M.; et al. Endocrine Therapy for Hormone Receptor–Positive Metastatic Breast Cancer: American Society of Clinical Oncology Guideline. *J. Clin. Oncol.* **2016**, *34*, 3069–3103. [CrossRef]
4. Hayes, E.; Nicholson, R.I.; Hiscox, S. Acquired endocrine resistance in breast cancer: Implications for tumour metastasis. *Front. Biosci.* **2011**, *16*, 838. [CrossRef]
5. Osborne, C.K.; Schiff, R. Mechanisms of Endocrine Resistance in Breast Cancer. *Annu. Rev. Med.* **2011**, *62*, 233–247. [CrossRef]
6. Rugo, H.S. Achieving Improved Survival Outcomes in Advanced Breast Cancer. *N. Engl. J. Med.* **2019**, *381*, 371–372. [CrossRef]
7. Cristofanilli, M.; Turner, N.C.; Bondarenko, I.; Ro, J.; Im, S.-A.; Masuda, N.; Colleoni, M.; DeMichele, A.; Loi, S.; Verma, S.; et al. Fulvestrant plus palbociclib versus fulvestrant plus placebo for treatment of hormone-receptor-positive, HER2-negative metastatic breast cancer that progressed on previous endocrine therapy (PALOMA-3): Final analysis of the multicentre, double-blind, phase 3 randomised controlled trial. *Lancet Oncol.* **2016**, *17*, 425–439. [CrossRef]
8. Dickler, M.N.; Tolaney, S.M.; Rugo, H.S.; Cortés, J.; Diéras, V.; Patt, D.; Wildiers, H.; Hudis, C.A.; O'Shaughnessy, J.; Zamora, E.; et al. MONARCH 1, a Phase ii Study of Abemaciclib, a CDK4 and CDK6 Inhibitor, as a Single Agent, in Patients with Refractory HR$^+$/HER2$^-$ Metastatic Breast Cancer. *Clin. Cancer Res.* **2017**, *23*, 5218–5224. [CrossRef]
9. Hortobagyi, G.N.; Stemmer, S.M.; Burris, H.A.; Yap, Y.S.; Sonke, G.S.; Paluch-Shimon, S.; Campone, M.; Blackwell, K.L.; André, F.; Winer, E.P.; et al. Ribociclib as First-Line Therapy for HR-Positive, Advanced Breast Cancer. *N. Engl. J. Med.* **2016**, *375*, 1738–1748. [CrossRef]
10. Hortobagyi, G.N. Ribociclib for the first-line treatment of advanced hormone receptor-positive breast cancer: A review of subgroup analyses from the MONALEESA-2 trial. *Breast Cancer Res.* **2018**, *20*, 123. [CrossRef]
11. Preusser, M.; De Mattos-Arruda, L.; Thill, M.; Criscitiello, C.; Bartsch, R.; Ruhstaller, T.; De Azambuja, E.; Zielinski, C.C. CDK4/6 inhibitors in the treatment of patients with breast cancer: Summary of a multidisciplinary round-table discussion. *ESMO Open* **2018**, *3*, e000368. [CrossRef]
12. Sledge, G.W.; Toi, M.; Neven, P.; Sohn, J.; Inoue, K.; Pivot, X.; Burdaeva, O.; Okera, M.; Masuda, N.; Kaufman, P.A.; et al. The Effect of Abemaciclib Plus Fulvestrant on Overall Survival in Hormone Receptor–Positive, ERBB2-Negative Breast Cancer That Progressed on Endocrine Therapy—MONARCH 2: A Randomized Clinical Trial. *JAMA Oncol.* **2019**, *6*, 116–124. [CrossRef]

13. Im, S.-A.; Lu, Y.-S.; Bardia, A.; Harbeck, N.; Colleoni, M.; Franke, F.; Chow, L.; Sohn, J.; Lee, K.-S.; Campos-Gomez, S.; et al. Overall Survival with Ribociclib plus Endocrine Therapy in Breast Cancer. *N. Engl. J. Med.* **2019**, *381*, 307–316. [CrossRef]
14. Gao, J.J.; Cheng, J.; Bloomquist, E.; Sanchez, J.; Wedam, S.B.; Singh, H.; Amiri-Kordestani, L.; Ibrahim, A.; Sridhara, R.; Goldberg, K.B.; et al. CDK4/6 inhibitor treatment for patients with hormone receptor-positive, HER2-negative, advanced or metastatic breast cancer: A US Food and Drug Administration pooled analysis. *Lancet Oncol.* **2020**, *21*, 250–260. [CrossRef]
15. Orlandi, A.; Aroldi, F.; Garutti, M.; Di Dio, C.; Garufi, G.; Iattoni, E.; Palazzo, A.; Indellicati, G.; Franceschini, G.; Cassano, A.; et al. Poor efficacy of palbociclib in second-line treatment of metastatic lobular breast cancer in a case series: Use before or never more? *Breast J.* **2019**, *26*, 1458–1460. [CrossRef]
16. Portman, N.; Alexandrou, S.; Carson, E.; Wang, S.; Lim, E.; Caldon, C.E. Overcoming CDK4/6 inhibitor resistance in ER-positive breast cancer. *Endocr.-Relat. Cancer* **2019**, *26*, R15–R30. [CrossRef]
17. Hortobagyi, G.N.; Noguchi, S.; Neven, P.; Puttawibul, P.; Heng, D.; Brechenmacher, T.; Ringeisen, F.P.; Saletan, S.; Bachelot, T. Everolimus plus exemestane in patients with advanced invasive lobular carcinoma: Efficacy and safety results from BOLERO-2. *J. Clin. Oncol.* **2014**, *32*, 152. [CrossRef]
18. Rugo, H.S.; Finn, R.S.; Diéras, V.; Ettl, J.; Lipatov, O.; Joy, A.A.; Harbeck, N.; Castrellon, A.; Iyer, S.; Lu, D.R.; et al. Palbociclib plus letrozole as first-line therapy in estrogen receptor-positive/human epidermal growth factor receptor 2-negative advanced breast cancer with extended follow-up. *Breast Cancer Res. Treat.* **2019**, *174*, 719–729. [CrossRef]
19. Teo, K.; Gómez-Cuadrado, L.; Tenhagen, M.; Byron, A.; Rätze, M.; Van Amersfoort, M.; Renes, J.; Strengman, E.; Mandoli, A.; Singh, A.A.; et al. E-cadherin loss induces targetable autocrine activation of growth factor signalling in lobular breast cancer. *Sci. Rep.* **2018**, *8*, 15454. [CrossRef]
20. Lau, M.-T.; Klausen, C.; Leung, P.C.K. E-cadherin inhibits tumor cell growth by suppressing PI3K/Akt signaling via b-catenin-Egr1-mediated PTEN expression. *Oncogene* **2011**, *30*, 2753–2766. [CrossRef]
21. Liu, X.; Su, L.; Liu, X. Loss of CDH1 up-regulates epidermal growth factor receptor via phosphorylation of YBX1 in non-small cell lung cancer cells. *FEBS Lett.* **2013**, *587*, 3995–4000. [CrossRef]
22. Pandey, K.; An, H.; Kim, S.K.; Lee, S.A.; Kim, S.; Lim, S.M.; Kim, G.M.; Sohn, J.; Moon, Y.W. Molecular mechanisms of resistance to CDK4/6 inhibitors in breast cancer: A review. *Int. J. Cancer* **2019**, *145*, 1179–1188. [CrossRef]
23. Turner, N.C.; Liu, Y.; Zhu, Z.; Loi, S.; Colleoni, M.; Loibl, S.; DeMichele, A.; Harbeck, N.; André, F.; Bayar, M.A.; et al. Cyclin E1 Expression and Palbociclib Efficacy in Previously Treated Hormone Receptor–Positive Metastatic Breast Cancer. *J. Clin. Oncol.* **2019**, *37*, 1169–1178. [CrossRef]
24. Yardley, D.A.; Noguchi, S.S.; Pritchard, K.I.; Burris, H.H.; Baselga, J.; Gnant, M.; Hortobagyi, G.N.; Campone, M.; Pistilli, B.B.; Piccart-Gebhart, M.; et al. Everolimus Plus Exemestane in Postmenopausal Patients with HR+ Breast Cancer: BOLERO-2 Final Progression-Free Survival Analysis. *Adv. Ther.* **2013**, *30*, 870–884. [CrossRef]
25. Piccart-Gebhart, M.; Hortobagyi, G.N.; Campone, M.; Pritchard, K.I.; Lebrun, F.; Ito, Y.; Noguchi, S.; Perez, A.; Rugo, H.S.; Deleu, I.; et al. Everolimus plus exemestane for hormone-receptor-positive, human epidermal growth factor receptor-2-negative advanced breast cancer: Overall survival results from BOLERO-2. *Ann. Oncol.* **2014**, *25*, 2357–2362. [CrossRef]
26. Pritchard, K.I.; Burris, H.H.; Ito, Y.Y.; Rugo, H.S.; Dakhil, S.S.; Hortobagyi, G.N.; Campone, M.; Csöszi, T.T.; Baselga, J.; Puttawibul, P.P.; et al. Safety and Efficacy of Everolimus With Exemestane vs. Exemestane Alone in Elderly Patients with HER2-Negative, Hormone Receptor-Positive Breast Cancer in BOLERO-2. *Clin. Breast Cancer* **2013**, *13*, 421–432.e8. [CrossRef]
27. Riccardi, F.; Colantuoni, G.; Diana, A.; Mocerino, C.; Lauria, R.; Febbraro, A.; Nuzzo, F.; Addeo, R.; Marano, O.; Incoronato, P.; et al. Exemestane and Everolimus combination treatment of hormone receptor positive, HER2 negative metastatic breast cancer: A retrospective study of 9 cancer centers in the Campania Region (Southern Italy) focused on activity, efficacy and safety. *Mol. Clin. Oncol.* **2018**, *9*, 255–263. [CrossRef]
28. Jerusalem, G.; Mariani, G.; Ciruelos, E.M.; Martin, M.; Tjan-Heijnen, V.C.G.; Neven, P.; Gavila, J.G.; Michelotti, A.; Montemurro, F.; Generali, D.; et al. Safety of EVE plus EXE in patients with hormone-receptor–positive, HER2–negative locally advanced or metastatic breast cancer progressing on prior non-steroidal aromatase inhibitors: Primary results of a phase IIIb, open-label, single-arm, expanded-access multicenter trial (BALLET). *Ann. Oncol.* **2016**, *27*, 1719–1725. [CrossRef]

29. Generali, D.; Venturini, S.; Rognoni, C.; Ciani, O.; Pusztai, L.; Loi, S.; Jerusalem, G.; Bottini, A.; Tarricone, R. A network meta-analysis of everolimus plus exemestane versus chemotherapy in the first- and second-line treatment of estrogen receptor-positive metastatic breast cancer. *Breast Cancer Res. Treat.* **2015**, *152*, 95–117. [CrossRef]
30. McCartney, A.; Migliaccio, I.; Bonechi, M.; Biagioni, C.; Romagnoli, D.; De Luca, F.; Galardi, F.; Risi, E.; De Santo, I.; Benelli, M.; et al. Mechanisms of Resistance to CDK4/6 Inhibitors: Potential Implications and Biomarkers for Clinical Practice. *Front. Oncol.* **2019**, *9*, 666. [CrossRef]

Publisher's Note: MDPI stays neutral with regard to jurisdictional claims in published maps and institutional affiliations.

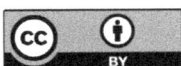

© 2020 by the authors. Licensee MDPI, Basel, Switzerland. This article is an open access article distributed under the terms and conditions of the Creative Commons Attribution (CC BY) license (http://creativecommons.org/licenses/by/4.0/).

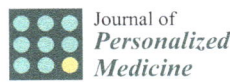

Review

Locoregional Surgery in Metastatic Breast Cancer: Do Concomitant Metabolic Aspects Have a Role on the Management and Prognosis in this Setting?

Maria Ida Amabile [1,*], Federico Frusone [1,†], Alessandro De Luca [1,†], Domenico Tripodi [1], Giovanni Imbimbo [2], Silvia Lai [2], Vito D'Andrea [1], Salvatore Sorrenti [1] and Alessio Molfino [2]

[1] Department of Surgical Sciences, Sapienza University of Rome, 00161 Rome, Italy; federico.frusone@gmail.com (F.F.); dr.aless.deluca@gmail.com (A.D.L.); domenico.tripodi@uniroma1.it (D.T.); vito.dandrea@uniroma1.it (V.D.); salvatore.sorrenti@uniroma1.it (S.S.)
[2] Department of Translational and Precision Medicine, Sapienza University of Rome, 00185 Rome, Italy; imbimbo.1638090@studenti.uniroma1.it (G.I.); silvia.lai@uniroma1.it (S.L.); alessio.molfino@uniroma1.it (A.M.)
* Correspondence: marida.amabile@gmail.com; Tel.: +39-06-499-72042
† These authors equally contributed to the work.

Received: 15 September 2020; Accepted: 11 November 2020; Published: 13 November 2020

Abstract: Although they cannot be considered curative, the new therapeutic integrated advances in metastatic breast cancer (MBC) have substantially improved patient outcomes. Traditionally, surgery was confined to palliation of symptomatic or ulcerating lumps. Data suggest, in some cases, a possible additive role for more aggressive locoregional surgical therapy in combination with systemic treatments in the metastatic setting, although a low level of evidence has been shown in terms of improvement in overall survival in MBC patients treated with surgery and medical treatment compared to medical treatment alone. In this light, tumor heterogeneity remains a challenge. To effectively reshape the therapeutic approach to MBC, careful consideration of who is a good candidate for locoregional resection is paramount. The patient's global health condition, impacting on cancer progression and morbidity and their associated molecular targets, have to be considered in treatment decision-making. In particular, more recently, research has been focused on the role of metabolic derangements, including the presence of metabolic syndrome, which represent well-known conditions related to breast cancer recurrence and distant metastasis and are, therefore, involved in the prognosis. In the present article, we focus on locoregional surgical strategies in MBC and whether concomitant metabolic derangements may have a role in prognosis.

Keywords: metastatic breast cancer; breast surgery; immune system; metabolic derangements; precision medicine; integrated therapies

1. Introduction

The prevalence of metastatic breast cancer (MBC) is about 3–6% in the United States [1], affecting 15,000 women annually [2], and it is estimated that 3–8% of patients with newly diagnosed breast cancer have distant metastases as an initial presentation [3]. Metastatic disease is particularly common in undeveloped countries, where up to 25% of patients present at stage IV at first diagnosis [4]. Interestingly, the median overall survival rate of MBC patients has improved over the last years (from 13 months in 1985 to 33 months in 2016), as well as the 5-year survival rate (from 10% in 1985 to 27% in 2016) [5].

The main goal in MBC treatment is to prolong survival and to maintain or improve the quality of life of the patient [6]. To achieve this, a large palette of anticancer treatments is at hand for use in the adjuvant and metastatic settings. Current therapeutic options for MBC management include radiotherapy, systemic treatments (i.e., hormonal therapy, monoclonal antibodies, chemotherapy, small molecule signal transduction inhibitors, antibody–drug conjugates), surgical treatment [7], as well as nutritional and metabolic interventions [8]. Regarding antineoplastic treatments, the choice is often based on the immunohistochemical characteristics of the breast cancer, according to receptor status [7]. This is an example of modern precision medicine in cancer patients, which relies on identifying key biomarkers driving tumor progression, representing novel therapeutic approaches [7], including genomic sequencing, which may help in the selection of personalized treatment as well as in assessing treatment resistance [9,10].

Although surgical treatment has usually been reserved for the palliative care of symptomatic MBC, i.e., patients with large exophytic masses or ulcerating breast lumps, recent data suggest a possibly expanding role for more aggressive locoregional therapy in combination with systemic therapy [7,11]. Khan et al. analyzed the data from the National Cancer Database of resections of the primary tumor in patients with MBC [12] and documented an improvement in 3-year survival in MBC patients undergoing surgery compared to those who did not. Moreover, patients with negative surgical margins presented the best prognosis [12]. Recent studies, conducted on homogeneous cohorts of MBC patients, have confirmed an improved survival rate after resection of the primary tumor, identifying several variables associated with the response to surgical resection, including younger age, having a single metastatic site, chemotherapy as first-line treatment, HER2-enriched tumor, and lower nodal burden [13,14]. Moreover, Rao et al. reported that MBC patients who had undergone breast surgery and the appropriate extent of axillary surgery had improved outcomes in terms of overall survival compared with patients who only had resection of the primary tumor and/or limited axillary surgery [15]. In this light, several clinical studies were conducted in the past few years to clarify the impact and role of locoregional surgical treatment in patients affected by MBC.

Moreover, it is clear that the treatment of MBC is rapidly evolving, driven by either a greater understanding of the biologic pathways underlying tumorigenesis and metastatic growth or the concept that immune surveillance supports and provides molecular mechanisms during tumor progression. A reduction of primary tumor volume determines a reduction of circulating tumor cells, and the role of the immune system has been hypothesized in promoting/suppressing metastatic growth [16].

An emerging clinically relevant aspect in the management of breast cancer is represented by metabolic and nutritional derangements before, during, and after anticancer therapies [8,17]. The majority of the data in the literature are available on specific risk factors (i.e., overweight/obesity, insulin-resistance) for tumorigenesis and cancer relapse [8].

However, the clinical management of metabolic derangements in MBC does not represent consolidated clinical practice, despite the available experimental and clinical evidence indicating their roles in negatively impacting the prognosis in the MBC setting.

In this light, in the present article, we focus on locoregional surgical strategies in MBC and whether concomitant metabolic derangements may have a role in clinical outcomes.

2. Breast Surgery in MBC: Where Are We Now?

2.1. Data from Retrospective Studies

Khan et al., in 2002, conducted a large retrospective study on more than 16,000 patients from the National Cancer Database and documented that women with MBC treated with locoregional treatment (mastectomy or local excision, both with R0 margins) had a better prognosis compared to patients with involved margins after locoregional surgery or who had not undergone surgical treatment [12] (Table 1). Lang et al. [13], in their study, found a significantly higher overall survival rate and progression-free survival in MBC patients who had undergone locoregional treatment when compared to patients who had not undergone surgery. The median survival of patients treated with surgery was 56.1 months compared to 37.1 months in patients who did not undergo surgical treatment. A higher overall survival was also associated with estrogen receptor positivity and having a single metastasis [13].

Table 1. Studies considered in the present article that were conducted to investigate the impact of locoregional treatment compared to systemic therapy in MBC on prognosis.

Author (Year)	N° Patients	Time Period	Surgery	Outcome: Mortality *	PMID
Khan (2002)	16023	1990–1993	57.2%	HR 0.61 [95% CI 0.58–0.65] better prognosis	12407345
Rapiti (2006)	300	1977–1996	42%	HR 0.6 [95% CI 0.4–1] reduced risk of death	16702580
Fields (2007)	409	1996–2005	46%	aHR 0.53 [95% CI 0.42–0.67] reduced risk of death	17687611
Gnerlich (2007)	9734	1988–2003	47%	aHR 0.63 [95% CI 0.60–0.66] reduced risk of death	17522944
Blanchard (2008)	395	1973–1991	61%	HR 0.71 [95% CI 0.56–0.91] reduced risk of death	18438108
Cady (2008)	622	1970–2002	38%	Increased survival ($p < 0.0001$)	18726129
Bafford (2009)	147	1998–2005	41%	HR 0.47 ($p = 0.003$) reduced risk of death	18581232
Le Scodan (2009)	581	1980–2004	55%	HR 0.70 [95% CI 0.58–0.85] reduced risk of death	19204198
Ruiterkamp (2009)	728	1993–2004	40%	HR 0.62 [95% CI 0.51–0.76] reduced risk of death	19398188
Khadakban (2013)	196	2004–2009	25%	[95% CI 16.69–36.57] reduced risk of death	24426700
Lang (2013)	208	1997–2002	35.6%	HR 0.58 [95% CI 0.35–0.98] reduced risk of death	23306905
Akay (2014)	172	1994–2009	46%	HR 0.9 [95% CI 0.2–0.6] reduced risk of death	24510381
Vohra (2018)	29916	1988–2011	51%	increased survival ($p < 0.0001$)	29498453
Lane (2019)	24015	2003–2012	43.8%	HR 0.56 [95% CI 0.52–0.61] reduced risk of death	29227346
Badwe (2015)	350	2005–2013	50%	HR 1.04 [95% CI 0.81–1.34] no improvement in overall survival	26363985
Soran (2018)	274	2007–2012	50%	HR 0.66 [95% CI 0.49–0.88] reduced risk of death	29777404

* HR (hazard ratio) is indicated if available in the mentioned article.

More recently, Vohra et al. considered 29,916 patients from the Surveillance, Epidemiology, and End Result program (SEER) database and found that MBC patients who had undergone primary tumor resection had a better median disease-specific survival compared to MBC patients who had not undergone locoregional treatment (34 versus 18 months) [18]. Other factors associated with better disease-specific survival were younger age, lower T and N stage, lower grade, luminal tumors, lower tumor grading, adjuvant radiotherapy, and surgery performed in the latter years [18], although no information was given on nutritional and metabolic status.

Lane et al. [11] presented, in 2019, the largest contemporary analysis to evaluate surgical resection of the primary tumor among women with MBC and its association with overall survival. The authors considered 24,015 stage IV breast cancer patients and found a survival improvement of patients who were undergone locoregional treatment, independent of treatment sequence. In fact, they had a median overall survival of 52.8 months in patients subjected to surgery after chemotherapy and a median overall survival of 49.4 months in patients subjected to surgical treatment before chemotherapy, compared to a median overall survival of 37.5 months in patients who underwent systemic treatment without surgery [11] (Table 1). Although these data suggest a benefit from surgery, it has to be considered that some patients may not be candidate for surgery, according to medical comorbidities or extension of the locoregional disease.

In the effort to further control for selection bias, the authors conducted an additional sensitivity subanalysis, considering only MBC patients in whom a diagnosis of clinical M1 disease and confirmation of known sites of metastatic disease were present, and this approach confirmed the initial results [11]. However, this is a retrospective study, which may limit the interpretation of the results obtained, and, to address these questions, some authors performed prospective randomized clinical trials. In the last few years, several randomized trials have investigated the role of locoregional treatment in stage IV breast cancer patients (Table 1).

2.2. Data from Prospective Studies

In 2015, Badwe et al. [19] conducted a randomized controlled trial on 350 patients with newly diagnosed MBC, who had responded to first-line chemotherapy, assigning them to two arms (locoregional treatment versus no-locoregional treatment). With a median follow-up of 23 months (IQR 12.2–38.7), the authors did not find significant differences in the two groups and thus no benefit of locoregional treatment. Moreover, the 2-year overall survival was 41.9% in the locoregional treatment and 43% in the no-locoregional treatment, and, furthermore, only 18% of patients who had undergone locoregional treatment required palliative surgery [19]. Finally, they found a reduction of progression-free survival in the group that had undergone locoregional treatment, hypothesizing that this was determined by the growth of the metastatic tumor as a result of the removal of the primary tumor, as showed by other preclinical studies [20–23]. The authors concluded that they did not find any evidence to support the use of surgical locoregional treatment to improve overall survival in MBC patients who responded to first-line chemotherapy and suggested not to consider this procedure in routine practice.

Conversely, Soran et al. later described results obtained by the MF07-1 trial, a multicenter, phase 3, randomized, controlled study that compared the locoregional treatment followed by systemic therapy with systemic therapy alone for newly diagnosed MBC patients [24]. The authors enrolled 274 patients and, despite the results documented by Badwe et al. [19], found that patients who had undergone locoregional treatment had a 34% lower hazard of death compared to systemic treatment alone, with a median follow-up of 54.5 months and 55 months, respectively. In particular, the survival rates were similar at 3 years (60% in the locoregional arm and 51% in the systemic therapy arm), but at 5 years, the percentage of alive patients was higher in the locoregional group (41.6% versus 24.4% of the systemic group) [24]. This is the first randomized study showing a significant improvement in the survival rate in patients with MBC treated with locoregional surgery, 5 years after treatment [24]. Analyzing the two groups, the authors found that particular subgroups of MBC patients were associated with higher overall survival after surgery, in particular, mainly luminal tumors, age <55 years, and solitary bone metastases. In this light, in patients with MBC, locoregional treatment might be an option to consider in a multidisciplinary setting according to age, performance status, tumor type, comorbidities, and metastatic tumor burden [24].

In particular, a debate exists due to the significant bias identified in these studies: (i) surgery may be a surrogate for more aggressive multimodal therapy, (ii) stage IV breast cancer patients may include women diagnosed either early by modern imaging or shortly after surgery, and (iii) MBC patients in better general condition are offered surgery, while patients with worse general status (i.e., presence of comorbidities, more frail) are not.

2.3. Data from the Cochrane Database and Ongoing Trials

A recent Cochrane systematic review [25] analyzed data on the effectiveness of breast surgery associated with medical treatment with respect to medical treatment alone in MBC patients. The authors have considered randomized clinical trials for the analyses, finally collecting only two studies involving a total of 624 women. The results did not show a clear improvement in survival in MBC patients treated with surgery and medical treatment compared to medical treatment alone, highlighting how the results were limited by a very low quality of evidence [25]. Further randomized clinical trials are needed to achieve more robust evidence and to better understand how the complex heterogeneity influences the prognosis.

In particular, in 2010, recruitment was initiated for the Eastern Cooperative Oncology Group (ECOG) E2108 randomized trial (https://clinicaltrials.gov/ct2/show/NCT01242800), including patients presenting with stage IV breast cancer. This is a 2-arm study (standard palliative therapy versus locoregional surgery on primary tumor), having as the primary end-point to determine if early locoregional surgical therapy improves overall survival and, as secondary end-points, to study the quality of life and control of chest wall disease. The results will potentially clarify these aspects and possibly change the management of patients with stage IV breast cancer disease.

3. Are There Other Factors Affecting the Choice for the Resection of the Primary Tumor in MBC?

Metastatic breast tumor management remains a challenge for physicians, and there is debate on the evidence that suggests that locoregional treatment of the primary tumor confers an overall survival advantage in this setting. Stage IV breast cancer represents a disease characterized by tremendous heterogeneity, as described by Lim and Hortobagyi [1]. In particular, differences in the underlying health status, i.e., age, comorbidities, performance status, and organ function, contribute to MBC presentation, affecting treatment decisions and patient outcomes [1].

There are gaps in the knowledge that may impact the decision-making process regarding who is a good candidate for locoregional resection in MBC. In this light, what risk factors need to be identified and thus treated to improve the prognosis of MBC patients remain unclear.

Treatment of MBC may target fundamentally different mechanisms than standard chemotherapeutic drugs, which are generally antiproliferative and, therefore, most efficiently eliminate rapidly growing cells.

Although a clinically apparent metastasis is usually associated with late stages of cancer development, micrometastatic dissemination may be an early phenomenon. Nonconclusive data are available on the molecular events, including changes in specific metabolic pathways underlying the development of metastatic disease, and this may impact the treatment's decision process and, in part, may influence the response to surgical locoregional treatment [26–28].

First, the impact of the immune system on metastatic colonization is still unclear. Authors have theorized that disseminated tumor cells could metastasize, evading the immune system (actively, performing a sort of "immunoediting" or remaining "dormant") [26,27]. Secondly, the destiny of disseminating tumor cells after the removal of the primary tumor is unclear. Despite the fact that retrospective clinical studies have demonstrated that complete resection of the primary tumor improves survival [11,18], experimental evidence has shown that ablation of the primary tumor accelerates the growth of disseminating tumor cells in metastatic sites [28,29], possibly due to systemic inflammatory response [30]. In contrast, in 2019, Piranlioglu et al. demonstrated in a mouse model that an innate and adaptive immune system, stimulated by the tumor (in particular CD8+ cells), may kill disseminating tumor cells after the complete resection of primary tumors, keeping an immunologic memory [16]. These results can be seen as a molecular explanation of improved overall survival in breast cancer patients, following primary tumor resections with clear margins.

In this light, the improvement in the survival rates of patients with MBC represents one of the major concerns in public health [1].

4. Emerging Metabolic Aspects: Do They Have a Key Role in MBC Management?

As previously shown, surgery in MBC represents a clinically relevant issue due to the controversial results obtained in different studies in terms of prognosis. In fact, some questions remain unanswered: (i) who is a target candidate for locoregional surgical during MBC? (ii) what are the risk factors related to MBC prognosis to be identified? (iii) Do metabolic changes affect the outcome(s) of MBC surgical procedure? (iv) Are specific metabolic interventions available in this setting?

We suggest that answers to these questions may derive from the implementation of precision (formerly called "personalized") medicine. This can be defined as the possibility of managing a patient with the same taxonomic (affected by the same disease) disease differently to another by means of a tailored strategy based on strong evidence [31].

It is well known that there are different types of breast cancer, and it is a mixture rather than a single disease. Personalized medicine is based on tumor molecular profiles, and it is currently applied at different stages of breast cancer, including, especially, the prediction of treatment efficacy. One typical example of personalized medicine is represented by therapies implemented among patients with HER2-positive breast cancer compared to HER2-negative [32]. Moreover, a great challenge remains for the treatment of triple-negative breast cancer. This subtype, which is the most aggressive one, presents extensive and heterogeneous molecular features that need to be investigated in order to develop combined targeted agents to improve the efficacy of the treatment and possibly reduce disease progression. [33]. Although different tailored strategies have already been developed in the management of breast cancer patients, a paucity of data is available on MBC to obtain guidelines on a tailored therapeutic strategy. The specific and complex pathophysiology of MBC and its relationship with metabolic aspects should be considered to build new tailored approaches. In particular, the growing interest in metabolic derangements is emphasized by the role of altered glucose metabolism in driving the response to cancer treatment, its role in therapy resistance, and in cancer progression and metastasis [34].

Breast cancer metastasis is the systemic dissemination and colonization of cancer cells from the primary tumor to a secondary site and represents a major cause of cancer-related deaths [35]. The event of a circulating breast tumor cell, forming a metastatic colony in a distant organ, is extremely low [36]. Most cells that leave the tumor often die because of the inability to infiltrate distant organs. However, once metastasis occurs, breast cancer becomes a systemic disease, and, as previously indicated, the survival rate at 5 years decreases to 20% [36]. The heterogeneity between patients influences the journey of the cancer disease, as well as the prognosis and the treatment decisions [1]. The patient's health conditions, which impact cancer progression and morbidity and their associated molecular targets, have to be considered for the treatment decisions and therapy development. Based on this, the metabolic syndrome represents a well-known condition related to breast cancer recurrence and distant metastasis and must, therefore, be accurately managed to improve the prognosis [37].

4.1. Metabolic Syndrome and Obesity

Metabolic syndrome is often associated with hormones and adipokines derangement, including changes in serum adiponectin, a polypeptide presenting properties related to glucose homeostasis and fatty acid oxidation [38,39]. In particular, adiponectin is involved in the pathogenesis of several obesity-related disorders and represents a potential therapeutic strategy for insulin resistance, type 2 diabetes, metabolic syndrome, and, more recently, carcinogenesis [40]. Clinical studies have linked obesity-related low adiponectin plasma levels with several types of cancer, including breast cancer [40–42], and with a more aggressive phenotype (i.e., larger size of tumor, high histological grade, and increased distant metastasis). In fact, in breast cancer, increased adiponectin levels may inhibit metastatic properties, including migration, adhesion, and invasion of cancer cells [43]. Accordingly, Taliaferro-Smith et al. have documented that adiponectin may block breast cancer cell invasion and migration, producing a profound modification in metastatic properties of breast cancer cells and thus presenting an antimetastatic effect [44].

There is significant epidemiologic evidence indicating that obesity promotes breast cancer development and progression [8] by secreting protumorigenic chemokines, growth factors, and fatty acids. However, the detailed mechanisms by which hypertrophic adipose tissue influences breast cancer cells are still not well understood. The peroxisome proliferator-activated receptors (PPARs) are ligand-activated transcription factors of the nuclear hormone receptor superfamily, regulating the expression of target genes involved in glucose and lipid metabolism and levels of inflammatory cytokines and adipokines. Data suggest that factors released by the adipose tissue may modify PPAR-regulated gene expression and lipid metabolism, inducing a more aggressive breast cancer cell phenotype. These effects are, at least in part, mediated by fatty acids provided by the adipose tissue [45].

Focusing on cancer-related risk factors associated with poor prognoses, such as obesity-related diseases and on their molecular pathways [8,45,46] (i.e., increasing adiponectin levels using adiponectin analogs, targeting specific PPAR-signaling), can potentially become an innovative personalized treatment for breast cancer patients and metastatic disease in improving the metabolic state and, therefore, response to systemic therapies, locoregional surgery, and overall survival.

4.2. Glucose Metabolism

Metabolic alterations in glucose metabolism in breast cancer are known to be associated with resistance towards conventional chemotherapy, and drugs modifying glucose metabolism have been identified to positively favor chemotherapy effects, possibly resensitizing the most aggressive breast cancer phenotypes, such as the triple-negative subtype, to novel treatments [34,47]. In this light, epidemiological studies showed that diabetic subjects on the metformin treatment regimen to control blood glucose levels had a lower risk of developing all type of cancers, and patients who were diabetic and on metformin treatment and were suffering from cancer, including breast cancer, had an improved response to chemotherapy, a better prognosis, and higher disease-free survival rates when compared to those who did not take metformin [47,48]. Metformin effects, which include inhibition of cell growth and proliferation-related pathways, as well as apoptotic cell death and reduction of tissue invasiveness and metastasis, may, in part, be related to the ability of metformin to reduce insulin resistance, insulin levels, and glucose circulation levels. In this light, adhering to an approach of precision medicine, including the treatment of well-known risk factors related to breast cancer recurrence and distant metastasis, may allow researchers to develop targeted combined therapies to improve the response to cancer therapies and prognosis.

4.3. MicroRNA Modulation

Interestingly, Farrè et al. have documented in experimental models that metabolic syndrome may influence the hyperactivation of C-terminal binding protein 1 (CTBP1), a corepressor of tumor suppressor genes, determining a crucial role in breast cancer progression through metastatic cascade activation (the regulation of multiple EMT-related genes and microRNAs) [37]. In this light, metabolic syndrome impacts breast cancer progression and the metastatic process, confirming that this condition has a key role to be considered in MBC patient's prognosis and management [37].

Moreover, in this study, the authors analyzed the effect of metabolic syndrome and CTBP1 on miRNA regulation, showing that CTBP1 modulated several microRNAs implicated in cell proliferation and tumor progression [37]. MicroRNAs are noncoding small RNA that can negatively modulate gene expression, and they were recently considered either for their biological role and for their potential in the diagnosis and treatment of breast cancer [49].

In particular, the expression of miR-381-5p was detected as reduced in breast cancer tissue, and it was able to suppress cell migration and invasion [50]. Metabolic syndrome and CTBP1 were able to modulate miR-381-5p levels in xenografts generated in mice, and, in particular, CTBP1 promoted cell adhesion and migration by miR-181-5 repression [37]. In this light, microRNA profiling represents a promising approach in the integrated management of breast cancer.

5. Conclusions

In breast cancer, the identification of the most appropriate therapeutic strategies and their implementation in clinical practice appear challenging in the management of metastatic breast malignancies. However, the data available appear promising in MBC, although some are preliminary or obtained in experimental models. Regarding the surgical aspect, studies are not conclusive as to the improved survival rates in MBC patients undergoing resection of the primary tumor with clear margins. Interestingly, the analysis of the metabolic and clinical phenotypes—including modulation of adipokines (i.e., adiponectin) and miRNAs regulating metabolism—underlying the development of metastatic disease, which remains the principal cause of breast cancer-related deaths, may lead to the identification of more effective targeted approaches to prevent and treat metastases. According to the implementation of novel personalized treatments, surgical and metabolic strategies, when synergic, appear to be a promising, targeted, and integrated treatment approach to breast cancer. Extensive clinical evidence is expected to clarify these important aspects of MBC.

Author Contributions: Each author has contributed to the conception and design of the work and has approved the submitted version. All authors have read and agreed to the published version of the manuscript.

Funding: This study was funded by Institutional Research Funding of the Department of Surgical Sciences, Sapienza University of Rome, Italy.

Conflicts of Interest: The authors declare no conflict of interest.

References

1. Lim, B.; Hortobagyi, G.N. Current challenges of metastatic breast cancer. *Cancer Metastasis Rev.* **2016**, *35*, 495–514. [CrossRef] [PubMed]
2. Barbie, T.U.; Golshan, M. De Novo Stage 4 Metastatic Breast Cancer: A Surgical Disease? *Ann. Surg. Oncol.* **2018**, *25*, 3109–3111. [CrossRef] [PubMed]
3. DeSantis, C.E.; Ma, J.; Gaudet, M.M.; Newman, L.A.; Mph, K.D.M.; Sauer, A.G.; Jemal, A.; Siegel, R.L. Breast cancer statistics, 2019. *CA A Cancer J. Clin.* **2019**, *69*, 438–451. [CrossRef] [PubMed]
4. Rivera-Franco, M.M.; Leon-Rodriguez, E. Delays in Breast Cancer Detection and Treatment in Developing Countries. *Breast Cancer Basic Clin. Res.* **2018**, *12*. [CrossRef] [PubMed]
5. Sundquist, M.; Brudin, L.; Tejler, G. Improved survival in metastatic breast cancer 1985–2016. *Breast* **2017**, *31*, 46–50. [CrossRef]
6. Kimbung, S.; Loman, N.; Hedenfalk, I. Clinical and molecular complexity of breast cancer metastases. *Semin. Cancer Biol.* **2015**, *35*, 85–95. [CrossRef]
7. Savard, M.-F.; Khan, O.; Hunt, K.K.; Verma, S. Redrawing the Lines: The Next Generation of Treatment in Metastatic Breast Cancer. *Am. Soc. Clin. Oncol. Educ. Book* **2019**, *39*, e8–e21. [CrossRef]
8. Molfino, A.; Amabile, M.I.; Monti, M.; Arcieri, S.; Fanelli, F.R.; Molfino, A. The Role of Docosahexaenoic Acid (DHA) in the Control of Obesity and Metabolic Derangements in Breast Cancer. *Int. J. Mol. Sci.* **2016**, *17*, 505. [CrossRef] [PubMed]
9. Bartucci, M.; Dattilo, R.; Moriconi, C.; Pagliuca, A.; Mottolese, M.; Federici, G.; Di Benedetto, A.; Todaro, M.; Stassi, G.; Sperati, F.; et al. TAZ is required for metastatic activity and chemoresistance of breast cancer stem cells. *Oncogene* **2015**, *34*, 681–690. [CrossRef] [PubMed]
10. Molfino, A.; Amabile, M.I.; Monti, M.; Muscaritoli, M. Omega-3 Polyunsaturated Fatty Acids in Critical Illness: Anti-Inflammatory, Proresolving, or Both? *Oxidative Med. Cell. Longev.* **2017**, *2017*, 5987082. [CrossRef] [PubMed]
11. Lane, W.O.; Thomas, S.M.; Blitzblau, R.C.; Plichta, J.K.; Rosenberger, L.H.; Fayanju, O.M.; Hyslop, T.; Hwang, E.S.; Greenup, R.A. Surgical Resection of the Primary Tumor in Women With De Novo Stage IV Breast Cancer: Contemporary practice patterns and survival analysis. *Ann. Surg.* **2019**, *269*, 537–544. [CrossRef] [PubMed]
12. Khan, S.A.; Stewart, A.K.; Morrow, M. Does aggressive local therapy improve survival in metastatic breast cancer? *Surgery* **2002**, *132*, 620–627. [CrossRef] [PubMed]
13. Lang, J.E.; Tereffe, W.; Mitchell, M.P.; Rao, R.; Feng, L.; Meric-Bernstam, F.; Bedrosian, I.; Kuerer, H.M.; Hunt, K.K.; Hortobagyi, G.N.; et al. Primary tumor extirpation in breast cancer patients who present with stage IV disease is associated with improved survival. *Ann. Surg. Oncol.* **2013**, *20*, 1893–1899. [CrossRef] [PubMed]
14. Gera, R.; Chehade, H.E.L.H.; Wazir, U.; Tayeh, S.; Kasem, A.; Mokbel, K. Locoregional therapy of the primary tumour in de novo stage IV breast cancer in 216 066 patients: A meta-analysis. *Sci. Rep.* **2020**, *10*, 1–11. [CrossRef] [PubMed]
15. Rao, R.; Feng, L.; Kuerer, H.M.; Singletary, S.E.; Bedrosian, I.; Hunt, K.K.; Ross, M.I.; Hortobagyi, G.N.; Feig, B.W.; Ames, F.C.; et al. Timing of Surgical Intervention for the Intact Primary in Stage IV Breast Cancer Patients. *Ann. Surg. Oncol.* **2008**, *15*, 1696–1702. [CrossRef]

16. Piranlioglu, R.; Lee, E.; Ouzounova, M.; Bollag, R.J.; Vinyard, A.H.; Arbab, A.S.; Marasco, D.; Guzel, M.; Cowell, J.K.; Thangaraju, M.; et al. Primary tumor-induced immunity eradicates disseminated tumor cells in syngeneic mouse model. *Nat. Commun.* **2019**, *10*, 1–13. [CrossRef]
17. Bhandari, R.; Kelley, G.A.; Hartley, T.A.; Rockett, I.R.H. Metabolic Syndrome Is Associated with Increased Breast Cancer Risk: A Systematic Review with Meta-Analysis. *Int. J. Breast Cancer* **2014**, *2014*, 189384. [CrossRef]
18. Vohra, N.; Brinkley, J.; Kachare, S.; Muzaffar, M. Primary tumor resection in metastatic breast cancer: A propensity-matched analysis, 1988-2011 SEER data base. *Breast J.* **2018**, *24*, 549–554. [CrossRef]
19. Badwe, R.; Hawaldar, R.; Nair, N.; Kaushik, R.; Parmar, V.; Siddique, S.; Budrukkar, A.; Mittra, I.; Gupta, S. Locoregional treatment versus no treatment of the primary tumour in metastatic breast cancer: An open-label randomised controlled trial. *Lancet Oncol.* **2015**, *16*, 1380–1388. [CrossRef]
20. Gunduz, N.; Fisher, B.; Saffer, E.A. Effect of surgical removal on the growth and kinetics of residual tumor. *Cancer Res.* **1979**, *39*, 3861–3865.
21. Braunschweiger, P.G.; Schiffer, L.M.; Betancourt, S. Tumour cell proliferation and sequential chemotherapy after primary tumour resection in C3H/hej mammary tumours. *Breast Cancer Res. Treat.* **1982**, *2*, 323–329. [CrossRef]
22. Fisher, B.; Gunduz, N.; Coyle, J.; Rudock, C.; Saffer, E. Presence of a growth-stimulating factor in serum following primary tumor removal in mice. *Cancer Res.* **1989**, *49*, 1996–2001. [PubMed]
23. Demicheli, R.; Retsky, M.W.; Swartzendruber, D.E.; Bonadonna, G. Proposal for a new model of breast cancer metastatic development. *Ann. Oncol.* **1997**, *8*, 1075–1080. [CrossRef] [PubMed]
24. Soran, A.; Ozmen, V.; Ozbas, S.; Karanlik, H.; Muslumanoglu, M.; Igci, A.; Canturk, Z.; Utkan, Z.; Ozaslan, C.; Evrensel, T.; et al. Randomized Trial Comparing Resection of Primary Tumor with No Surgery in Stage IV Breast Cancer at Presentation: Protocol MF07-01. *Ann. Surg. Oncol.* **2018**, *25*, 3141–3149. [CrossRef] [PubMed]
25. Tosello, G.; Torloni, M.R.; Mota, B.S.; Neeman, T.; Riera, R. Breast surgery for metastatic breast cancer. *Cochrane Database Syst. Rev.* **2018**, *3*, 011276. [CrossRef] [PubMed]
26. Liu, Y.; Cao, X. Immunosuppressive cells in tumor immune escape and metastasis. *J. Mol. Med.* **2015**, *94*, 509–522. [CrossRef] [PubMed]
27. Schreiber, R.D.; Old, L.J.; Smyth, M.J. Cancer Immunoediting: Integrating Immunity's Roles in Cancer Suppression and Promotion. *Science* **2011**, *331*, 1565–1570. [CrossRef]
28. Zhang, Y.; Zhang, N.; Hoffman, R.M.; Zhao, M. Surgically-Induced Multi-organ Metastasis in an Orthotopic Syngeneic Imageable Model of 4T1 Murine Breast Cancer. *Anticancer. Res.* **2015**, *35*, 4641–4646.
29. Al-Sahaf, O.; Wang, J.H.; Browne, T.J.; Cotter, T.G.; Redmond, H.P. Surgical Injury Enhances the Expression of Genes That Mediate Breast Cancer Metastasis to the Lung. *Ann. Surg.* **2010**, *252*, 1037–1043. [CrossRef]
30. Krall, J.A.; Reinhardt, F.; Mercury, O.A.; Pattabiraman, D.R.; Brooks, M.W.; Dougan, M.; Lambert, A.W.; Bierie, B.; Ploegh, H.L.; Dougan, S.K.; et al. The systemic response to surgery triggers the outgrowth of distant immune-controlled tumors in mouse models of dormancy. *Sci. Transl. Med.* **2018**, *10*, eaan3464. [CrossRef]
31. Yan, J.; Liu, Z.; Du, S.; Li, J.; Ma, L.; Li, L. Diagnosis and Treatment of Breast Cancer in the Precision Medicine Era. *Methods Mol. Biol.* **2020**, *2204*, 53–61. [CrossRef] [PubMed]
32. Jeibouei, S.; Akbari, M.E.; Kalbasi, A.; Aref, A.R.; Ajoudanian, M.; Rezvani, A.; Zali, H. Personalized medicine in breast cancer: Pharmacogenomics approaches. *Pharm. Pers. Med.* **2019**, *12*, 59–73. [CrossRef] [PubMed]
33. Le Du, F.; Eckhardt, B.L.; Lim, B.; Litton, J.K.; Moulder, S.; Meric-Bernstam, F.; Gonzalez-Angulo, A.M.; Ueno, N.T. Is the future of personalized therapy in triple-negative breast cancer based on molecular subtype? *Oncotarget* **2015**, *6*, 12890–12908. [CrossRef] [PubMed]
34. Varghese, E.; Samuel, S.M.; Lišková, A.; Samec, M.; Kubatka, P.; Büsselberg, D. Targeting Glucose Metabolism to Overcome Resistance to Anticancer Chemotherapy in Breast Cancer. *Cancers* **2020**, *12*, 2252. [CrossRef]
35. Dillekås, H.; Rogers, M.S.; Straume, O. Are 90% of deaths from cancer caused by metastases? *Cancer Med.* **2019**, *8*, 5574–5576. [CrossRef]
36. Yardley, D.A. Visceral Disease in Patients With Metastatic Breast Cancer: Efficacy and Safety of Treatment With Ixabepilone and Other Chemotherapeutic Agents. *Clin. Breast Cancer* **2010**, *10*, 64–73. [CrossRef]

37. Farré, P.L.; Scalise, G.D.; Duca, R.B.; Dalton, G.N.; Massillo, C.; Porretti, J.; Graña, K.; Gardner, K.; De Luca, P.; De Siervi, A. CTBP1 and metabolic syndrome induce an mRNA and miRNA expression profile critical for breast cancer progression and metastasis. *Oncotarget* **2018**, *9*, 13848–13858. [CrossRef]
38. Díez, J.J.; Iglesias, P. The role of the novel adipocyte-derived hormone adiponectin in human disease. *Eur. J. Endocrinol.* **2003**, *148*, 293–300. [CrossRef]
39. Ohashi, K.; Ouchi, N.; Matsuzawa, Y. Anti-inflammatory and anti-atherogenic properties of adiponectin. *Biochimie* **2012**, *94*, 2137–2142. [CrossRef]
40. Kelesidis, I.; Mantzoros, C.S. Adiponectin and cancer: A systematic review. *Br. J. Cancer* **2006**, *94*, 1221–1225. [CrossRef]
41. Barb, D.; Pazaitou-Panayiotou, K.; Mantzoros, C.S. Adiponectin: A link between obesity and cancer. *Expert Opin. Investig. Drugs* **2006**, *15*, 917–931. [CrossRef] [PubMed]
42. Mantzoros, C.; Petridou, E.; Dessypris, N.; Chavelas, C.; Dalamaga, M.; Alexe, D.M.; Papadiamantis, Y.; Markopoulos, C.; Spanos, E.; Chrousos, G.; et al. Adiponectin and Breast Cancer Risk. *J. Clin. Endocrinol. Metab.* **2004**, *89*, 1102–1107. [CrossRef] [PubMed]
43. Saxena, N.K.; Sharma, D. Metastasis suppression by adiponectin: LKB1 rises up to the challenge. *Cell Adhes. Migr.* **2010**, *4*, 358–362. [CrossRef] [PubMed]
44. Taliaferro-Smith, L.; Nagalingam, A.; Zhong, D.; Zhou, W.; Saxena, N.K.; Sharma, D. LKB1 is required for adiponectin-mediated modulation of AMPK–S6K axis and inhibition of migration and invasion of breast cancer cells. *Oncogene* **2009**, *28*, 2621–2633. [CrossRef] [PubMed]
45. Blucher, C.; Iberl, S.; Schwagarus, N.; Muller, S.; Liebisch, G.; Horing, M.; Hidrobo, M.S.; Ecker, J.; Spindler, N.; Dietrich, A.; et al. Secreted factors from adipose tissue reprogram tumor lipid metabolism and induce motility by modulating PPARα/ANGPTL4 and FAK. *Mol. Cancer Res.* **2020**. [CrossRef]
46. Molfino, A.; Amabile, M.I.; Mazzucco, S.; Biolo, G.; Farcomeni, A.; Ramaccini, C.; Antonaroli, S.; Monti, M.; Molfino, A. Effect of Oral Docosahexaenoic Acid (DHA) Supplementation on DHA Levels and Omega-3 Index in Red Blood Cell Membranes of Breast Cancer Patients. *Front. Physiol.* **2017**, *8*, 549. [CrossRef]
47. Samuel, S.M.; Varghese, E.; Kubatka, P.; Triggle, C.R.; Büsselberg, D. Metformin: The Answer to Cancer in a Flower? Current Knowledge and Future Prospects of Metformin as an Anti-Cancer Agent in Breast Cancer. *Biomolecules* **2019**, *9*, 846. [CrossRef]
48. DeCensi, A.; Puntoni, M.; Goodwin, P.; Cazzaniga, M.; Gennari, A.; Bonanni, B.; Gandini, S. Metformin and Cancer Risk in Diabetic Patients: A Systematic Review and Meta-analysis. *Cancer Prev. Res.* **2010**, *3*, 1451–1461. [CrossRef]
49. McGuire, A.; Brown, J.A.L.; Kerin, M.J. Metastatic breast cancer: The potential of miRNA for diagnosis and treatment monitoring. *Cancer Metastasis Rev.* **2015**, *34*, 145–155. [CrossRef]
50. Xue, Y.; Xu, W.; Zhao, W.; Wang, W.; Zhang, D.; Wu, P. miR-381 inhibited breast cancer cells proliferation, epithelial-to-mesenchymal transition and metastasis by targeting CXCR4. *Biomed. Pharmacother.* **2017**, *86*, 426–433. [CrossRef]

Publisher's Note: MDPI stays neutral with regard to jurisdictional claims in published maps and institutional affiliations.

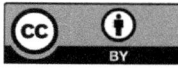

© 2020 by the authors. Licensee MDPI, Basel, Switzerland. This article is an open access article distributed under the terms and conditions of the Creative Commons Attribution (CC BY) license (http://creativecommons.org/licenses/by/4.0/).

MDPI
St. Alban-Anlage 66
4052 Basel
Switzerland
Tel. +41 61 683 77 34
Fax +41 61 302 89 18
www.mdpi.com

Journal of Personalized Medicine Editorial Office
E-mail: jpm@mdpi.com
www.mdpi.com/journal/jpm

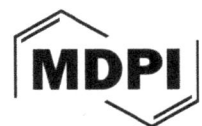